Case Studies in Emergency Medicine

Case Studies in Emergency Medicine

Edited by

Rebecca Jeanmonod

Michelle Tomassi

Dan Mayer

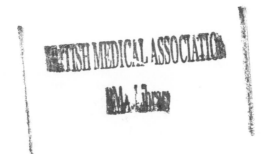

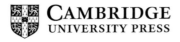

CAMBRIDGE
UNIVERSITY PRESS

CAMBRIDGE UNIVERSITY PRESS
Cambridge, New York, Melbourne, Madrid, Cape Town, Singapore,
São Paulo, Delhi, Dubai, Tokyo, Mexico City

Cambridge University Press
The Edinburgh Building, Cambridge CB2 8RU, UK

Published in the United States of America by
Cambridge University Press, New York

www.cambridge.org
Information on this title: www.cambridge.org/9780521736480

First published 2010

Printed in the United Kingdom at the University Press, Cambridge

*A catalogue record for this publication is available from the
British Library*

ISBN 978-0-521-73648-0 Paperback

Contents

Preface

Welcome to *Case Studies in Emergency Medicine*. This case-based book is designed to help medical students, physicians-in-training, and practicing clinicians learn many of the fundamentals of emergency medicine in a chief complaint, case-based format. Each of the ten chapters corresponds to one of the top ten chief complaints seen in emergency medicine, and is filled with cases of patients presenting with that chief complaint. The cases are presented as "unknowns," and the reader is provided with the information necessary to evaluate and treat each patient in a manner similar to that which occurs in clinical practice. Each case is then followed by information regarding the presentation, evaluation, treatment, and follow-up of patients with the disease described.

The cases in this book are all real, written by the healthcare providers who saw these patients. Because of this, the cases are not "textbook" cases, but contain the subtle clinical nuances and diagnostic challenges of real practice. The authors of the cases come from a broad range of specialties, and include physicians-in-training, academicians, and clinical physicians.

Through this format, you will gain an appreciation of the variety of presentations of disease processes, a good understanding of the pathophysiology of common acute disease entities, and a rational approach to the evaluation of the major complaints seen in the emergency department. Additionally, you will have the opportunity to read many interesting, educational, and sometimes eye-opening cases of real patients evaluated in the emergency department. Enjoy!

How to use this book

Background: There are many case-based books out there, both for emergency medicine and for other disciplines. Most of the time, these books are organized by organ system, with chapters on cardiac complaints, chapters on gastrointestinal complaints, and the like. This is a great way to learn pathophysiology. However, it's a lousy way to learn clinical medicine. This method presupposes that the healthcare provider or student already knows the organ system involved when approaching a patient (i.e. I know it's a pulmonary complaint, because the patient's case is in the pulmonary chapter). Anyone in clinical medicine knows that patients haven't read the books, and often present in an atypical manner. Patients with the same disease process can present in different ways. Patients with the same chief complaint can have different disease processes. These simple facts are the reason why deductive and inductive reasoning are so important to medicine in general and emergency medicine in particular, and they are why we wrote this book.

Book structure: Rather than organizing these cases by organ systems, we have organized them by chief complaint. This structure approximates real-life emergency medicine, where you don't know the answer before you walk in the room. It also is illustrative of how diverse diseases can present with the same complaint, and how the clinician can work through the differential diagnosis to arrive at the correct conclusion. There are ten chapters in this book, each representing one of the top ten chief complaints encountered in the emergency department. Each chapter contains ten to 12 cases with different etiologies of that chief complaint to cover the majority of common and dangerous diseases presenting to the emergency department. The top ten chief complaints encountered in the emergency department are abdominal pain, fever, chest pain, breathing difficulties, traumatic injuries, complaints of the eyes, ears, nose and throat, pelvic discomfort, headache, back pain, and altered mental status.

Case structure: Each case in each chapter follows a standard format that mimics the format of the medical record. It is this same format that clinicians use when presenting patients to one another during sign-over or consultation, and is therefore a format worth learning. The case begins with the history of present illness, past medical history, medications, allergies, and social history. Physical exam findings come next, as well as the results of pertinent ancillary tests.

We encourage the reader to pause after reading the case to ponder the "Questions for thought" provided. When seeing a patient, a healthcare provider gathers information and then needs to synthesize this information to diagnose, manage, and care for the patient. These questions for thought are designed to simulate that process. Following the questions for thought, the patient's diagnosis is given. There is discussion about the epidemiology, patho-physiology, and treatment of the disease, and there is a follow-up of the clinical course of the patient. Each case ends with a short list of references for further reading.

About the cases: All of the diagnoses in this book are either common or dangerous, making them critical to the knowledge base of an emergency medical provider. In addition, the cases in this book are real. Sometimes the patients are misdiagnosed, sometimes mismanaged, and sometimes there are psychosocial issues that complicate the patient's care. Emergency medicine providers take care of anyone, anytime, regardless of complaint or ability to pay. This leads to a rich clinical environment from which to draw teaching material. These cases are written by the emergency medicine providers who saw these patients.

The algorithms: Because any given chief complaint may be caused by multiple organ systems, at the end of each chapter there is a basic algorithm to aid in the approach to a patient with a given chief complaint. These algorithms focus on the inductive reasoning used in generating a differential diagnosis and the deductive reasoning used to come up with a final diagnosis. These are not meant to be comprehensive, but rather should be used as a tool to help the reader understand the importance of considering multiple organ systems when faced with a chief complaint prior to narrowing down diagnostic possibilities. The algorithms for approach to the patient with a given chief complaint can be read and used before, during, or after reading the cases.

Index: At the end of the book, there is an index of disease processes. We included this so that the reader could choose to read several presentations for the same disease process, or look up a disease to review the pathophysiology. Since cases and chapters are titled by chief complaint only, the index is the only way to identify the final diagnoses prior to reading the cases.

So we hope you find this book enjoyable, but more importantly, we hope you find it educational. This is emergency medicine in its fundamentals, truly: an enjoyable career where you learn something every day.

Chief complaint: abdominal pain

Donald Jeanmonod, Dan Mayer, Chad S. Lewis, John Schleicher Jr., Marco Tomassi, Michelle Tomassi, Dan Pauze, Luke T. Day, Roman Petrov

Case #1

History

The patient is a 43-year-old female with abdominal pain for the past week. The patient describes the pain as being underneath where her bra fits and also complains of some back pain. The patient states that the pain started less intensely in the last week, but has since increased in intensity to the point where it is unbearable. The patient reports that she has not eaten anything for the past 4 days because every time that she does eat, she vomits undigested food and the pain increases dramatically. When she does not eat, the pain is less intense. The patient reports that the pain is sharp and intermittent in nature and increases when she is supine. The patient also notes some back pain. She has noticed decreased urine output and subjective fever. The patient reports no blood in her urine or stool. The patient denies having any chest pain or shortness of breath. The patient has no complaints of constipation or diarrhea. She denies headache and visual changes. The patient had seen her primary care physician 2 days ago for her complaints and had a barium swallow done earlier on the day of presentation that showed a hiatal hernia.

Past medical history

The patient's past medical history includes migraine headaches, GERD, appendectomy, ton-sillectomy, and motor vehicle accident (which led to head trauma and reparative rhinoplasty). The patient has two teenage children.

Medications

The patient takes omeprazole and sumatriptan.

Case Studies in Emergency Medicine, ed. R. Jeanmonod, M. Tomassi and D. Mayer.
Published by Cambridge University Press © Cambridge University Press 2010.

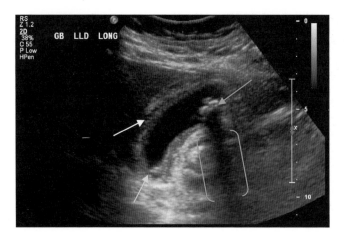

Figure 1.1. The patient's right upper quadrant ultrasound (long axis) shows that the liver is of normal size and echogenicity. There is a positive sonographic Murphy's sign (right upper quadrant tenderness when the gallbladder is compressed with the ultrasound probe). Multiple stones are present within the gallbladder lumen (upper right arrow), including a single stone within the gallbladder neck (lower left arrow). The stones produce an acoustic shadow (brackets). There is a thin rim of pericholecystic fluid (upper left arrow) surrounding the gallbladder.

Allergies

The patient is allergic to penicillin.

Physical exam and ancillary studies

- *Vital signs:* the patient's temperature is 37.9°C, her heart rate is 95, her blood pressure is 120/69, her respiratory rate is 18, and her room air oxygen saturation is 100%.
- *General:* the patient is awake, alert, and appears mildly uncomfortable. She is obese.
- *Head and neck:* the patient's pupils are equally round and reactive to light. Her cranial nerves are intact. The patient's mucous membranes are moist. Her neck is supple with a midline trachea.
- *Cardiovascular:* the patient's heart has regular rate and rhythm, without murmurs, rubs, or gallops.
- *Lungs:* her lungs are clear to auscultation bilaterally. There are no wheezes, rales, or rhonchi.
- *Abdomen:* the patient has positive bowel sounds. Her abdomen is soft and obese with diffuse generalized tenderness to palpation, most focally in the epigastrum and right upper quadrant. The patient has a positive Murphy's sign, with no rebound tenderness or guarding.
- *Extremities and skin:* the patient has no edema, clubbing, or calf tenderness.
- *Pertinent labs:* the patient's white blood cell count is 18.3, alkaline phosphatase is 80, AST 363, ALT 339, amylase 1946, and lipase 2386.

Questions for thought

- What further diagnostic modalities could you use to evaluate this patient?
- What are the typical laboratory findings in this condition?
- What are the typical ultrasound findings?
- What treatments should be initiated in the emergency department?
- What is definitive treatment of this condition?

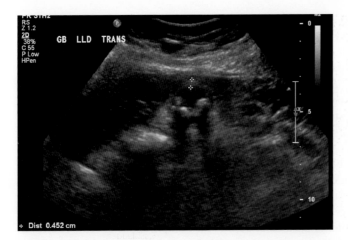

Figure 1.2. The patient's right upper quadrant ultrasound (transverse view) demonstrates thickening of the gallbladder wall at 4.5 mm. Gallbladder wall thickness of greater than 3 mm is consistent with acute cholecystitis.

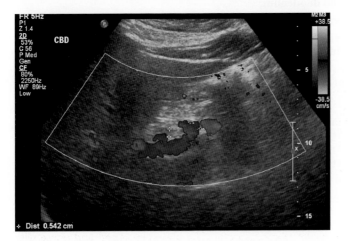

Figure 1.3. Ultrasound of the patient's common bile duct measures 5.4 mm, also consistent with acute cholecystitis. The diameter of the common bile duct should normally be about 1 mm per decade of life, therefore our 43-year-old patient should have a common bile duct of roughly 4.3 mm.

Diagnosis

Acute cholecystitis with acute pancreatitis.

Discussion

- *Epidemiology:* acute cholecystitis is an acute inflammatory disease of the gallbladder. It is often associated with gallstones, but can potentially be secondary to other causes including decreased gallbladder perfusion or motility disorders. Ninety to ninety-five percent of cases of acute cholecystitis are associated with gallstones, but approximately 5–10% of cases will be acalculous. Cholelithiasis is a relatively common condition affecting 25 million Americans annually with an additional 1 million new cases diagnosed each year. The majority of patients with cholelithiasis will remain asymptomatic, but approximately 30% of patients with gallstones will develop symptoms. Acute cholecystitis accounts for 3–10% of patients presenting with abdominal pain and results in approximately 500 000–700 000 cholecystectomies yearly. Risk factors for acute cholecystitis are referred to as the "4 Fs" (female, fertile, fat, forty). Females are more than twice as likely to develop gallstones as males. Although the majority of cases occur in adults, the rate in the pediatric population is 1.3 cases per 1000 adult cases and pediatric patients account for 4% of all cholecystectomies. The incidence of gallbladder disease in children is on the rise, in association with childhood obesity.

- *Pathophysiology:* in the majority of patients, gallstones play a central role in the development of acute cholecystitis. Gallstones blocking the neck of the gallbladder result in increased pressure within the gallbladder as it continues to fill, but cannot empty. If the obstruction is temporary or partial, the patient experiences biliary colic. If complete and unrelenting, the gallbladder becomes distended and edematous over the course of 2–4 days. As the gallbladder distends, the wall experiences increased pressure which subsequently leads to decreased capillary perfusion and gallbladder wall necrosis over 3–5 days. The third stage of acute cholecystitis involves suppuration of the areas of necrosis, with translocation of bacteria at days 7–10. Complications of acute cholecystitis include perforation, biliary peritonitis, pericholecystic abscess, and biliary fistula between the gallbladder and duodenum.
- *Presentation:* the usual presentation of acute cholecystitis includes nausea and vomiting, right upper quadrant or epigastric pain, and fever. The patient will frequently describe episodes of preceding right upper quadrant abdominal pain, often following fatty meals, which represent previous episodes of biliary colic. The patient may describe right shoulder pain from irritation of the diaphragm. Jaundice from common bile duct obstruction is only rarely seen. On physical exam, the patient will usually have right upper quadrant tenderness and one might be able to elicit a Murphy's sign (pain +/− associated inspiratory arrest upon palpation of right upper quadrant). Rebound and guarding (signs of peritonitis) are usually absent.
- *Diagnosis:* acute cholecystitis is usually referring to a clinical syndrome including the appropriate clinical history, exam findings, and laboratory values with supporting evidence from radiologic studies. Lab studies have insufficient sensitivity and specificity to reliably rule in or rule out disease. Ultrasound remains the most commonly used test to evaluate for acute cholecystitis. A meta-analysis found that ultrasound has a sensitivity of 88% (95% confidence interval 74–100%) and a specificity of 80% (95% confidence interval 62–98%) when adjusted for verification bias. HIDA scan has a higher sensitivity of approximately 95% but is more expensive and difficult to obtain from the emergency department.
- *Treatment:* although the majority of cases of acute cholecystitis are only inflammatory, most patients will get treated with antibiotics that cover polymicrobial infections of *E. coli*, *Klebsiella*, *Enterobacter*, and *Enterococcus* species. Ultimately, the patient will require surgical treatment. Possible approaches include laparoscopic cholecystectomy, open cholecystectomy, and percutaneous drainage if the patient is unable to tolerate a full surgical procedure.

Clinical course

The keys to this patient's diagnosis are careful attention to her history, physical exam, and ancillary studies.

Historical clues	Physical findings	Ancillary studies
• Presence of risk factors (obese, female, forty)	• Fever	• Elevated liver function tests (alkaline phosphatase/AST/ALT)
• Right upper quadrant pain	• Right upper quadrant tenderness	• Gallstones on U/S
• Nausea	• Positive Murphy's sign	• Gallbladder wall thickening
• Vomiting		• Dilated common bile duct

This patient had the combination of acute cholecystitis and acute gallstone pancreatitis. The patient was started on intravenous fluid therapy and broad-spectrum antibiotics. The patient remained NPO and the following day underwent an ERCP. During the procedure, a ductal stone was identified and retrieved. Five days later, the patient underwent an uncomplicated laparoscopic cholecystectomy.

Further reading

Strasburg SM. Clinical practice. Acute calculous cholecystitis. *N Engl J Med* 2008;**358**:2804–11.

Trowbridge RL, Rutkowski NK, Shojania KG. Does this patient have acute cholecystitis? *JAMA* 2003;**289**:80–6.

Portincasa P, Moschetta A, Petruzzelli M, et al. Gallstone disease: symptoms and diagnosis of gallbladder stones. *Best Pract Res Clin Gastroenterol* 2006;**20**:1017–29.

Shah K, Wolfe RE. Hepatobiliary ultrasound. *Emerg Med Clin North Am* 2004;**22**:661–73.

Case #2

History

A 74-year-old woman arrives to the emergency department by taxi at 8:00 a.m. on a Saturday morning complaining of severe abdominal pain. She states that her pain began a few hours earlier and is incredibly "bad," in fact it is the worst pain she has ever felt. However, she appears to be fairly comfortable and the treating nurses and physicians initially state that she "doesn't look like she is in pain." Her initial abdominal examination reveals a fairly soft abdomen. The patient does have some nausea associated with her abdominal pain and has vomited once today. She does not have any chest pain, shortness of breath, leg pain, fever or chills, and has had normal bowel movements without any blood up until today. She has not had a bowel movement as of yet today.

Past medical history

The patient has a history of poorly controlled hypertension and hypercholesterolemia. She fractured her foot several years earlier and waited approximately 3 days before going to the doctor for an evaluation as she "thought it would get better by itself."

Social history

The patient lives alone. She has smoked 1 to $1\frac{1}{2}$ packs per day for 30 years.

Medications

The patient's medications are metoprolol and hydrochlorothiazide.

Allergies

The patient has no known drug allergies.

Physical exam and ancillary studies

- *Vital signs:* the patient's temperature is 36.8°C, her heart rate is 116 bpm, her blood pressure is 183/99, her respiratory rate is 24, and her room air oxygen saturation is 98%.
- *General:* the patient is awake and alert, but irritable. She is lying quietly on the stretcher in no acute distress. She is able to speak in three-word sentences.
- *Head and neck:* the patient's pupils are equal, round, and reactive to light. Her mucous membranes are dry.
- *Cardiovascular:* the patient has a regular heart beat without rubs, murmurs, or gallops. Her peripheral pulses are decreased throughout.
- *Lungs:* the patient's lungs are clear to auscultation bilaterally, with slightly diminished breath sounds. She has scattered bibasilar rales.

- *Abdomen:* the patient's abdomen is soft with minimal tenderness in the epigastrium. Her bowel sounds are markedly diminished. There is no guarding or rebound tenderness. The patient is found to be guaiac negative on digital exam, although her rectal vault is empty.
- *Extremities and skin:* the patient has no edema, clubbing, or calf tenderness. She has normal capillary refill.
- *Pertinent abnormal labs:* the patient's white blood cell count is 18.0, hemoglobin 12.8, hematocrit 38.6, and bicarbonate 20. The remainder of the patient's blood work, including cardiac markers, is normal.

Questions for thought

- What are the appropriate initial actions to take to stabilize this patient?
- Once the patient has been stabilized, are there any other diagnostic tools that are required to make the diagnosis?
- What immediately life and limb threatening conditions are present in this patient?
- Why is the patient's abdominal examination benign?

Diagnosis

Acute superior mesenteric artery (SMA) infarction.

Discussion

- *Epidemiology:* acute mesenteric ischemia is an uncommon but life-threatening clinical entity that leads to certain death if not diagnosed and treated in a timely manner. The morbidity and mortality are quite high and have not decreased markedly over the past 30 years.
- *Pathophysiology:* acute mesenteric ischemia (AMI) is the result of poor blood flow to or from the small intestine (in contrast to ischemic colitis, which is the result of poor blood flow to the colon). The classic pain "out of proportion" to physical exam is thought to occur because in the early stages of disease, the ischemic tissue involves the poorly innervated mucosal side of the bowel. Approximately 70% of AMI is secondary to an acute thrombotic or embolic arterial occlusion (most likely the SMA or one of its terminal branches). Non-occlusive events – low cardiac output or local vasospasm – account for 20% of cases. Less than 10% of AMI is associated with venous thromboses. Bowel infarction is the common pathologic pathway, regardless of the underlying cause. Bowel damage begins with reversible ischemia and can proceed to transmural infarction with resultant bowel necrosis, perforation, and septic shock.
- *Presentation:* the index of suspicion for acute mesenteric ischemia should be high for patients presenting with acute onset of severe abdominal pain that is "out of proportion" to the physical findings on abdominal exam. Patients particularly at risk for this problem are those with significant atherosclerotic disease (with concomitant diabetes, hypertension, hypercholesterolemia) or patients at risk for vascular embolic disease (those with atrial fibrillation, cardiac prostheses, hypercoagulable states). The presence of severe acute abdominal pain with few findings on examination in any patient with these risk

factors should be considered to indicate mesenteric infarction until proven otherwise. Following diagnosis of AMI, immediate surgical intervention is necessary to minimize morbidity and mortality.

- *Diagnosis:* the finding of pain "out of proportion" to the physical examination in a person older than 50 years should prompt immediate surgical consultation for AMI. The white blood cell count is elevated in 98% of patients with this disease. Serum lactate is present in about 90% of patients and has been used to make this diagnosis, but a negative test does not rule out the diagnosis. A low, compensating bicarbonate with no other explanation may be considered a surrogate marker for acidosis. Stool may be positive for occult blood, but once again a negative test does not rule out the diagnosis. CT angiography is the imaging modality of choice for AMI, with a sensitivity of 71–96% and specificity of 92–94%. CT scan may show bowel wall thickening, portal venous air, pneumatosis intestinalis, and solid organ infarction. The most common finding on CT scan is bowel wall edema. Although CT may identify the diseased bowel segment, differentiating an arterial occlusion from a venous one can be challenging even with a contrast-enhanced study. Arterial occlusion may be evidenced by vessel cutoff, whereas venous occlusion shows as a portal or superior mesenteric vein thrombus. In the end, abdominal visceral angiography remains the gold standard for diagnosis.
- *Definitive therapy:* when AMI is diagnosed, immediate fluid resuscitation and surgical revascularization is the therapy of choice. This can be accomplished percutaneously via angiography-directed catheters to remove or dissolve thrombus/embolus from the SMA (with or without arterial stenting). If angiography fails to revascularize, the next surgical option is a mesenteric bypass procedure. Medical anticoagulation is the standard therapy for venous occlusive disease. It should be noted that, in the setting of worsening acidosis or sepsis, an exploratory laparotomy is indicated to identify infarcted bowel and ascertain whether the degree of intestinal infarction is ultimately survivable.

Clinical course

The keys to this patient's diagnosis are careful attention to her history, physical exam, and ancillary studies.

Historical clues	Physical findings	Ancillary studies
• Severe pain	• Relatively benign abdominal examination	• None
• Sudden onset	• Decreased bowel sounds	• Elevated WBCs
• History of hypertension or vascular disease		• Elevated WBCs

A surgical consultation was requested and a CT angiogram of the abdomen and pelvis was obtained. The study was read as negative by radiology; however, the patient continued to deteriorate over the following 6 hours. Ultimately, the patient was taken for surgery, where laparotomy revealed no SMA pulse and less than 50 centimeters of viable bowel, findings not compatible with life. The patient's abdomen was closed, she was placed on comfort care, and died 2 days later.

Case #3

History

A 19-year-old incarcerated male presents stating that over the last week, he has been having increased urination, unquenchable thirst, and hunger. When the patient woke up this morning, he was having generalized abdominal pain and felt very dizzy as if he was "going to pass out." He currently has nausea, but denies vomiting or diarrhea. Despite the nausea, the patient states he is hungry. He has lost 10 pounds over the last 2 weeks, even with adequate food intake. The patient denies any fevers or chills. He denies any headache, acute visual changes, sore throat, shortness of breath, or chest pain. He has not experienced any dysuria or flank pain with his polyuria.

Past medical history

The patient denies any past medical history. He had operative repair of a tibial fracture 5 years ago. He does not know his family history. He is a one pack per day smoker.

Medications

The patient does not take any medications.

Allergies

The patient has no known drug allergies.

Physical exam and ancillary studies

- *Vital signs:* the patient's temperature is 38.3°C, his heart rate is 133 bpm, his blood pressure is 139/78, his respiratory rate is 28, and his room air oxygen saturation is 96%. The patient's finger stick blood glucose is read as "high."
- *General:* the patient is awake and alert. He is in mild respiratory distress, but speaks in full sentences.
- *Head and neck:* the patient's pupils are equally round and reactive to light. His cranial nerves are intact and his mucous membranes are dry. The patient's neck is supple with a midline trachea. There is no jugular venous distension.
- *Cardiovascular:* the patient's heart has regular rhythm, with normal heart sounds. There are no murmurs, rubs, or gallops. The patient's radial pulses are 2+ bilaterally.
- *Lungs:* the patient has equal breath sounds. He has no wheezes, rales, or rhonchi. There are no appreciable retractions.
- *Abdomen:* the patient's abdomen is soft and non-distended, with normoactive bowel sounds. There is tenderness to palpation in the epigastrium. There are no peritoneal signs or CVA tenderness.

- *Extremities and skin:* the patient has no edema, clubbing, cyanosis, or calf tenderness. He has normal capillary refill.
- *Neurologic:* the patient is alert and oriented. His speech is normal. Motor strength is 5/5 and sensation is intact. There are no focal neurologic deficits.
- *Pertinent abnormal labs:* the patient's sodium is 137, potassium 5.4, bicarbonate 10, glucose 606, anion gap 25, and amylase 134. The patient's venous blood gas shows a pH of 7.21. His urinalysis demonstrates large ketones and glucose, with a specific gravity of 1.040.
- *Radiologic studies:* the patient's chest X-ray is read as negative, with no signs of infection.

Questions for thought

- Why does this patient have abdominal pain?
- What are the appropriate initial actions to take to stabilize this patient?
- Once stable, what is needed to make a diagnosis?
- How does one treat this condition in the emergency department?
- What should be the disposition of this patient?

Diagnosis

Abdominal pain secondary to new-onset diabetic ketoacidosis.

Discussion

- *Epidemiology:* diabetic ketoacidosis (DKA) is mainly a disease of Type 1 (insulin-dependent) diabetes mellitus. DKA accounts for an estimated 25% of all diabetes-associated admissions in the United States, with an incidence of 15 in 1000 patients. Approximately one-third of DKA admissions are for new-onset diabetes. Some of the more common precipitating factors include noncompliance with insulin regimen, infection, stroke, myocardial infarction, trauma, pregnancy, hyperthyroidism, pancreatitis, surgery, and steroid use.
- *Pathophysiology:* DKA is the body's response to cellular glucose starvation. Insulin deficiency results in the body's inability to transport glucose across cellular membranes. Despite hyperglycemia, the body is in a state of relative starvation with accelerated glycogenolysis, gluconeogenesis, proteolysis, and lipolysis. The continued increase in glucose and the inability to use it as a fuel source leads to osmotic diuresis, dehydration, and electrolyte deficiencies. The body turns to fatty acid for fuel utilization, and the breakdown of free fatty acids leads to the production of ketoacidemia. The primary ketones produced are beta-hydroxybutyric acid and acetoacetic acid (AcAc). Acetone, a by-product of AcAc, also contributes to the acidosis of DKA.
- *Presentation:* early signs of DKA are the traditional triad of polyuria, polydipsia, and polyphagia. As the metabolic acidosis progresses, there is a compensatory increased respiratory rate. These patients can develop a characteristic fruity odor to their breath,

which is from acetone. The accumulation of ketones leads to headache, nausea, vomiting, and abdominal pain. Gastric distension, ileus, and pancreatitis can also contribute to abdominal pain in DKA patients. Poor skin turgor, hypotension, and tachycardia result from volume depletion and lipolysis-mediated prostaglandin production. Mental confusion and coma are rare, but can occur in the presence of high serum osmolarity. Kussmaul respirations (paroxysms of deep, rapid breathing) are a sign of severe acidosis.

- *Diagnosis:* initial studies should include a finger stick blood glucose and urine dip looking for ketones and glucosuria. An electrocardiogram should be obtained to evaluate for signs of acute myocardial ischemia and electrolyte derangements (such as hyperkalemia or hypokalemia). Once hyperglycemia and ketonuria are established, a complete blood count, venous blood gas, basic metabolic panel (including calcium, magnesium, phosphorus), and serum osmolarity should be drawn. If abdominal pain is present, pancreatic enzymes can be included. One should consider cardiac biomarkers in patients with risk factors for coronary artery disease. In addition, a sepsis workup including blood cultures, urine culture, and chest X-ray should be obtained to assess for infection (since fever may not be present in patients with DKA). In general, the patient with DKA has a blood glucose > 250 mg/dL, bicarbonate < 15 mEq/L, pH < 7.3, and presence of ketonemia. DKA is an anion gap acidosis. The anion gap should be elevated, with normal range between 4 and 12.

- *Treatment:* the first step for patients with DKA is to initiate fluid resuscitation. Two liters of isotonic fluid (preferably normal saline) should be given over the first 2 hours, as most patients will have a water deficit between 5 and 10 liters. This will help lower the glucose and ketone concentration in the serum. Once the potassium level is determined, an insulin drip can be started at 0.1 units per kg per hour. As the acidosis corrects, the potassium will shift back into the cells and become depleted. Replacement potassium should be administered when the level is below five, as patients will initially show a mildly elevated level. Normal saline should be changed to a dextrose-containing solution when the glucose level is 250 to 300 mg/dL. Finger stick blood glucose should be assessed every hour for the first 4 hours and electrolytes should be checked every 2 hours for the first 6 hours, in order to follow the anion gap. All electrolytes should be repleted and any underlying disease treated.

- *Disposition:* since DKA patients need close monitoring and careful electrolyte replacement, they often require a bed in the intensive care unit.

Clinical course

The keys to this patient's diagnosis are careful attention to his history, physical exam, and ancillary studies.

Historical clues	Physical findings	Ancillary studies
• Polyuria	• Tachycardia	• Hyperglycemia of 606 mg/dL
• Polydypsia	• Hypotension	• pH of 7.21
• Polyphagia with weight loss	• Dry mucous membranes	• Bicarb of 10 mEq/L
• Report of orthostasis	• Tachypnea	• Potassium 5.4
		• Anion gap acidosis

This gentleman was diagnosed with new-onset diabetes mellitus. His anion gap was reduced to 17 at the 2-hour mark. The patient was deemed appropriate for a hospital floor bed, based on his response to treatment in the emergency department. He remained stable while in the hospital and was started on subcutaneous insulin. The patient was discharged back to the correctional facility on ultralente insulin as well as rapid-acting insulin before every meal.

Case #4

History

> The patient is a 5-year-old male sent in from his pediatrician's office for further testing. He has had 2 days of vague abdominal pain, anorexia, and maximum fever of 38.2°C. The patient's parents state that the child has been less playful and more irritable than normal, while frequently complaining of pain in the right side of his abdomen. He has been passing normal stools, which have not improved his pain. The child has had several days of a non-productive cough, with two episodes of post-tussive emesis. No other family members have had gastrointestinal complaints, but the patient's older brother had an upper respiratory infection last week that has resolved. The child and parents relate no further complaints of ear pain, congestion, sore throat, rash, or urinary symptoms.

Past medical history

The patient has mild developmental delay and has had frequent ear infections requiring bilateral tympanostomy tubes. He was born at full-term without complications via normal spontaneous vaginal delivery. All childhood vaccinations are up-to-date.

Medications

The patient takes one multivitamin with iron daily.

Allergies

The patient has an allergy to penicillin, which causes him hives.

Social history

The child is in a preschool program for children with developmental delay. He lives in a two-parent household with a nine-year-old brother. The patient's father is employed as an engineer and his mother stays at home to care for her children.

Physical exam

- *Vital signs:* the patient's rectal temperature is 38.1°C, his heart rate is 138 bpm, his blood pressure is 95/49, his respiratory rate is 30 breaths per minute, and his room air oxygen saturation is 95%.
- *General:* the patient is well-groomed and alert. He is in mild respiratory distress lying in bed on his father's lap.
- *HEENT:* the patient's pupils are equal, round, and reactive to light, without scleral icterus. There is no conjunctival injection. The patient's mucous membranes are moist. His oropharynx is normal without tonsillar hypertrophy, erythema, or exudates. The patient's external auditory canals are clear with minimal cerumen. His tympanic membranes have

tympanostomy tubes in place without signs of otitis media. There is mild clear rhinorrhea with no sinus tenderness to palpation.

- *Cardiovascular:* the patient has a regular rate and rhythm. He has normal S1 and S2 heart sounds without murmurs, rubs, or gallops. There is no S3 or S4. Capillary refill is brisk.
- *Lungs:* the patient's lungs are clear to auscultation bilaterally without adventitious breath sounds. There is slight accessory muscle use, with abdominal breathing. Deep inspiration causes paroxysmal coughing.
- *Abdomen:* the patient's abdomen is non-distended on inspection. Bowel sounds are normoactive on auscultation. There is marked tenderness to both superficial and deep palpation, most pronounced in the right lower quadrant. The abdomen is firm, without rebound tenderness or guarding.
- *Neurological:* there are no gross neurologic deficits.
- *Skin:* the patient's skin turgor is normal. There are no rashes.
- *Genitourinary:* the child is circumcised with non-tender bilaterally descended testes.
- *Pertinent abnormal labs:* the patient's white blood cell count is 16.55 with 10% bands.
- *Radiologic studies:* the patient's chest X-ray shows poor inspiratory effort with no acute abnormalities.
- *CT scan abdomen and pelvis with oral and intravenous contrast:* there is right lung base consolidation consistent with lobar pneumonia. The liver, spleen, and small intestines are normal. The appendix is well visualized and normal. There is a large volume of stool in the rectum.

Questions for thought

- What is the differential diagnosis for this patient?
- What clinical signs may help to consider the correct diagnosis?
- What laboratory or imaging modalities would help to make a diagnosis?
- Are there any interventions that would be appropriate at this time?
- What is the appropriate treatment?

Diagnosis

Community-acquired right lower lobe pneumonia.

Discussion

- *Epidemiology:* pneumonia is a very common disease seen in the ED and accounts for up to 10% of hospital admissions in the United States. Pneumonia can present during any time of year. It is found in patients of all ages, although the causative agents vary with age, comorbidities, and living situations. Diagnosing pneumonia in a child can be particularly challenging because the disease can have variable presentations, including abdominal pain as was seen in this case. While pneumococcal vaccinations and influenza vaccinations are commonplace, they do not preclude the development of pneumonia.

Recently hospitalized, incarcerated, and nursing-home patients are of particular concern because they tend to be at risk for pseudomonal and other more resistant infections.

- *Pathophysiology:* pneumonia can be caused by several types of microorganisms. Aspiration of oropharyngeal secretions is the primary mechanism of infection. Preceding viral upper respiratory infection, such as influenza, can leave the lung tissue vulnerable to superinfection by bacterial pathogens. Once infection has been established, the body's inflammatory response leads to cough, fever, and malaise. If the infection crosses from the alveoli into the bloodstream, sepsis can result. Certain population subsets are more vulnerable to infection. Alcoholic and debilitated patients have increased risk of aspiration. Smokers have impaired mucociliary transport. AIDS patients and other immunosuppressed patients are susceptible to opportunistic pathogens. Patients with cystic fibrosis are predisposed to pneumonia due to their inability to adequately clear secretions.

- *Presentation:* the typical presentation of a person with pneumonia is several days of fever, cough, and dyspnea. Some patients may report chills, chest pain, nausea, or generalized weakness. Infants and children tend to present with atypical findings – decreased feeding, increased irritability, dehydration, or abdominal pain. It is important to consider other historical clues including recent hospitalization, sick contacts, smoking history, underlying lung disease, immunosuppression, and overall health when diagnosing pneumonia. Close attention should be given to vital-sign abnormalities – particularly tachycardia, tachypnea, fever, and hypoxia. Other signs of pneumonia may be locally decreased breath sounds, rhonchi heard on auscultation, whispered pectoriloquy, and egophony. Some patients may present in extremis with hypotension, altered level of consciousness, or even respiratory arrest.

- *Treatment:* bacterial pneumonia is treated with antibiotics, and supportive care as needed. Most patients can be treated as an outpatient on oral agents. First-line treatment for community-acquired pneumonia in patients older than 4 is usually a macrolide antibiotic, such as azithromycin. In patients with comorbidities and exposure to resistant pathogens, respiratory fluoroquinolones (such as levofloxacin) are recommended. More seriously ill patients may require admission and intravenous antibiotics. In severely ill patients, mechanical ventilation may be required. If the patient is hypotensive, aggressive IV hydration with inotropic support may be necessary. Ideally, antibiotic therapy should be selected based on blood and sputum cultures. In practice, broad-spectrum antibiotics are typically initiated followed by more directed treatment based on cultures and sensitivity.

Clinical course

The keys to this child's diagnosis are careful attention to his history, physical exam, and ancillary studies.

Historical clues	Physical findings	Ancillary studies
• Cough	• Fever	• Leukocytosis
• Fever	• Tachypnea	• Bandemia
• Sick contact	• Hypoxia	• Radiographic evidence of infiltrate

The child was given a dose of weight-based oral acetaminophen to control his fever. He was also started on oral azithromycin in the emergency department and provided a prescription to continue at home. Vital signs were rechecked prior to discharge with a defervescence to 37.2°C and a room air oxygen saturation of 98%. The referring pediatrician was called and informed of the diagnosis. Follow-up was arranged for the next day at the pediatrician's office. At that visit, the child was back to baseline behavior with normal appetite and activity level. The patient's parents reported a decrease in cough and fever, with resolution of the patient's abdominal pain. A follow-up chest X-ray 2 weeks later showed no evidence of residual infiltrate.

Further reading

Marx J, Hockberger R, Walls R. *Rosen's Emergency Medicine*, 6th edition. St Louis, MO: Mosby Elsevier, 2006, pp. 1128–41.

Tintinalli J, Kelen G, Stapczynski S. *Emergency Medicine: A Comprehensive Study Guide*, 6th edition. New York: McGraw-Hill, 2004, pp. 446–8.

Rivers C, Howell J, Barkin R. Pneumonia chapter. In *Preparing for the Written Board Exam in Emergency Medicine*, 5th edition. Columbus, OH: Emergency Medicine Educational, 2006, pp. 323–4.

Case #5

History

> A 7-year-old male is brought in by his parents with the chief complaint of abdominal pain. He woke up this morning with pain in his epigastrium, as well as associated nausea. He has vomited twice today. The patient states that after the second episode of emesis, his throat started to feel raw and now it hurts when he swallows. The patient's mother reports a low-grade tactile fever at home but no chills. The patient denies photophobia, otalgia, rhinorrhea, cough, neck stiffness, chest pain, shortness of breath, diarrhea, or urinary symptoms.

Past medical history

The patient denies any past medical history. His mother states his vaccinations are up-to-date.

Medications

The patient takes no medications.

Allergies

The patient has no known drug allergies.

Physical exam and ancillary studies

- *Vital signs:* the patient's tympanic temperature is 38.8°C, his heart rate is 115 bpm, his blood pressure is 100/78, his respiratory rate is 18, and his room air oxygen saturation is 98%.
- *General:* the patient is awake and alert. He speaks in full sentences, but looks mildly uncomfortable when trying to swallow.
- *Head and neck:* the patient's pupils are equally round and reactive to light, cranial nerves are intact. There is no trismus or facial asymmetry. The patient's mucous membranes are moist. The tonsils are equally hypertrophic and erythematous, with pharyngeal exudates present bilaterally. The patient's uvula is midline. His neck is supple with a midline trachea. Right anterior cervical lymphadenopathy is present, with two palpable tender lymph nodes measuring more than 1 cm each.
- *Cardiovascular:* the patient has regular rhythm, but is tachycardic at 115. Normal S1 and S2 are present. There are no murmurs, rubs, or gallops appreciated. Radial pulses are 2+ bilaterally.
- *Lungs:* the patient has no retractions. He has equal breath sounds. There are no wheezes, rales, or rhonchi.
- *Abdomen:* the patient's abdomen is soft and non-distended, with normoactive bowel sounds. There is no reproducible tenderness to deep palpation or peritoneal signs. The patient has no costovertebral angle tenderness.

- *Extremities and skin:* there is no edema, clubbing, or cyanosis present. The patient has no calf tenderness. He has good capillary refill.

Questions for thought

- What is the differential diagnosis for this patient?
- What clinical signs may help to make the correct diagnosis?
- What laboratory or imaging modalities would help to make a diagnosis?
- Are there any interventions that would be appropriate at this time?
- What is the appropriate treatment?

Diagnosis

Abdominal pain secondary to streptococcal pharyngitis.

Discussion

- *Epidemiology:* group A streptococcal (GAS) pharyngitis accounts for up to 30% of all cases of pharyngitis in children between the ages of 4 and 11 years, with viral etiologies being the most common cause. GAS is a rare cause of fever in children under 3 years of age. Peak incidence is between January and May, with a higher than average incidence seen at the beginning of the school year as well.
- *Pathophysiology:* GAS causes an exudative pharyngitis due to overgrowth of bacteria in the posterior pharynx. Lymphatic drainage of the bacteria leads to cervical lymphadenopathy. Bacterial overgrowth becomes the source of fever. The exact reason for abdominal pain as a presenting complaint is not certain. It is probably due to microingestion of exudates, which has a direct toxic effect on the gastric mucosa.
- *Presentation:* patients with the diagnosis GAS will typically have acute sore throat with low-grade fever. Erythema and exudate of the tonsils and pharynx, as well as edema and erythema of the uvula, can be seen. Patients may also have petechiae of the palate and tender anterior cervical lymphadenopathy.
- *Diagnosis:* the diagnosis of strep throat can be made clinically. Patients who exhibit pharyngeal erythema, edema, or exudates on physical examination, with fever and tender anterior cervical lymphadenopathy, have up to an 85% chance of a positive GAS etiology. The gold standard for diagnosis of any bacterial pharyngitis is a throat culture. However, rapid strep tests have such a high specificity that if positive, cultures are usually not necessary. Nevertheless, the sensitivity is not as high as the specificity and false negative tests can be seen in up to 10–35% of all rapid strep screening exams.
- *Treatment:* treatment for GAS is directed at preventing the extension of the pharyngitis into surrounding tissues. This helps to prevent sinusitis and otitis media, as well as abscesses of the retropharyngeal and peritonsillar spaces. Treatment also aids in averting rheumatic fever. Penicillin is first-line treatment for GAS pharyngitis. Macrolides are reserved for those patients who are penicillin allergic. Steroids may be necessary if the patient's airway is compromised.

Clinical course

The keys to this child's diagnosis are careful attention to his history and physical exam.

Historical clues	Physical findings	Ancillary studies
• Fever	• Exudative pharyngitis	• None
• Sore throat	• Cervical lymphadenopathy	• None
• Lack of URI symptoms		

Clinically this patient presented with GAS pharyngitis, which was confirmed by throat culture. The patient was started on ibuprofen (as both an antipyretic and an anti-inflammatory) and penicillin in the ED. On reassessment, the patient was found to be afebrile and able to tolerate oral liquids. He was sent home with a prescription for penicillin and instructions to follow up with his pediatrician the following day.

Further reading

Wald ER, Green MD, Schwartz B, Barbadora K. A streptococcal score card revisited. *Pediatr Emerg Care* 1998;**14**:109.

McIsaac WJ, Kellner JD, Aufricht P, et al. Empirical validation of guidelines for the management of pharyngitis in children and adults. *JAMA* 2004;**291**:1587.

Case #6

History

A 63-year-old male patient presents stating he has not been feeling well over the last 3 to 4 days. The patient states that he has been having episodes of nausea, vomiting, and diarrhea. He is "unable to keep anything down." He also states that he has diffuse belly pain, most pronounced over the suprapubic region. He has not urinated over the past day and a half. The patient denies any fevers or chills. He has no shortness of breath at rest, but experiences dyspnea on exertion. The patient denies chest pain. He describes bilateral swelling in his legs over the last couple of days. He denies any dizziness or headache.

Past medical history

The patient denies any previous medical history. He states he does not like doctors and has not seen a health professional for 20 years.

Medications

The patient does not take any medication.

Allergies

The patient has no known drug allergies.

Physical exam and ancillary studies

- *Vital signs:* the patient's temperature is 36.4°C, his heart rate is 113 bpm, his blood pressure is 179/112, his respiratory rate is 16, and his room air oxygen saturation is 99%.
- *General:* the patient is awake and alert, but somewhat uncomfortable. He speaks in full sentences.
- *Head and neck:* the patient's pupils are equally round and reactive to light, cranial nerves are intact. The patient's mucous membranes are dry. His neck is supple with a midline trachea. There is no jugular venous distension.
- *Cardiovascular:* the patient has regular rhythm and is tachycardic at 113. He has normal S1 and S2 heart sounds. There are no appreciable murmurs, rubs, or gallops. Peripheral pulses are 2+ throughout.
- *Lungs:* the patient has normal expansion and equal breath sounds. There are no retractions, wheezes, or rhonchi. Bibasilar rales are present.
- *Abdomen:* the patient's abdomen is mildly distended. He has normoactive bowel sounds. There is tenderness to palpation in all four quadrants, with a large palpable mass in the suprapubic region. There is no hepatosplenomegaly and no palpable aneurysm.
- *Extremities and skin:* there is bilateral pitting edema to the distal knee joints, with no clubbing or calf tenderness. There is normal capillary refill throughout.

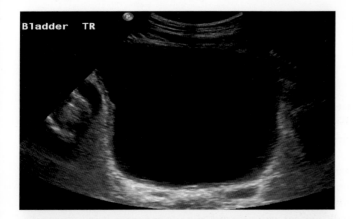

Figure 1.4. The patient's bladder ultrasound shows significant distension, with no appreciable masses.

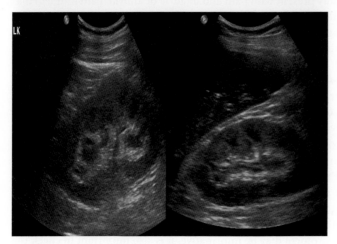

Figure 1.5. Bilateral renal ultrasound confirms hydronephrosis.

- *Pertinent abnormal labs:* the patient's white blood cell count is 15. His BUN is 213 and creatinine is 25. The patient's sodium is 133, potassium 5.8, chloride 94, and bicarbonate 12. The patient's urinalysis is negative for infection.
- *EKG:* the patient's electrocardiogram shows sinus tachycardia at 110, with no acute ischemic changes.
- *Further imaging:* bedside ultrasound is shown above.

Questions for thought

- What are the appropriate initial actions to take to stabilize this patient?
- Once stable, what other tools can be used to make the diagnosis?
- What medications should be avoided in this patient?
- How does one urgently treat this condition in the emergency department?
- What is definitive treatment of this condition?
- Why does this patient have abdominal pain?

Diagnosis

Abdominal pain secondary to bladder obstruction with acute renal failure.

Discussion

- *Pathophysiology:* urinary tract obstruction is a relatively common problem. Causes of obstruction depend on the age of the patient. Anatomic abnormalities account for the majority of cases in children. Young adults typically present with urolithiasis. Prostatic hypertrophy or carcinoma, pelvic or retroperitoneal cancers, urethral strictures, and urolithiasis are the primary causes in older patients. Pharmacological agents, such as sympathomimetics or anticholinergics, can also cause bladder outlet obstruction with stimulation of the α-agonistic fibers of the bladder neck.
- *Presentation:* patients usually present with pain and oliguria or anuria. Pain is due to distension of the bladder, collecting system, or renal capsule. Severe pain may be seen with acute complete obstruction. It also occurs when there is acute bladder dilatation, after a fluid load increases the urine output to a level greater than the flow rate through the area of obstruction. The site of obstruction determines the location of pain. Upper ureteral or renal pelvic lesions lead to flank pain or tenderness, whereas lower ureteral obstruction causes pain that may radiate to the ipsilateral groin. Obstruction of the bladder neck or other distal structures can lead to a palpable suprapubic mass. A digital rectal exam should be performed to evaluate the prostate.
- *Diagnosis:* if the diagnosis of bladder obstruction is in question, the best exam in the emergency department is bedside ultrasonography. This permits visualization of the bladder to measure the volume of actual retained urine. For the oliguric patient, a post-void residual can be helpful. Serum tests should include renal function and electrolytes. An EKG in the anuric patient is important in order to assess for hyperkalemia. In the patient with complaints of renal colic, nausea, vomiting, and hematuria a spiral CT with renal stone protocol may be informative. It is also important to check the urine for blood, infection, and cytology in assessing for possible etiology of the bladder obstruction.
- *Treatment:* initial treatment should start with placement of a 16-French Foley catheter, which will relieve the distended bladder and kidneys. Patients with urethral strictures may require a 16-French Coudé (angulated) catheter to facilitate drainage of the bladder. In patients with significant obstruction, a suprapubic catheter may be required. Mucosal edema of the bladder wall can be seen with chronic distension, leading to transient gross hematuria which usually resolves spontaneously. Post-bladder decompression syncope is sometimes seen and can be treated symptomatically.
- *Definitive therapy:* although the main etiology for post-renal azotemia in the older male population is benign prostatic hypertrophy, it is important to rule out a malignant source. Leaving a catheter in for the short term is important to prevent a repeat episode of obstruction. A CT of the abdomen and pelvis, along with a prostate specific antigen (PSA) level, should be included in the workup. In addition, medications that help to increase urinary flow, such as tamsulosin, can be started. A thorough review of the patient's medication list may identify the possibility of drug-induced urinary retention.

Clinical course

The keys to this patient's diagnosis are careful attention to his history, physical exam, and ancillary studies.

Historical clues	Physical findings	Ancillary studies
• Abdominal pain with anuria	• Palpable mass in the suprapubic abdominal region	• Markedly elevated renal function
• Bilateral lower extremity edema	• Pitting edema to the lower extremities	• Anion gap acidosis
	• Bibasilar rales	• Large, fully distended bladder on ultrasound
		• Hydronephrosis on ultrasound

The patient had a Foley catheter placed in the emergency department which drained almost nine liters of clear yellow urine. After the first two liters were drained, the patient had gross hematuria. He was admitted to the hospital for observation of his acute renal failure. During the patient's hospital stay, his creatinine dropped from 25 to 1.6. Urine culture was negative. The PSA was found to be elevated. He was later discharged home with instructions to follow-up with urology to further investigate his elevated PSA.

Case #7

History

A 48-year-old woman presents to the ED complaining of sudden sharp right-sided abdominal pain which awoke her from sleep at 4:45 a.m., 1 hour prior to arrival. She states the pain has been persistent since it began and now is radiating diffusely throughout her abdomen. It is associated with nausea, although the patient has not vomited. She had a late dinner of lasagne at midnight before going to bed. The patient denies fever, shortness of breath, urinary symptoms, or vaginal discharge. The patient reports multiple episodes of similar symptoms over the last year. She had an outpatient right upper quadrant ultrasound done 1 year ago which was negative to her knowledge.

Past medical history

The patient has a history of chronic abdominal pain and menorrhagia secondary to endometriosis, for which she has had a left salpingo-oophorectomy and two diagnostic laparoscopies. The patient also had a dilatation and curettage; she is a G1P0. Her last menstrual period was 2 years ago. She works as a PACU assistant nurse manager, smokes, and lives with her husband of many years. The patient's father is deceased from an abdominal aortic aneurysm. Her mother is living and suffers from previous stroke, atrial fibrillation, hypertension, dementia, and arthritis. The patient has seven siblings, two of whom are sisters who had cholecystectomies.

Medications

The patient has been taking Prempro over the last year for menopausal symptoms.

Allergies

The patient has no known drug allergies.

Physical exam and ancillary studies

- *Vital signs:* the patient's oral temperature is 36.4°C, her heart rate is 100 bpm, her blood pressure is 148/91, her respiratory rate is 20, and her room air oxygen saturation is 99%. The patient weighs 135 pounds.
- *General:* the patient is awake and alert, acutely distressed secondary to pain, clutching her abdomen, lying in the right lateral decubitus position.
- *Head and neck:* the patient's pupils are equally round and reactive to light, cranial nerves are intact. There is no nasal discharge. The patient's mucous membranes are dry. Her neck is supple.

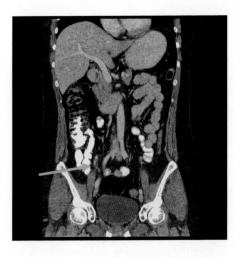

Figure 1.6. The patient's reformatted coronal image of CT of the abdomen and pelvis with oral and IV contrast indicates an enlarged appendix with an edematous wall (arrow). An appendicolith is located within the lumen.

- *Cardiovascular:* the patient has regular rate and rhythm, normal S1S2. Her radial and dorsalis pedis pulses are 2+/2+.
- *Lungs:* the patient has regular expansion and equal breath sounds, with no retractions, wheezes, rales, or rhonchi.
- *Abdomen:* the patient's abdomen is soft and non-distended. She has hyperactive bowel sounds, with tenderness to palpation at McBurney's point. There are positive Rovsing's, positive iliopsoas, and negative obturator signs. There is no rebound tenderness or guarding. The patient has a negative Murphy's sign. There are no appreciable masses or hernias. The patient has no hepatosplenomegaly or costovertebral angle tenderness (CVAT).
- *Extremities and skin:* the patient has full range of motion and no edema. Her skin is warm and dry, with normal capillary refill.
- *Pertinent abnormal labs:* the patient's white blood cell count is 14.4 with a left shift (segmented neutrophils 75%, bands 14%). The remaining lab tests including liver function tests, amylase, lipase, and urinalysis are within normal limits.

Questions for thought

- What other tests are needed to make the diagnosis?
- What are the differential diagnoses of this condition?
- What treatment should be given in the emergency department?
- What are the potential complications of this condition?
- What is the definitive treatment of this condition?
- What are the alternative treatment courses available?

Diagnosis

Acute appendicitis.

Discussion

- *Epidemiology:* the lifetime prevalence of appendicitis in the United States and Europe is between 5 and 10%, but it is almost non-existent in developing nations. A highly processed diet has been offered as a putative explanation for this difference. People of all ages suffer from appendicitis, but some patients typically present later in the course of their disease (age > 65 years, infants, immunosuppressed) and need to be evaluated with a higher degree of suspicion for the diagnosis.
- *Pathophysiology:* the pathologist Reginald Fitz first described inflammation of the vermiform appendix in 1886. The inciting event of appendicitis is an occlusion of the appendiceal lumen, which prevents normal drainage of the distal appendiceal contents. The resultant increased intraluminal pressure is transmitted to the appendiceal wall, causing venous congestion. As the venous congestion worsens over the next 48 to 72 hours, the appendiceal wall becomes necrotic and can ultimately perforate. After perforation, the patient may develop peritoneal signs from gross spillage of enteric contents into the peritoneum. Patients may also contain the perforation and develop a focal abscess.
- *Presentation:* the classic presentation of acute appendicitis is well described. Traditionally, the first symptom is abdominal pain, which begins as a dull ache in the periumbilical area or epigastrium. Then, as the inflamed appendix rubs against the parietal peritoneum (and its somatic nerve fibers), the pain becomes sharper and more focal in the right lower quadrant (RLQ). Nausea and anorexia follow the pain, after which the patient's abdomen becomes tender to palpation. Finally, the patient will characteristically develop a low-grade fever and mild leukocytosis (11 000–15 000), which both become more marked (greater than 38°C and 16 000) after appendiceal perforation. The presence of diarrhea, sick contacts, urinary or gynecologic symptoms, or similar prior episodes all speak against a diagnosis of appendicitis.
- *Physical exam:* McBurney's point is two-thirds of the distance from the umbilicus to the right anterior superior iliac spine (ASIS). It frequently overlies the appendiceal base and is the most common point of maximal tenderness in acute appendicitis. Historically, the appendix has been said to shift to the right upper quadrant in pregnant patients because the gravid uterus pushes the mobile cecum superiorly. Oto et al. recently disproved this aphorism in a series of patients who underwent abdominal MRIs to diagnose appendicitis. Although the study confirmed that the appendix tended to migrate superiorly from the first to third trimester, the appendiceal base only moved an average of two inches relative to the ASIS.
- Physical signs of peritoneal inflammation in appendicitis include RLQ hyperesthesia (the earliest sign of peritonitis), involuntary guarding or tense musculature, rebound tenderness, as well as the Rovsing's sign (which is referred RLQ tenderness upon left lower quadrant palpation). Rectal exam is important to identify whether the patient has guaiac-positive diarrhea (negatively predictive) or right-sided tenderness (positively predictive). Finally, the psoas and obturator signs indicate the presence of an inflamed, retrocecal appendix sitting upon the pelvic side wall muscles. The psoas test is performed by gently hyperextending the right hip. Obturator flexion is performed by medially rotating the right thigh. Either sign is positive if it reproduces abdominal pain.
- *Diagnosis:* an astute clinician can correctly identify only about 85–90% of patients with acute appendicitis, which corresponds to a negative surgical exploration rate of 10–15%.

Table 1.1. Alvarado's clinical scoring system for appendicitis

Clinical parameter	Score
Migration of pain	1
Anorexia	1
Nausea or vomiting	1
Right iliac fossa tenderness	2
Rebound tenderness	1
Temperature > 37.3°C	1
WBC > 10 000	2
Left shift > 75% PMNs	1
Total	10

Alvarado's score is a 10-point clinical scoring system designed to predict appendicitis based on clinical parameters, and is a good reminder of the important historical and physical clues for appendicitis. An Alvarado score of 8 or greater is about 96% sensitive for appendicitis, while a score of less than 5 usually rules out the diagnosis.

- Clinical diagnostic accuracy is lower in women, patients older than 50 years, and immunosuppressed patients, all of whom have more possible diagnoses than young male patients. CT imaging with oral contrast is very helpful in these difficult patients. Routine use of preoperative contrast-enhanced CT or MR can decrease the rate of negative surgical exploration from 15% to about 5%. Moreover, a negative CT or MR has a negative predictive value of about 98%, effectively ruling out a diagnosis of acute appendicitis.
- *Treatment:* surgical intervention is the standard of care for acute appendicitis in the United States. Open or laparoscopic appendectomies are basically equivalent in terms of operative time, length of hospital stay, post-operative pain, and time to return to work. In the ED, patients should receive intravenous fluids, pain control, and preoperative antibiotics to cover normal skin and colonic flora. Perforated appendicitis is a separate clinical entity and may not require surgery at all. If patients are stable clinically, they may be treated with bowel rest, IV antibiotics, and possible percutaneous drainage of defined abscesses. Interestingly, some European groups will treat all cases of acute appendicitis with antibiotics primarily, leaving surgical interventions to treat failures of medical therapy.
- *Follow-up:* in the setting of simple operative management of appendicitis, a single routine surgical post-operative visit is required to assess wound healing and to review pathology. Approximately 1% of pathology specimens will show malignant disease in the resected appendix, and these patients may require additional surgery. In the case of non-operatively managed appendicitis, the prevalence of recurrent appendicitis is reported at 5–10%. Based on the chance of recurrence or underlying malignancy, many US surgeons recommend a prophylactic appendectomy 6–12 weeks after initial presentation.

Clinical course

The keys to this patient's diagnosis are careful attention to her physical exam and ancillary studies, particularly since her history is suspicious for biliary colic.

Historical clues	Physical findings	Ancillary studies
• Acute onset	• Acute distress	• Normal LFTs, amylase, and lipase
• Symptoms awoke patient from sleep	• Hyperactive bowel sounds	• Normal EKG
• Unremitting abdominal pain	• Tenderness at McBurney's point	
• Nausea	• + Rovsing's, iliopsoas signs	
• Negative outpatient right upper quadrant ultrasound	• Negative Murphy's sign	
	• No CVAT	

In our patient, a dual contrasted CT of the abdomen and pelvis was consistent with a diagnosis of acute appendicitis. There was a fecolith in the appendix, with distal dilation of the tip to 1.1 cm and associated periappendiceal stranding. Prior to diagnosis, the patient received two liters of intravenous normal saline, anti-emetics, and narcotic analgesics with some relief of her symptoms. She received piperacillin-tazobactam en route to the operating room, where she underwent a laparoscopic appendectomy. The appendix was acutely inflamed with surrounding suppuration. Pathology showed an acute nonperforated appendicitis with no underlying tumors. The patient tolerated the surgery well and sustained a full recovery.

Further reading

Silen W. *Cope's Early Diagnosis of the Acute Abdomen*, 20th edition. New York: Oxford University Press, 2000, pp. 65–103.

Oto A, et al. Revisiting MRI for appendix location during pregnancy. *Am J Roentgenol* 2006;**186**(3): 883–7.

Yildirim E, et al. Alvarado scores and pain onset in relation to multislice CT findings in acute appendicitis. *Diagn Interv Radiol* 2008;**14**:14–18.

Raman SS, et al. Effect of CT on false positive diagnosis of appendicitis and perforation. *N Eng J Med* 2008;**358**(9):972–3.

Case #8

History

A 27-year-old man presents to the ED complaining of abdominal pain, nausea, and diarrhea over the past 3 days. The pain is located in the patient's upper abdomen. It is described as a dull and boring sensation, which has no change with position or food. The patient has some associated fevers, mild nausea, and generalized fatigue. He denies extensive alcohol, aspirin, or NSAID use. He has no melena, hematochezia, or gross red blood per rectum. He also denies any urinary complaints.

Past medical history

The patient had a tooth extraction last week and was placed on clindamycin. He drinks occasional alcohol and is not a smoker.

Medications

The patient's medications include clindamycin.

Allergies

The patient has no known drug allergies.

Physical exam and ancillary studies

- *Vital signs:* the patient's temperature is 38.2°C, his heart rate is 110 bpm, his blood pressure is 121/74, his respiratory rate is 24, and room air oxygen saturation is 98%.
- *General:* the patient is awake and alert. He appears fatigued and uncomfortable.
- *Head and neck:* the patient's head is normocephalic and atraumatic. He has anicteric sclera and dry mucous membranes. His neck is supple with a midline trachea.
- *Cardiovascular:* the patient has a rapid and regular heart rate without murmurs, rubs, or gallops. Distal pulses are all intact.
- *Lungs:* the patient's lungs are clear to auscultation bilaterally.
- *Abdomen:* the patient's abdomen is soft with some midepigastric fullness and tenderness. There is no guarding or rebound. There are no peritoneal signs. The patient has a negative Murphy's sign.
- *Extremities and skin:* the patient has no clubbing, cyanosis, or edema. His skin is warm and dry, without lesions.
- *Pertinent abnormal labs:* the patient's white blood cell count is 21, with 35% bands. His glucose is 454 and his lipase 780.

Questions for thought

- What are the appropriate initial actions to take to manage this patient?
- What are some diagnostic tools you can use to make a diagnosis?
- What are the main risk factors for this disease process?
- How does one treat this condition in the emergency department?
- What is definitive treatment of this condition?
- What are some of the complications of this disease process?

Diagnosis

Necrotizing pancreatitis.

Discussion

- *Epidemiology:* the age of onset of pancreatitis depends on its etiology. Pancreatitis is typically first seen in middle-aged patients. Males are more commonly affected than females, due to a higher incidence of alcoholic pancreatitis.
- *Pathophysiology:* pancreatitis is thought to be caused by destruction or malfunction of the pancreatic acinar cells, causing inflammation and enzymatic degradation of the surrounding tissue. It is most commonly caused by alcohol or biliary disease, but may also be caused by medications, hypercalcemia, hypertriglyceridemia, infection, trauma, procedures, and rarely by scorpion bite.
- *Presentation:* patients often have upper abdominal pain, most commonly in the mid-epigastric region and radiating to the back. Nausea and vomiting may be associated. Diarrhea can also be a common complaint, as was the case in this patient. His pancreatic machinery was damaged to the point of preventing adequate enzymatic release and gastrointestinal absorption, which in turn resulted in diarrhea. Depending on the cause and extent of the disease, the patient may also have systemic complaints, such as fever, respiratory complaints, or hepatic involvement. Hemorrhagic pancreatitis may exhibit ecchymotic areas on the flank or near the umbilicus.
- *Diagnosis:* this diagnosis can often be made on history and physical alone; however, elevated lipase and amylase levels help to confirm clinical suspicion. Imaging is not necessary in mild cases, but if there is severe disease a CT scan is necessary to elucidate any necrosis, hemorrhage, or fluid collection. If gallstone pancreatitis is suspected, an ultrasound will be helpful to determine biliary pathology.
- *Treatment:* mild pancreatitis is often successfully treated with supportive measures, such as bowel rest and fluid resuscitation. Patients with severe or necrotizing pancreatitis will need aggressive fluid therapy and intensive supportive treatment, especially if there is multisystem organ involvement. In the case of significant necrosis, prophylactic antibiotic therapy can reduce the incidence of infection. Early surgery or procedural intervention is reserved for decompensating patients, those with abscess formation, and patients with obstructive jaundice and biliary sepsis from gallstone pancreatitis.
- *Definitive therapy:* causative agents and underlying pathology contributing to the disease process need to be treated. Cholestatic disease needs to be addressed through procedural

intervention or surgery. Cessation of any alcohol use is imperative. Offending medications should be stopped and electrolyte abnormalities corrected.

- *Complications:* while most cases of pancreatitis are mild and resolve in less than 1 week, severe or necrotizing pancreatitis can be life-threatening. Infection, hemorrhage, and irreversible destruction of pancreatic tissue can occur. The patient may develop severe end-organ damage and multisystem involvement. Loss of pancreatic tissue may require the patient to be insulin-dependent and digestive-enzyme-dependent.

Clinical course

The keys to this patient's diagnosis are careful attention to his history, physical exam, and ancillary studies.

Historical clues	Physical findings	Ancillary studies
• Midepigastric abdominal pain	• Fever	• Elevated white blood cell count
• Nausea and vomiting	• Tachycardia	• Elevated glucose
• Diarrhea	• Midepigastric fullness	• Elevated pancreatic enzymes
• Fatigue	• Midepigastric tenderness	

This patient was recognized to have very severe pancreatitis. He was placed on a monitor, aggressively rehydrated, and his pain was controlled. A CT scan was performed showing necrosis of a large portion of the pancreas and a surrounding fluid collection. The patient was therefore given prophylactic imipenem. He symptomatically improved in the ED, and was eventually found to have a gallstone pancreatitis. The patient had a prolonged hospital course, involving a sphincterotomy and subsequent cholecystectomy, and is now reliant on digestive enzymes and insulin therapy.

Case #9

History

A 19-year-old Latino male presents to the ED with the chief complaint of 6 hours of abdominal pain and two episodes of vomiting. The pain awoke him from sleep, and has been persistently increasing over time. He describes the pain as sharp and crampy, and states that it comes in waves. Initially the paroxysms of pain occurred every 10 minutes. But now they are occurring every 3 or 4 minutes, and are increasing in length and intensity. The patient has had four episodes of emesis over the last 3 hours. The vomit initially consisted of the contents of the previous evening's dinner, but subsequently became yellow and then greenish-brown, though non-bloody. The patient states he had one "massive" explosive bowel movement and now has the intense urge to have another, but has not been able to even pass gas.

Past medical history

The patient's history is significant for an urgent laparotomy last year after a gunshot wound to his abdomen. He underwent resection of 18 inches of ileum, with an ileocecal anastomosis.

Medications

The patient's medications include clindamycin for a dental infection.

Allergies

The patient has no known drug allergies.

Physical exam and ancillary studies

- *Vital signs:* the patient's tympanic temperature is 37.8°C, his heart rate is variable between 90 bpm and up to 130 bpm during a painful episode, his respiratory rate is 20, his blood pressure is 142/100 mmHg, and his room air oxygen saturation is 98%.
- *General:* the patient is awake, alert, and appropriate. He is resting in bed comfortably until waves of pain cause him to double over and clutch his abdomen.
- *Head and neck:* the patient's mucous membranes are moist. His neck is supple without jugular venous distension or bruit. The patient's sclerae are non-icteric.
- *Cardiovascular:* the patient's heart is tachycardic without murmurs, rubs, or gallops. He has 2+ distal pulses in all four extremities.
- *Lungs:* the patient's breath sounds are equal and lungs are clear bilaterally without wheezes, rales, or rhonchi.
- *Abdomen:* the patient's abdomen demonstrates a midline surgical scar, well healed. The right upper and lower abdominal quadrants are more distended than the left, with

occasional observable peristaltic waves. The bowel sounds are initially normoactive, but during auscultation a high-pitched sound with a "rush" is heard. There is slight tenderness to palpation without rebound or guarding in the right lower quadrant. There are no masses or organomegaly.

- *Extremities and skin:* the patient's skin is dry without rashes. There is no peripheral edema. The patient's legs are of equal size, with no palpable cords.
- *Neurologic:* the patient's cranial nerves II–XII are grossly intact. He has 5/5 strength and reflexes are 2+ in the upper and lower extremities.
- *Pertinent abnormal labs:* the patient has a mildly elevated white count at 12 000, but without left shift. His chemistry profile is significant for hypochloremia at 97 and a low bicarbonate at 18.
- *Radiographs:* the patient's chest X-ray is unremarkable, with no free air below the diaphragm. His flat and upright abdominal films show distended loops of small bowel, no free air in the biliary tree, no air fluid levels, and no large bowel distension.

Questions for thought

- What are the appropriate initial actions to take to stabilize this patient?
- What are the differential diagnoses?
- What are other ways to make the diagnosis?
- What is the definitive treatment of this condition?

Diagnosis
Small bowel obstruction.

Discussion
- *Epidemiology:* small bowel obstruction (SBO) is one of the most common abdominal surgical emergencies, with an incidence of up to 300 000 cases per year in the United States. The condition was classically and still can be caused by hernias (inguinal or femoral). However, with the increased incidence and survival of patients undergoing planned and urgent laparotomies, the overwhelming cause of more than three-fourths of cases is now surgical adhesions. In the future, this number may diminish due to heightened use of laparoscopy, but there are currently no data to support this hypothesis. The condition is also common among patients with Crohn's disease due to the frequent occurrence of strictures. SBO can result from intussusception in young children and bowel cancers in older patients.
- *Pathophysiology:* bowel obstruction occurs when there is failure of intestinal contents to pass through the lumen of the gut. This can be secondary to loss of intestinal motility (also known as ileus) due to peritonitis, recent surgery, electrolyte abnormalities, or chronic opioid use. Actual obstruction occurs as a result of intra- or extraluminal obstruction and compression. Mechanical obstruction occurs in the setting of surgical adhesions, which act as a lead point around which the gut can coil and kink. Other lead points include

Meckel's diverticulum in children and polyps, lymphoma, and colonic adenocarcinoma in adults. Hernias can directly block the passage of bowel contents and, if severe enough, can also compromise vascular supply, leading to "strangled" bowel. SBO tends to occur among psychiatric patients by formation of a bezoar (clump of indigestible organic or vegetable matter, such as hair) or by formation of a sigmoid volvulus from use of psychiatric medications with anticholinergic properties. If a bowel obstruction progresses to its natural end point, the intraluminal pressure will become greater than the pressure within the vascular and lymphatic bed, ceasing drainage and causing ischemia. This in turn permits spontaneous translocation of bacteria across the bowel wall into the bloodstream and peritoneum, leading to sepsis and shock.

- *Presentation:* the presentation of bowel obstruction can be somewhat nonspecific, and is almost purely a clinical diagnosis. Although it is possible to estimate where in the gut the obstruction has occurred, this is notoriously inaccurate. All patients' initial symptom is pain, which is generally described as severe and intermittent if the patient has a mechanical obstruction or less severe and more constant if the patient has an aperistaltic ileus. The pain is generally not reproducible by palpation, as the peritoneum is not involved until late in the disease course. Vomiting occurs with obstruction in the proximal GI tract, and classically progresses in color and feculence from light to dark. Constipation tends to present with a more distal obstruction. Bowel sounds may be normal, but are classically described as high-pitched or "rushing." Laboratory tests are generally nonspecific for SBO. The CBC may demonstrate an elevated white count if infection has set in, but, as sepsis is a late and hopefully avoided complication of intestinal obstruction, the lack of a leukocyte count should not rule this condition out. There may be electrolyte abnormalities caused by the vomiting (hypochloremic alkalosis), but this generally takes hours to days to develop. The objective is early diagnosis prior to these changes. Plain radiographs should be performed in all cases of suspected obstruction. Abdominal films can confirm the diagnosis, and illustrate free air under the diaphragm in the case of viscus rupture. However, X-rays cannot rule out obstruction, and the gold standard for radiographic diagnosis is an abdominal CT with oral and IV contrast. Bedside ultrasound can be useful for ruling in, but never for ruling out bowel obstruction.
- *Treatment:* in treating the patient with small and large bowel obstructions, the final common pathway often occurs in the surgical suite. Notification of the on-call surgical team should not be delayed. In the ED, it is important to initiate treatment with intestinal decompression. This is achieved via a large-bore nasogastric tube, which may avert the need for surgical intervention. The risk of infection due to bacterial septicemia and peritonitis is high in these patients, and they should be empirically started on broad-spectrum antibiotics. Zosyn (piperacillin-tazobactam) or Unasyn (ampicillin-sulbactam) are appropriate choices. If the patient is penicillin allergic, treatment can consist of a combination of clindamycin, gentamicin, metronidazole, vancomycin and/or third- or fourth-generation cephalosporins. All patients should receive IV fluids, and should be typed and crossed in anticipation of a trip to the operating suite.

Clinical course

The keys to this patient's diagnosis and eventual treatment were careful attention to his history and physical exam, with ancillary radiographic studies.

Historical clues	Physical findings	Ancillary studies
• Previous history of abdominal surgery	• Distended abdomen	• Radiograph with distended loops of small bowel
• Vomiting	• Rushing bowel sounds	
• Inability to pass stool or air	• Tenderness on abdominal exam	
	• Tachycardia	

This patient was suspected of having a small bowel obstruction based on the nature and time course of his symptoms, his history of recent abdominal surgery, and a physical exam significant for notable intestinal peristalsis. Abdominal radiograph confirmed the diagnosis. A nasogastric tube was placed, immediately draining 500 mL of brown feculent liquid. Intravenous hydration, broad-spectrum antibiotics, and pain medications were initiated. The surgeons quickly evaluated the patient and brought him to the operating theater. Within 2 hours, they discovered and corrected a cecal volvulus at the ileocecal junction, restoring blood flow to the affected intestine. The patient sustained a full recovery.

Further reading

Vicaro S, Price T. Intestinal obstruction. *Tintanelli's Emergency Medicine*, 6th edition. New York: McGraw-Hill, 2004.

Silen W. *Cope's Early Diagnosis of the Acute Abdomen*, 20th edition. New York: Oxford University Press, 2000.

Tierney L., ed. *Current Medical Diagnosis and Treatment*, 41st edition. New York: Lange Medical Books/McGraw-Hill, 2002.

Case #10

History

A 30-year-old female is brought into the emergency department by ambulance with complaints of severe constant abdominal pain. The pain initially started on her left side and slowly spread out and has since become diffuse. She states she has had similar pain during childbirth but denies any chance of pregnancy now, as she has had a tubal ligation. She denies nausea, vomiting, and dysuria. She has no vaginal discharge. She denies trauma to her abdomen or forceful sex. The patient admits to trying a substance she believes was heroin for the first time 1 day before the pain started.

Past medical history

The patient has a history of asthma. She had a tubal ligation several years ago.

Medication

The patient takes albuterol when needed.

Allergies

She has no known allergies.

Physical exam and ancillary studies

- *Vital signs:* the patient's temperature is 37.1°C, her pulse is 85 bpm, her blood pressure is 129/88, her respirations are 20, and her oxygen saturation is 99% on room air.
- *General:* the patient is in obvious distress secondary to abdominal discomfort. She is lying quietly in bed since any movement exacerbates the pain.
- *Head and neck:* the patient has moist mucous membranes. Her neck is supple without lymphadenopathy.
- *Cardiovascular:* the patient's heart has a regular rate and rhythm with no murmur.
- *Respiratory:* her breath sounds are equal and clear bilaterally.
- *Abdomen:* the patient's abdomen is diffusely tender to palpation, greatest in the right upper quadrant. Her bilateral lower quadrants are tender with equal severity. She has no peritoneal signs. She has no McBurney's point tenderness, Rovsing's or obturator signs. She has no abdominal pain on heel tap. Her rectal exam shows no masses, tenderness, or blood.
- *Pelvic exam:* the patient has no cervical discharge or tenderness. There are no adnexal masses.

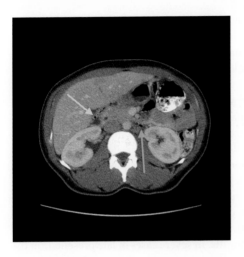

Figure 1.7. This abdominal CT shows multiple foci of air, concerning for an extraluminal location along the posterior edge of the left hepatic lobe (upper left arrow) and in the left retroperitoneal region. There is also air in the left mid-abdomen (right arrow), concerning for duodenal perforation.

- *Musculoskeleta/neurologic:* the patient's extremities are without tenderness, clubbing, or cyanosis. Her neurologic exam is intact.
- *Skin:* the patient's skin has no lesions or rashes.
- *Pertinent labs:* the patient's complete blood cell count is remarkable for a white blood cell count of 11.3, a hematocrit of 30.3%, and normal liver function tests. All other lab studies are negative or normal.
- *Radiographs:* the patient's upright abdominal X-ray shows no free air or air fluid levels. A representative slice of her computed tomography is shown in Figure 1.7.

Questions for thought

- What is the most appropriate initial intervention in this patient?
- Once stable, what are other diagnostic tools you can use to make a diagnosis?
- What medications should be avoided in this patient?
- What is the most appropriate ER intervention in this patient?
- What is the definitive treatment of this condition?
- Why does this patient have abdominal pain?

Diagnosis

Acute abdomen with suspicion of hollow viscus perforation.

Discussion

- *Epidemiology:* an acute abdomen is a frequent presentation in the emergency department. Multiple disease processes can lead to this clinical picture. Inflammatory processes in abdominal organs, such as appendicitis, cholecystitis, diverticulitis and pancreatitis can cause an acute abdomen. Other causes include hollow organ perforation, bowel obstruction, or referred pain from other organs such as the heart, lung, or kidney. One of the most dramatic presentations is in patients with perforated hollow viscus. The most common causes of perforation are peptic duodenal or gastric ulcers or diverticulitis. Other, more rare causes are perforated lymphatic patches in patients with salmonella typhi, Borhaave's syndrome, and acute ulcer perforation in patients with cocaine abuse.

- *Pathophysiology:* initial inflammation of intraperitoneal organs and visceral peritoneum causes visceral pain, which is perceived by patients as an undifferentiated, vague pain in the mid-abdomen. This pain is poorly localized. Later, with involvement of parietal peritoneum (which is innervated by somatic, intercostal nerves) pain becomes localized to the area of the pathological process. Irritation of the parietal peritoneum causes significant pain, adynamia of the bowels and protective contraction of the overlying abdominal musculature referred as passive guarding. Due to vagal activation, bradycardia can be evident during the first few hours of symptoms, especially in cases of perforation. With progression of pain, dehydration secondary to third spacing, and eventual sepsis, the patient develops tachycardia and progresses to peritonitis. In severe cases of late presentation the patient can be toxic, with unstable vital signs. Mentation can be depressed. At this stage, the patient's abdomen is usually firm due to peritoneal irritation, oftentimes described as "board-like."

- *Presentation:* the presentation of patients with acute abdomen depends on the specific derangement causing the pain. Many will initially have vague and ill-defined pain. The pain may be crampy in cases of bowel obstruction or biliary colic. In inflammatory processes, such as cholecystitis, it is usually constant, becoming worse over time. Pancreatitis pain is epigastric in location and extremely intense, secondary to somatic innervation and retroperitoneal location. Leaking of gastrointestinal contents into the peritoneal cavity from a perforation leads to significant irritation, causing severe pain and adynamia of bowels. Usually patients with "true" surgical acute abdomen and peritoneal irritation appear toxic. They typically lie very still in bed since every movement causes aggravation of their pain. Dyspepsia, such as nausea, emesis and anorexia, is common in surgical patients but usually evolves after the pain.

- *Diagnosis:* diagnosis of acute abdomen is primarily clinical and involves careful analysis of patient history and physical exam. Additional studies oftentimes can be done to rule out other pathology. Chest X-ray and electrocardiogram can be performed in patients with SOB and upper limit of age to rule out pneumonia or myocardial infarction. Chest radiograph also allows evaluation of free air under the diaphragm in cases of suspected perforation. Computed tomography is the most sensitive readily available study to evaluate for most causes of intraabdominal pathology, with sensitivity and specificity approaching 99% for some disease processes.

- *Treatment:* ultimately, patients with an acute abdomen will require prompt surgical evaluation. Surgical consultation should be obtained as soon as the diagnosis is suspected. Initial interventions in the ED should include fluid resuscitation. The patient should not be allowed to take anything by mouth until the treatment plan has been agreed upon in concert with surgery. Patients with emesis and nausea, especially those with suspected small bowel obstruction or requiring surgery, will benefit from nasogastric tube placement. Pain medication should be provided, as numerous studies have shown that providing analgesia does not hinder physical diagnosis. Finally, if the clinician suspects perforation, broad spectrum antibiotics should be administered.

- *Definitive therapy:* patients with a perforated hollow viscus require prompt surgical intervention.

Clinical course

The keys to this patient's diagnosis are careful attention to her history, physical exam, and ancillary studies.

Historical clues	Physical findings	Ancillary studies
• Use of drugs	• Diffusely tender abdomen	• Mild leukocytosis
• Abdominal pain, initially epigastric, spreading to entire abdomen	• Normal pelvic exam	• CT findings suspicious for free air

This patient was suspected of having an acute abdomen based on her history and exam, and underwent rapid CT of her abdomen, which supported her working diagnosis of hollow viscus perforation. On repeat questioning, the patient admitted to taking cocaine and not heroin, which was probably the predisposing factor in her duodenal perforation. She was fluid-resuscitated and received broad-spectrum antibiotics and narcotic analgesics. She was taken urgently to the operating room by the surgical team and underwent diagnostic laparoscopy for suspected perforated ulcer. However, no perforation was found. That led the surgeons to perform an exploratory laparotomy – and again no pathology was found after careful inspection of the abdominal cavity. Intraoperative esophagogastroduodenoscopy and injection of methylene blue did not reveal perforation, either. The patient's surgical wound was closed and she was admitted to the hospital, where she underwent uneventful recovery and was discharged on post-operative day 5.

This case reinforces the difficulties in diagnosis and management of acute abdomen, even with the most experienced of physicians. This patient may have had a perforation that closed on its own, or possibly had transient ischemia related to cocaine use, but no definitive cause was ever found.

Further reading

Humphries R, Russel A. Chapter 13. Abdominal pain. In Stone CK Humphries RL, eds., *Current Emergency Diagnosis and Treatment*, 5th edition. New York: McGraw-Hill, 2004, pp. 257–82.

Doherty G, Boey J. The acute abdomen. In Way L Doherty G, eds., *Current Surgical Diagnosis and Treatment*, 11th edition. New York: McGraw-Hill/Appleton & Lange, 2003, pp. 503–17.

Soybel D, Delcore R. Acute abdominal pain. In Souba WW, et al., eds., *ACS Surgery: Principles & Practice* WebMD Professional Publishing, 2008.

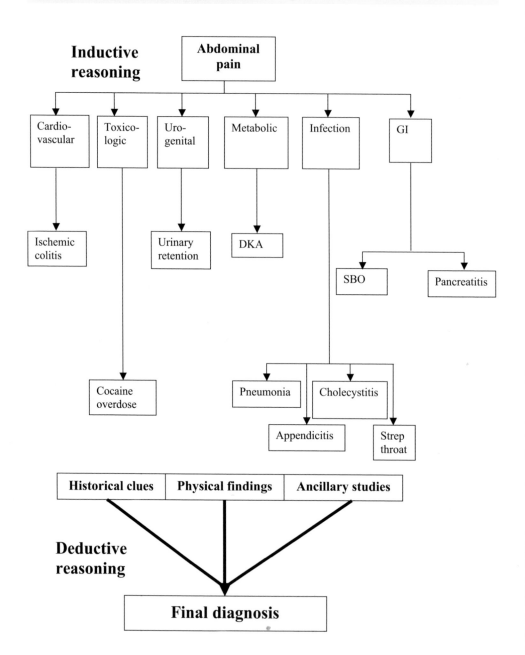

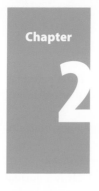

Chapter 2

Chief complaint: fever

Shellie Asher, Nicole M. Cicchino, David Conti, Luke Day, Wendy DeMartino, Kevin Jones, Leon Kushnir, Dimitrios Makridis, P. J. Miller, Joseph C. Piccione, Taylor Spencer, Aixa Toledo

Case #1

History

A 21-year-old Caucasian male presents to the ED complaining of a 1-week history of intermittent chills without rigors, with measured temperatures at home of 38.0°C to 38.3°C, mostly at bedtime. He denies any rash, fatigue, anorexia, or weight loss. He also denies any night sweats, headache, cough, diarrhea, dysuria, or ill contacts.

He initially contacted his primary care doctor, who ordered a complete blood count. He was told that this was "essentially normal." He also had chemistry studies and was told he had a mild elevation of his liver enzymes. He was advised to come to the ED if the fever continued.

Past medical history

The patient has a history of moderate to severe inflammatory acne, for which he sees a dermatologist. He also has a history of a left meniscal tear after sports-related trauma, and has had arthroscopy.

Medications

The patient has been taking minocycline ER 90 mg p.o. daily for the last 2 weeks, which was prescribed by his dermatologist. He also takes a multivitamin.

Allergies

The patient has no drug allergies.

Physical exam and ancillary studies

- *Vital signs:* the patient's temperature is 38.3°C, his heart rate is 61 bpm, his blood pressure is 105/50 mmHg, his respiratory rate is 16, and his room air oxygen saturation is 98%.

Case Studies in Emergency Medicine, ed. R. Jeanmonod, M. Tomassi and D. Mayer.
Published by Cambridge University Press © Cambridge University Press 2010.

- *General:* he is awake and alert and in no distress. He has an athletic build.
- *Head and neck:* his pupils are equally round and reactive to light, and his cranial nerves are intact. He has no scleral icterus. His mucous membranes are moist, without petechiae or intraoral lesions. His neck is supple, and there is no cervical, supraclavicular, or axillary adenopathy. His face is scarred from acne.
- *Cardiovascular:* the patient's heart has a regular rate and rhythm, without any murmur, rub, or gallop.
- *Lungs:* his lungs are clear to auscultation bilaterally, without wheezes or rhonchi.
- *Abdomen:* the patient's abdomen is soft, non-tender, and not distended. He has normal bowel sounds. The patient's liver edge is palpable at 7 cm below the costal margin. He has no splenomegaly.
- *Extremities and skin:* he has no peripheral edema. Other than the changes secondary to acne, his skin has no lesions.
- *Genital exam:* the patient has normal-size testicles without tumors, a normal penis without discharge, and no inguinal adenopathy. His rectal exam is unremarkable.
- *Neurologic exam:* he is alert and oriented, without any focal deficits. The patient's reflexes are normal bilaterally. His gait is normal.
- *Pertinent labs:* the patient's white blood cell count is 9.8, with a normal differential except for 10% eosinophils. His ALT is 105 and his AST is 85. His urinalysis is unremarkable.
- *EKG:* his EKG is in a normal sinus rhythm, without ST or axis changes.
- *Radiographs:* the patient's chest X-ray is read as normal.

Questions for thought

- What is the differential diagnosis in this patient?
- Does the patient need admission to the hospital?
- How should this patient be managed?

Diagnosis

Drug fever.

Discussion

- *Epidemiology:* febrile response to a drug is a common, often unrecognized, event. It occurs in 3–5% of general medicine patients, and in up to 10% of inpatients. Drug fever is defined as a fever coinciding with the administration of a drug that disappears after the discontinuation of the drug. It may be accompanied by cutaneous manifestations.
- *Pathophysiology:* multiple factors are implicated in the pathogenesis of drug fever, including hypersensitivity reactions, altered thermoregulatory mechanisms, fever directly related to administration of the drug, fever caused by direct extension of the pharmacologic action of the drug, and idiosyncratic reactions. Virtually all drugs have fever in their side-effect profile.
- *Presentation:* the timing of onset of fever secondary to a drug can range from less than 24 hours to many months after exposure, and does not help differentiate between other

causes of fever. Some patients with this entity may feel and look well despite the fever, whereas others have a dramatic pattern of spiking fevers, chills, and even rigors. A useful, though relatively uncommon, clinical hint is that patients with drug fever may have a relative bradycardia.

In hypersensitivity reactions, fever may be the only manifestation. Associated findings, such as rash or urticaria, hepatic or renal dysfunction, pulmonary involvement, mucosal ulceration, and hematologic abnormalities (such as eosinophilia), may increase the level of suspicion for this entity. Drug fever due to minocycline may manifest in association with elevation of liver function tests, rash, arthralgia, or interstitial nephritis. Hypersensitivity to anticonvulsants can present with a mononucleosis-like syndrome, lymphadenopathy, a morbilliform rash, or even Stevens-Johnson syndrome (especially with lamotrigine). Beta-lactam antibiotics and sulfonamides usually cause rash as an associated feature of drug fever.

Exogenous thyroid hormone can increase basal metabolic rate and heat production, and drugs with anticholinergic activity such as tricyclic antidepressants and phenothiazines can cause fever or hyperthermia especially when taken in combination. Amphetamines or illicit drugs such as cocaine or MDMA (ecstasy) can present with hyperthermia, seizures, and rhabdomyolysis secondary to marked vasodilatation due to their sympathomimetic properties and direct effects on hypothalamic function.

Idiosyncratic reactions causing fever include malignant hyperthermia and neuroleptic malignant syndrome, and these usually present with a very high temperature (>39.4°C). Patients with fever from this etiology often also have muscle rigidity, mental status changes, metabolic acidosis, and autonomic dysfunction.

- *Treatment:* discontinuation of the potential culprit drug is the only way to know whether it was really causing the fever, and in these situations fever should usually subside in 3 to 4 days. Although re-challenge with the same drug may cause fever again, which would confirm the diagnosis, this is rarely done in practice. Supportive care for other associated symptoms, such as pneumonitis, is usually all that is necessary.
- *Definitive therapy:* documentation of the medication reaction in the patient's chart, especially in reactions that clinically seem to be due to hypersensitivity or idiosyncratic factors, is critical to avoiding recurrence. Patients should be informed of the reaction and encouraged to avoid the drug in the future.

Clinical course

The key to this patient's diagnosis was careful attention to history, physical exam, and ancillary studies. Drug fever is ultimately a diagnosis of exclusion, and this patient underwent an extensive evaluation to rule out other potential causes of his fever.

Historical clues	Physical findings	Ancillary studies
• Recent new medication	• Hepatomegaly	• Eosinophilia
• Drug known to cause drug fever	• Relative bradycardia	• Mildly elevated LFTs
• No other obvious symptoms to account for fever	• No other fever source on exam	• No other fever source identified with ancillary studies
• No risk factors for occult infection		

This young and previously healthy patient's physical exam was unrevealing of any acute infectious or connective tissue or malignant disease process, and he had no risk factors for sexually transmitted, travel-related, or exposure-related fever. His laboratory exam was normal except for eosinophilia and mild transaminasemia. After review of the clinical and laboratory data, decision was made to discharge the patient home with the instruction to withhold the minocycline.

His symptoms completely resolved over the next 2 days. He was asymptomatic when he followed up with his primary care doctor 10 days later and his liver function tests and eosinophils had returned to normal.

Further reading

Roush MK, Nelson KM. Understanding drug-induced febrile reactions. *Am Pharm* 1993;**NS33**:39.

Tabor PA. Drug-induced fever. *Drug Intell Clin Pharm* 1986;**20**:413.

Johnson DH, Cunha BA. Drug fever. *Infect Dis Clin North Am* 1996;**10**:85.

Gorard DA. Late-onset drug fever associated with minocycline. *Postgrad Med J* 1990;**66**:404.

Sitbon O, Bidel N, Dussopt C, et al. Minocycline pneumonitis and eosinophilia. *Arch Intern Med* 1994;**154**:1633.

Case #2

History

> An 88-year-old woman presents to the ED brought in by ambulance during a heat wave. The prehospital providers report that the patient's mail carrier was concerned because she had not retrieved her mail in 3 days. He called the police, who forcibly entered the patient's city apartment and found her stuporous. The ambient temperature in the apartment was 38.9°C.

Past medical history

The patient has a history of hypertension.

Medications

The patient's medications include atenolol and furosemide.

Allergies

She has no known drug allergies.

Social history

The patient lives alone in a city apartment, which does not have air conditioning. She has no family nearby, and lives on public assistance.

Physical exam and ancillary studies

- *Vital signs:* the patient's vital signs are remarkable for a temperature of 41°C, a heart rate of 92 bpm, a blood pressure of 85/40 mmHg, a respiratory rate of 28, and a room air oxygen saturation of 96%.
- *General:* the patient is lethargic. She responds only to painful stimuli.
- *Head and neck:* her head shows no signs of trauma. Her sclerae are non-icteric. The patient's mucous membranes are very dry.
- *Cardiovascular:* the patient's heart is slightly tachycardic, with a normal S1 and S2. Her rhythm is regular. She has no murmurs. Her distal pulses are decreased but equal in all four extremities.
- *Lungs:* her lungs are clear to auscultation, and she has good air entry throughout.
- *Abdomen:* the patient's abdomen is soft, and not apparently tender. She has no palpable masses.
- *Extremities and skin:* the patient's skin is hot and dry. She has no rash. Her extremities are without cyanosis or edema. Her muscle tone is decreased.
- *Neurologic:* the patient opens her eyes and withdraws to painful stimuli. She has no obvious focal findings.

- *Pertinent labs:* the patient's complete blood count is remarkable for a white blood cell count of 23.2 and a hematocrit of 48.2%. Her chemistries are remarkable for a sodium of 152, a potassium of 5.5, a blood urea nitrogen of 65, a creatinine of 3.2, and a glucose of 42. Her ALT is 155 and her AST is 140. The remainder of blood counts, electrolytes, and coagulation studies are normal. Her urinalysis reveals positive protein and hemoglobin, with a specific gravity of 1.030.
- *EKG:* the patient's EKG shows sinus tachycardia, with no evidence of ischemia or severe electrolyte abnormality.
- *Radiographs:* the patient's chest X-ray is read as normal. The patient's head CT shows no acute abnormality.

Questions for thought

- What are the appropriate initial actions to take to stabilize this patient?
- What medications should be avoided in this patient?
- How does one urgently treat this condition in the emergency department?
- What is the definitive treatment of this condition?
- What is the prognosis for this patient?

Diagnosis

Hyperpyrexia secondary to exogenous heat and inability to autoregulate (heatstroke).

Discussion

- *Definition:* heat exhaustion is associated with mild to moderate dysfunction of temperature autoregulation, with associated dehydration and salt depletion. Heatstroke is severe dysfunction, with temperatures greater than 40°C with systemic inflammation and central nervous system (CNS) involvement.
- *Epidemiology:* exact numbers are unknown, but it is estimated that thousands of patients seek treatment each year for heat illnesses in the United States. The Centers for Disease Control report 4780 heat-related deaths over a 20-year period. The incidence is directly related to ambient temperature. Patients who are very young, very old, medically debilitated, or who are taking medications which blunt compensatory mechanisms are more susceptible to heat illnesses. Mortality may be up to 70% in patients presenting with CNS symptoms and a delay to treatment.
- *Pathophysiology:* passive heat exhaustion or heatstroke occurs in patients who cannot avoid extremes of temperature and have poor autoregulatory abilities. In normal cases, rising body temperature stimulates compensatory mechanisms which increase the body's ability to dissipate heat, primarily through radiation and evaporation. These compensatory mechanisms include shunting of blood to the peripheral circulation, increased minute ventilation, and increased sweating. Cellular damage begins to occur as early as 45 minutes with core temperatures of 42°C. In addition, the body mounts an acute-phase inflammatory response to hyperpyrexia resembling sepsis.

- *Presentation:* patients early in the course of illness may present with vague symptoms such as nausea or vomiting, fatigue, weakness, lightheadedness, headache, and myalgias. Progression to heatstroke results in hyperthermia above 40°C and CNS involvement which may include altered behavior, psychosis, lethargy, confusion, disorientation, seizure, delirium, or coma. Anhidrosis may or may not be present, and is usually a late finding. Tachycardia will be present in patients able to mount this response. Vital signs also reveal tachypnea and increased pulse pressure. Associated disseminated intravascular coagulation may result in purpura, conjunctival hemorrhages, gastrointestinal bleeding, or hematuria. Acute renal failure may result in oliguria or anuria. Decreased muscular tone distinguishes heatstroke from malignant hyperthermia or neuroleptic malignant syndrome.
- *Treatment:* mainstays of treatment are immediate cooling and support of end-organ oxygenation, perfusion, and function. Prehospital care includes removing the patient from the hot environment and removing excessive clothing. Airway, breathing, and circulation should be closely monitored and issues addressed as needed. Emergency department care includes cooling measures such as misting the patient and fan evaporation, cooling blankets, or ice packs to the neck, groin, and axillae. Alternative methods include immersion in ice water or internal cooling such as ice water gastric, bladder, rectal, peritoneal or thoracic lavage. These methods, however, have significant drawbacks and are therefore used sparingly. Intravenous fluid support should be instituted, with replacement of one-half of the total body water deficit in the first few hours. Antipyretics are not useful. Patients in frank rhabdomyolysis should receive sodium bicarbonate to alkalinize the urine.
- *Definitive therapy:* patients with heatstroke, or those with heat exhaustion who have significant electrolyte abnormalities or evidence of end-organ dysfunction, should be admitted to the hospital with cardiac monitoring. There should also be a low threshold for admitting elderly or debilitated patients. Fluid and electrolyte abnormalities should be corrected carefully. Prognosis is directly related to the height and duration of temperature. With appropriate cooling measures and prompt treatment, probability of survival is 90%. Mortality increases with severe liver damage, prolonged CNS symptoms, acute renal failure, and hyperkalemia.

Clinical course

The keys to this patient's diagnosis are careful attention to history, physical exam, and ancillary studies.

Historical clues	Physical findings	Ancillary studies
• Elderly patient	• Severe hyperthermia	• Electrolyte imbalance
• High ambient temperature	• Altered mentation	• Acute renal failure
• Medications which blunt adaptive mechanisms	• Evidence of dehydration	• Evidence of hepatic damage

This elderly patient was suspected to have acute heatstroke based upon her presentation of extreme hyperthermia and altered mental status. Based upon this, active external cooling was initiated. The patient's labs later provided adjunctive evidence of end-organ damage, including renal failure and liver abnormalities, as well as severe dehydration. Her electrolyte and fluid abnormalities were corrected slowly. The patient was admitted to the medical inten-sive care unit for close neurologic and hemodynamic monitoring. She did not fully recover to her previous baseline, and was eventually discharged to a long-term care facility.

Further reading

Hoppe J. Heat exhaustion and heatstroke. Retrieved from eMedicine.com on April 8, 2008.

Case #3

History

A 12-month-old male who was noted to have a slight fever at home today presents to the emergency department. His mother states that he has had a runny nose and cough that has been ongoing for several days. He has not had any shortness of breath. He has not had any vomiting. He was tolerating normal feedings until today when he had decreased intake. He did not have any diarrhea and has had a normal amount of wet diapers. He was slightly irritable last night, and with development of the fever, Mom got concerned and decided to bring him into the ED. He has had sick contacts, as several people around him have had upper respiratory tract infections.

Past medical history

He is a full-term baby, with no health problems. He is up to date on his immunizations.

Past surgical history

The child has had no surgeries.

Medications

He takes no medications.

Allergies

This patient has no known drug allergies.

Physical exam and ancillary studies

- *Vital signs:* the patient has a temperature of 37.2°C, a heart rate of 125 bpm, a respiratory rate of 24, a BP of 89/60 mmHg, and an oxygen saturation of 97% on room air.
- *General:* he is awake and alert, and is non-toxic in appearance. He has no respiratory distress at this time.
- *Head and neck:* the patient has no signs of trauma. His pupils are equal, round, and reactive to light. He has moist oral mucosa. His neck is supple and his trachea is midline. His tympanic membranes are clear bilaterally.
- *Cardiovascular:* the patient's heart has a regular rate and rhythm, with normal S1 and S2. He has no murmurs, rubs, or gallops.
- *Lungs:* his lungs are clear to auscultation bilaterally. He has no wheezes, rales, or rhonchi.
- *Abdomen:* his abdomen is soft, non-tender, and non-distended. He has normoactive bowel sounds.
- *Extremities and skin:* the patient has no petechiae or rashes. His skin is warm and dry.
- *Radiology:* the patient's chest X-ray is shown in Figure 2.1.

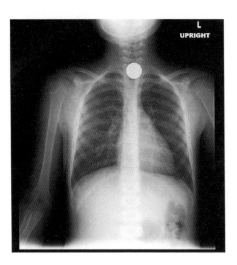

Figure 2.1. This chest X-ray shows a radio-opaque foreign body in the esophagus, probably a coin.

Questions for thought

- How do you tell on X-ray whether a foreign body is in the esophagus or the trachea?
- Should all foreign bodies be removed?
- What are the risks of not removing a foreign body?
- Who should remove the foreign body?

Diagnosis

Foreign body in esophagus.

Discussion

- *Epidemiology:* according to reports to the American Poison Control Center, 111 000 ingestions of foreign bodies occurred in children under the age of 19 in 2005. In young children the male to female ratio is 1:1. The greatest incidence is in children aged 6 months to 4 years of age. Children primarily swallow radio-opaque items such as coins, toys, crayons, pins, screws, button batteries, and pen caps. Most objects will pass spontaneously. Only 10–20% require intervention.
- *Pathophysiology:* there are five areas of constriction in the esophagus of a pediatric patient. The most common area for a foreign body to lodge is at the narrowing at C6 (cricopharyngeal sling). Other areas of constriction are T1 (the thoracic inlet), T4 (the aortic arch), T6 (tracheal bifurcation), T10–11 (hiatal narrowing). A study by Waltzman et al. showed that asymptomatic children are more likely to spontaneously pass the object and that most of the asymptomatic foreign bodies were in the distal esophagus. While most symptomatic foreign body ingestions in children result in obstruction of the proximal esophagus, obstruction can occur anywhere in the digestive tract. Large or irregularly shaped materials are unlikely to pass spontaneously. Objects that are longer than 6 cm and wider than 2 cm will not be able to pass into the pylorus. Objects that have sharp edges or an

irregular shape have an increased likelihood of causing an obstruction rather than spontaneously passing. Some complications of retained foreign bodies include airway obstruction, aspiration, stricture, mechanical or chemical erosion, peritonitis, perforation, mediastinitis, cardiac tamponade, paraesophageal abscess, and aortotracheoesophageal fistula.

- *Presentation:* children with an esophageal foreign body may be asymptomatic. Some common signs and symptoms include refusal to eat, vomiting, hematemesis, gagging, choking, stridor, neck or throat pain, inability to swallow, increased salivation, a foreign body sensation, red throat, dysphagia, palatal abrasions, fever, anxiety, respiratory distress and peritoneal signs. X-ray of the neck and/or abdomen is the initial test of choice. This will help localize the foreign body and direct further management. Coins in the esophagus lie in the frontal plane with the flat side visible on an AP X-ray and are seen as a disk on the film. Coins in the trachea will lie in the sagittal plane and are seen from the side on an AP film. Metal detectors may be used to localize metallic objects.
- *Treatment:* if the object has passed through the pylorus, expectant management is appropriate. Serial X-rays will confirm complete passage of the object. It is reasonable to have an 8 to 16 hour observation period of asymptomatic children, as 27% in Waltzman's study spontaneously passed the foreign body on their own during that time without complications. In symptomatic patients there are four management options. First, the patient may be observed. This will depend on the patient's clinical appearance, history and location of foreign body. There are three methods of removing foreign bodies. The Foley catheter method requires a Foley to be inserted past the foreign body. It is then inflated and gently withdrawn, allowing the foreign body to be removed with it. This is used for witnessed ingestions of blunt objects in healthy children less than 24 hours prior to the procedure. This procedure may also be done under fluoroscopy. The Bougienage method allows blunt objects with witnessed ingestion in healthy children less then 24 hours prior to the procedure to be pushed into the stomach. The child sits upright as a lubricated bougie is inserted into the esophagus and the object is gently pushed distally. Finally pediatric gastroenterologist, ENT, or pediatric surgeons may perform endoscopy to retrieve the object.

Clinical course

The key to this patient's diagnosis is maintaining a broad differential and doing a complete workup for his complaint.

Historical clues	Physical findings	Ancillary studies
• Cough	• Absence of any source for fever	• X-ray showing esophageal foreign body
• Low-grade fever		
• Decreased appetite		

This patient had a chest X-ray done as part of the evaluation for his fever and cough, and it revealed his esophageal foreign body. His mother had no recollection of him putting a coin in his mouth or having access to a coin. The patient's symptoms had been ongoing for a few days, so it was unclear how long the foreign body had been in his esophagus. Therefore, it was determined that observation was not a prudent option. Otolaryngology was consulted regarding the patient's care, and they took the little boy to the operating room for removal of his foreign body. He was discharged from the hospital after the procedure and had no complications.

Further reading

Barclay L. Conservative management appropriate for coin ingestion. *Pediatr Radiol* 2003:**33**:859–63.

Conners G. Management of asymptomatic coin ingestion. *Pediatrics* 2005:**116**(3):752–3.

Conners G. Pediatrics, foreign body ingestion. Emedicine. Topic 379. Jun 25, 2007.

Gaasch W, Barish R. Swallowed foreign bodies. *Tintinalli's Emergency Medicine: A Comprehensive Study Guide*. 6th edition. New York: McGraw-Hill, 2004, pp. 513–16.

Soprano J, Mandl K. Four strategies for the management of esophageal coins in children. *Pediatrics* 2000;**105**(1):e5.

Case #4

History

A 63-year-old male presents to the ED with fever and chills. He states that his symptoms have been ongoing for about 4 days, and he has also had painful swallowing. Approximately 2 weeks ago, he had a consolidation therapy for acute promyelocytic leukemia with chemotherapy including idarubicin. He was first diagnosed with leukemia 1 month ago. For his fevers, he had been taking occasional acetaminophen without relief. Due to his odynophagia he also has had decreased appetite. The patient currently denies nausea, vomiting, shortness of breath, chest pain, dyspnea on exertion, or any other associated symptoms. He reports that his fevers have not been improving. When he was describing the difficulty swallowing he positioned his fingers over the center of his chest and expressed a burning sensation that occurs with eating. He has sensitivity to hot and cold liquids as well as solid foods. He tolerates liquids better when they are at room temperature.

Past medical history

The patient has a history of acute promyelocytic leukemia which has been treated with idarubicin and all-trans retinoic acid. He has had follow-up bone marrow studies which showed remission. He also has a history of non-insulin-dependent diabetes mellitus and hypertension. He does not smoke or drink, and denies recreational drug use.

Medications

The patient takes amlodipine, furosemide, metoprolol, and insulin.

Allergies

The patient has anaphylaxis to penicillin.

Physical exam and ancillary studies

- *Vital signs:* the patient's temperature is 38.7°C, his blood pressure is 144/74 mmHg, his pulse is 102 bpm, his respiratory rate is 18, and his room air oxygen saturation is 95%.
- *General:* the patient is in no acute distress. He is alert and oriented to person, place, and time. He looks comfortable in bed.
- *Head and neck:* the patient's head and neck have no evidence of trauma. His oropharynx has no erythema or exudates. He has no lymphadenopathy. His sclerae are anicteric, and his conjunctivae are not injected.
- *Cardiovascular:* the patient's heart has a regular rate and rhythm, without murmurs or gallops.
- *Abdomen:* his abdomen is soft, non-tender, and non-distended. He has positive bowel sounds. There is no hepatosplenomegaly.

- *Lungs:* the patient has decreased breath sounds overall, but his lungs are clear to auscultation in all lung fields. He has no wheezing, rales, or rhonchi.
- *Extremities and skin:* the patient has normal pulses throughout. He has no extremity clubbing, cyanosis, or edema. His skin is warm to touch, without rashes or other lesions. There is no bruising or bleeding noted.
- *Pertinent labs:* the patient's complete blood count is remarkable for a white blood cell count of 0.3, a hematocrit of 24%, and a platelet count of 8000. The differential of his white cell count shows 100% lymphocytes. His chemistries show normal electrolytes. He has a bilirubin of 1.7, a uric acid of 3.8, a lactate dehydrogenase of 104, and normal LFTs. His urinalysis is unremarkable.
- *EKG:* the patient's EKG shows a sinus tachycardia, with no evidence of ischemia or pericarditis.
- *Radiographs:* The patient's chest X-ray is unremarkable. His CT scan of his chest shows a diffusely thickened esophagus.

Questions for thought

- What are the appropriate initial actions to take?
- What are other diagnostic tools you can use to make a diagnosis?
- What medications should be started in this patient?
- How does one urgently treat this condition in the emergency department?
- Why is this patient neutropenic?

Diagnosis

Neutropenic fever with esophagitis.

Discussion

- *Epidemiology:* neutropenic fever is a single temperature of >38.3°C (101.3°F), or a sustained temperature >38°C (100.4°F) for more than 1 hour in a patient with an absolute neutrophil count (ANC) of less than 500 cells/μL. The ANC can be calculated by multiplying the total white blood cell count by the percentage of neutrophils plus bands. Neutropenic fever is classically associated with cancer patients undergoing chemotherapy, but it can also be associated with patients with neutropenia from other causes. The incidence of this entity is unknown.
- *Pathophysiology:* neutropenic fever typically results from infection in a patient with neutropenia. The infection classically evolves through disruption of skin and mucosal barriers in patients with a low neutrophil count, which means that the patient has little ability to fight infection. Both the chemotherapy itself as well as the primary underlying malignancy may play a role in development of infection in the neutropenic patient. It is common to see chemotherapy-induced mucositis affecting the gastrointestinal system and seeding the bloodstream with gastrointestinal flora. Chemotherapy decreases the number of neutrophils, and affects their chemotactic and phagocytic capabilities.

Multiple myeloma causes abnormal antibody production and/or abnormal clearing of immune complexes. Both chronic lymphocytic leukemia (CLL) patients and splenectomized patients are at risk of infections with encapsulated organisms. Patients with malignancies causing T cell deficiencies such as Hodgkin lymphoma are at risk for infection with intracellular pathogens. Patients with acute lymphocytic leukemia (ALL), central nervous system tumors, and patients on high-dose steroids are at increased risk for *Pneumocystis carinii* pneumonia. Long-term indwelling lines increases the risk for Gram-positive infections. Overall, an infectious etiology for neutropenic fever is identified 30% of the time.

- *Presentation:* patients with neutropenic fever may present with a fever and no other symptoms, or they may present with focal findings related to the infectious source. They may seem minimally ill, or they may be toxic-appearing. The history and physical exam are important. Since neutropenic patients may have minimal localizing signs, a careful evaluation is necessary to determine the fever source. The perianal area should be inspected for cellulitis and abscess, but digital rectal examination should be avoided, as this may cause bacteremia. All intravenous line sites should be inspected for signs of infection. A lumbar puncture should be performed if there are mental status changes. Blood cultures should be performed, including from each intravenous port and from peripheral blood. A chest X-ray should be performed even if the patient has no pulmonary symptoms. Chest CT scanning is helpful when the patient continues to be febrile and the chest X-ray is clear. Chest CT is more sensitive than chest X-ray in finding pneumonia, particularly in the immunosuppressed patient.

- *Treatment:* fever in a neutropenic patient is considered a medical emergency. It is important to cover the patient broadly with antibiotics. Generally, Gram-negative pathogens are covered because of their virulence and associated risk of sepsis. The routine use of Gram-positive antibiotic coverage is not recommended unless there is hypotension, mucositis, skin or catheter site infection, history of methicillin-resistant *Staph. aureus* colonization, recent quinolone prophylaxis, or overall clinical deterioration and persistent fever despite empiric antibiotics. Linezolid is an alternative for patients intolerant to vancomycin. Anaerobic coverage is usually not necessary unless there is evidence of necrotizing mucositis, sinusitis, periodontal abscess, perirectal abscess, cellulitis, intraabdominal or pelvic infection, typhlitis (necrotizing neutropenic colitis), or anaerobic bacteremia. The risk for invasive fungal infections increases with the duration and severity of neutropenia, prolonged antibiotic use, and number of chemotherapy cycles. Viral infections, especially human herpes viruses, are very common. These often present as esophagitis. Reactivation of other human herpes viruses such as CMV or EBV can also occur. Neutropenic patients are also at risk for respiratory syncytial virus and influenza.

- *Definitive therapy:* if an infectious source is identified, antibiotics should be continued for 14 days. With no known source, the timing of the discontinuation of antibiotics is usually dependent on resolution of fever and neutropenia. If the ANC increases to greater than 500 cells/μL and the patient becomes afebrile, antibiotics may be stopped, although some recommend treating for a minimum of 7 days. In the patient without an identified source who becomes afebrile but remains neutropenic, it is suggested to treat for 14 days. If fever persists after 5 to 7 days, empiric antifungal therapy is usually started. In addition to antibiotics, catheter removal is recommended if there is evidence of catheter-related candidemia or bacteremia.

Clinical course

The keys to this patient's diagnosis are careful attention to his history, physical exam, and ancillary studies.

Historical clues	Physical findings	Ancillary studies
• Recent chemotherapy	• Fever	• Complete blood count showing ANC less than 500 cells/μL
• Dysphagia	• Tachycardia	• CT with evidence of esophagitis
• Odynophagia		
• Continued fever with first line of treatment		

The patient was identified on presentation as being high risk for having neutropenic fever, based on his recent chemotherapy. Blood and urine cultures were sent. Urinalysis, CBC, comprehensive metabolic panel, and chest X-ray were ordered. The patient's symptoms suggested mucositis and therefore a Gram-positive source, so he was empirically started on aztreonam and vancomycin, as he was allergic to penicillin. Because his symptoms and his CT scan were consistent with esophagitis, he was also started on esomeprozole. Esophagogastroduodenoscopy is the test of choice for esophagitis, but this was deferred until the patient's neutrophil count increased to prevent further bacteremia. Despite treatment with aztreonam and vancomycin, the patient continued to spike fevers on a daily basis. Diflucan and acyclovir were added to cover for the possibility of candidal or herpes esophagitis. Blood cultures and urine cultures remained negative. Twenty-four hours after the change to the antibiotic regimen, the patient became afebrile and remained afebrile for the rest of his hospital stay. His neutrophil count improved slowly but steadily. The patient's antibiotics were stopped, and he was discharged home on valacyclovir and diflucan for several more weeks. He also continued on a proton pump inhibitor. On discharge, he had no solid or liquid food intolerance, and was feeling well. He was planned for follow-up for upper endoscopy to delineate the extent of his esophageal inflammation.

Further reading

Braunwald E, et al., eds. Fever of unknown origin. In *Harrison's Principles of Internal Medicine*, 15th edition. New York: McGraw-Hill, 2004, pp. 804–5.

Sipsas NV, Bodey GP, Kontoyiannis DP. Perspectives for the management of febrile neutropenic patients with cancer in the 21st century. *Cancer* 2005;**103**:1103.

Paul M, Borok S, Fraser A, et al. Empirical antibiotics against Gram-positive infections for febrile neutropenia: systematic review and meta-analysis of randomized controlled trials. *J Antimicrob Chemother* 2005;**55**:436.

Rolston KV, Manzullo EF, Elting LS, et al. Once daily, oral, outpatient quinolone monotherapy for low-risk cancer patients with fever and neutropenia: a pilot study of 40 patients based on validated risk-prediction rules. *Cancer* 2006;**106**:2489.

Pizaro JJ. Management of the febrile neutropenic patient: a consensus conference. *Clin Infect Dis* 2004;**39**(1): e1–e12.

Robbins GK. Fever in the neutropenic adult patient with cancer. www.uptodate.com.

Case #5

History

An 18-year-old college freshman was brought to the university health service with a chief complaint of fever and headache, and from there was transferred to the ED. This occurred early in the morning one weekend, when the patient was found in bed by his roommate, who feels that the patient might have caught "what that girl down the hall got." There had been a recent outbreak of bacterial meningitis within the college community, and everyone has been on the lookout for this disease. The patient was sweaty and palpably hot to the touch, speaking nonsensically, and restlessly moving about in his bed. He was initially drowsy but verbal, and confirmed that he had received the meningococcal vaccine before coming to college that fall. The previous evening he had taken "five or six" methylphenidate tablets that belonged to one of his friends. He had washed them down with two energy drinks prior to going out to a party. Though initially responsive, the patient quickly became stuporous, with eye opening to pain only, confused speech, and motor localization to painful stimuli. His skin was flushed and sweaty, and he began shaking violently. His eyes were noted to be "scanning" back and forth.

Past medical history

According to school health records, the patient is in good health. He only has a history of mild depression.

Medications

The patient takes paroxetine for his depression.

Allergies

The patient has no known drug allergies.

Physical exam and ancillary studies

- *Vital signs:* the patient's temperature is 38.7°C, his pulse is 140 bpm, his respiratory rate is 22, his blood pressure is 159/76 mmHg, and his oxygen saturation is 94% on 6 liters of oxygen by nasal cannula.
- *General:* the patient is awake but non-responsive to direct questioning. He is making noises but is not speaking in sentences. He seems agitated.
- *HEENT:* the patient has no evidence of head trauma. His pupils are 8 mm, and are sluggishly reactive. He has rapid horizontal nystagmus. His neck is supple.
- *Cardiovascular:* the patient has a regular tachycardia. His pulses are intact.
- *Lungs:* his lungs are clear to auscultation bilaterally.

- *Abdomen:* the patient has hyperactive bowel sounds. His abdomen is non-tender and non-distended.
- *Extremities and skin:* the patient's skin is red, flushed, and diaphoretic. He has no rash or cyanosis.
- *Neuro:* the patient's Glasgow coma scale is 9 (E2, V3, M5). His neurologic exam is symmetric.
- *Pertinent labs:* the patient's laboratory data notes a respiratory acidosis on his ABG (pH of 7.3, pCO_2 of 52, pO_2 of 108), no electrolyte derangements, and a creatine kinase fraction of 8000 U/L. Other laboratory data including toxicology screen and complete blood count are unremarkable.
- *EKG:* the patient's EKG shows sinus tachycardia without morphology or interval changes.

Questions for thought

- What is the initial approach to the patient with delirium and fever?
- What condition does this history suggest?
- Does this patient warrant treatment, and how would one treat this condition in the ED?
- Does this patient require admission?

Diagnosis

Serotonin syndrome.

Discussion

- *Epidemiology:* serotonin syndrome is an odd but characteristic iatrogenic toxicological emergency increasingly seen within emergency practice. Along with its cousin the carcinoid syndrome, serotonin syndrome characterizes a spectrum of nonspecific signs, most notable in its severest throes for systemic autonomic dysfunction, neuromuscular impairment, and severe alterations in mental status. With the increased prescription by primary practitioners and psychiatrists of proserotonergic drugs, including many with occult agonistic effects, it is thought that serotonin syndrome is becoming more common. However, the broad range of manifestations and nonspecific nature of the presentation allows the disorder to masquerade as any of a number of other conditions, and it may be under-diagnosed, and therefore under-treated.
- *Pathophysiology:* serotonin toxicity occurs after ingestion of proserotonergic drugs, of which selective serotonin reuptake inhibitors (SSRIs) are the prototypical agents. The central nervous system (CNS) effect is to inhibit presynaptic uptake of the neurotransmitter serotonin (5-HT) in the raphe nuclei of the midbrain and brainstem, which promotes wakefulness, emotional behavior, hunger, pain sensation, and motor tone. In the peripheral nervous system (PNS) serotonin maintains intestinal motility and vascular tone. Alhough generally SSRIs are considered to be a safe monotherapy, when combined with other drugs with serotonin agonism the condition is increasingly possible. Generally

this condition presents after the addition of one drug (monoamine oxidase inhibitors and opiates are regularly implicated) to the regular use of another, especially the commonly prescribed SSRI antidepressants, although monotherapy cases have been reported. The number of prescription, illicit, and herbal substances with known proserotonergic properties is vast, and includes heterocyclic antidepressants, mixed reuptake inhibitors (for example, bupropion and duloxetine), mood stabilizers (lithium), triptan headache agents, opiates (for example, hydrocodone and meperidine), amphetamines (methylphenidate), illicit drugs (cocaine, LSD, MDMA, mescaline), anti-parkinsonian agents (levodopa), and antibiotics (linezolid).

- *Presentation:* the description of this patient is typical for the condition, but is also illustrative of the protean and nonspecific nature of the disorder. Symptoms can range from mild autonomic dysfunction (hypertension, diarrhea) to moderate (hyperreflexia, muscular clonus, rigidity) to severe (hyperthermia $> 41^{\circ}$C), and are generally rapid in onset. The most specific findings include hyperreflexia in the lower extremities, horizontal ocular clonus (nystagmus), and muscle rigidity so severe it may overwhelm the other findings. Other symptoms include altered mental status, diaphoresis, hyperthermia, hyperactive bowel sounds and incontinence. The constant agitation and tremors can lead to widespread muscle breakdown, which overwhelms the kidneys with muscle breakdown products and can cause rhabdomyolysis.

  The other causes of hyperthermia and delirium, including infectious sources and metabolic derangements, should be considered in the differential. Other similar presentations can occur in anticholinergic toxicity, malignant hyperthermia, neuroleptic malignant syndrome, and the carcinoid syndrome. Malignant hyperthermia is a rare reaction to anesthetic neuromuscular blockade, and neuroleptic malignant syndrome is due to dopaminergic blockade by antipsychotic medications. Carcinoid syndrome is a serotonin syndrome variant caused by vasoactive neurotransmitter release from gastric malignancies. These disorders can be distinguished based on key characteristics; anticholinergic toxicity demonstrates the classic toxidrome including *dry* skin and *hypoactive* bowel sounds, malignant hyperthermia demonstrates *mottled* skin and *hyporeflexia*, and neuroleptic malignant syndrome develops over a *longer period* (days to weeks) and has a marked *decrease* in movement with a "lead-pipe" rigidity.

- *Treatment:* treatment can range from supportive (active cooling, benzodiazepines to control agitation) to active neuromuscular sedation and intubation, especially in patients with severe hyperthermia. The mainstay of pharmacologic intervention is cyproheptadine, a centrally acting H1-antagonist, with a prominent peripheral 5-HT2A antagonism at smooth muscle. The drug is only available orally, and if the patient is unable to swallow, it should be administered nasogastrically. Diphenhydramine and chlorpromazine have also been utilized in the treatment of this condition. As in any overdose, Poison Control remains a wealth of information and support.

Clinical course

The keys to this patient's diagnosis and eventual treatment were careful attention to his history and physical exam, with ancillary laboratory studies to assess metabolic derangements and rule out other toxicologic pathology.

Historical clues	Physical findings	Ancillary studies
• History of SSRI use	• Hyperthermia	• Respiratory acidosis
• Co-ingestion of medication with proserotonergic properties	• Hyperreflexia	• Elevated creatine kinase
	• Agitation	• Negative toxicology screen
	• Nystagmus	• No electrolyte abnormalities
	• Diaphoresis	

The patient was suspected to have a toxic cause for his symptoms. Serotonin syndrome is a clinical diagnosis, and this patient had history and exam findings suggestive of this entity. It is prudent to check for other ingestions, such as acetaminophen and aspirin, as the incidence of co-ingestions in poisonings is very high. In this patient, these studies were negative. In the setting of serotonin syndrome, it is also important to rule out rhabdomyolysis and secondary renal failure. This patient had evidence of rhabdomyolysis, with a creatine kinase level of 8000, but his renal function was still intact. It was important in this case not to get confused by the red herring of a recent outbreak of bacterial meningitis within his college community, as the diagnostic workup for that disease, including blood studies and lumbar puncture, would add patient discomfort and even morbidity, without furthering the diagnosis.

The patient's condition degenerated within a brief period. Based upon the working diagnosis of serotonin syndrome, the physician instituted appropriate therapy immediately, before more serious sequelae developed. Had the patient not been found by his roommate, his condition might well have deteriorated further and been fatal.

The patient was hydrated in the ED with 2 liters of normal saline. He underwent external cooling with axillary icepacks, and he received a total of 4 mg of lorazepam for agitation. His fluids were then switched to sterile water with dextrose plus three ampules of sodium bicarbonate to assist in renal clearance of muscle breakdown products. The patient was given 8 mg of cyproheptadine, a centrally acting H1-antagonist with additional serotonin antagonism. The patient was transferred to a cardiac telemetry unit, and continuous cardiac monitoring showed no evidence of dysrhythmias. He received symptomatic care with diazepam 10 mg IV every 4 hours to decrease his tremors. Over the next 12 hours the patient's temperature, tachycardia, and tremors decreased, as did his creatine kinase, while his pH rose and his mental status improved back to a tired, but oriented, baseline.

Further reading

Boyer E, Shannon M. Current concepts: the serotonin syndrome. *N Engl J Med* 2005;**352**:1112–23.

Martin T. Serotonin syndrome. *Ann Emerg Med* 1996;**28**:520–6.

Mason PJ, Morris VA, Balcezak TJ. Serotonin in the literature. *Medicine(Baltimore)* 2000;**79**:201–9.

Case #6

History

A 5-year-old boy is brought to the ED by his parents for fever. His parents state that he has had a fever for the last few days. In addition, he has had progressively worsening abdominal and back pain over the past 2 days. His abdominal pain is severe and "all over." He has middle and lower back pain which is not well localized. His review of systems is significant for a decrease in appetite and oral intake for 1 day. He has had normal stools. He has had no episodes of emesis or dysuria. He has not had any symptoms of upper respiratory infection, cough, or difficulty breathing.

Past medical history

The patient was diagnosed with sickle cell disease by newborn screen and has been admitted several times for vaso-occlusive pain crises. He also has a history of mild persistent asthma.

Medications

His medications include folic acid, prophylactic penicillin, inhaled budesonide and albuterol as needed.

Allergies

The patient has no known drug allergies.

Physical exam and ancillary studies

- *Vital signs:* the patient's temperature is 39.2°C, his heart rate is 135 bpm, his respiratory rate is 30, his blood pressure is 128/72 mmHg, and his oxygen saturation is 96% on 2 liters of oxygen by nasal cannula.
- *General:* the patient is awake and alert. He is in mild respiratory distress, and is moaning in pain.
- *Head and neck:* the patient's head is normocephalic and atraumatic. His pupils are equally round and reactive to light. He has some scleral icterus. His tympanic membranes are intact. His oral mucosa is moist, and he has no pharyngeal erythema or exudate.
- *Cardiovascular:* the patient's heart is tachycardic, without murmurs, rubs, or gallops.
- *Lungs:* the patient has decreased breath sounds throughout. There are no rales, rhonchi, or wheezes heard.
- *Abdomen:* the patient's abdomen is soft and distended. He has normal bowel sounds. There is diffuse tenderness to palpation in all quadrants with some voluntary guarding. His liver edge is palpable 2 cm below his costal margin.
- *Extremities and skin:* the patient's extremities are warm and well-perfused with 2+ femoral pulses bilaterally.

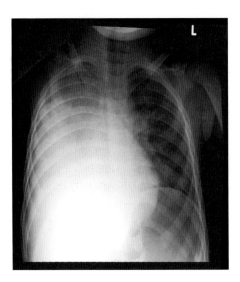

Figure 2.2. This X-ray shows evidence of extensive infiltration of the right lower and middle lung. This could be consistent with pneumonia, but also could be consistent with acute chest syndrome.

- *Pertinent labs:* the patient's complete blood count is remarkable for a white blood cell count of 10.4 and a hematocrit of 21.6%. He has a reticulocyte count of 14.3.
- *Radiographs:* the patient's chest X-ray is shown in Figure 2.2.

Questions for thought

- What actions should be taken prior to initiating further diagnostic investigation in this patient?
- What diagnosis must be considered for any patient with sickle cell disease who presents with fever and/or pain?
- Why is fever important to recognize in patients with sickle cell disease?
- What factors are important in determining whether this child should be admitted to the hospital?
- What treatment should be initiated?

Diagnosis

Vaso-occlusive pain crisis with acute chest syndrome in sickle cell anemia.

Discussion

- *Epidemiology:* sickle cell disease is one of the most common inherited hemoglobinopathies worldwide. It has a prevalence of 1 in 375 births among African Americans.
- *Pathophysiology:* patients with sickle cell disease have an autosomal recessive genetic defect involving a single nucleotide substitution on the beta-globin gene on chromosome 11, which substitutes valine for glutamic acid. This creates multiple polymers that deform and distort the classic bi-concave shape of the red blood cell into "sickled" cells. Sickle cells can cause vascular occlusion, organ ischemia and chronic end-organ damage when

provoked by hypoxia, dehydration, or illness. Acute chest syndrome is defined by the radiological appearance of a new pulmonary infiltrate and fever. The cause of acute chest syndrome is identified only 40% of the time. Infection accounts for about 33% of cases, and fat embolism causes 10% of cases. It is important to remember that patients with sickle cell disease are immunosuppressed. Chronic hypersplenism results in eventual loss of spleen function and secondary immunosuppression. Therefore, sepsis is a common cause of mortality.

- *Presentation:* characteristic manifestations of sickle cell disease include dactylitis in infancy, priapism, splenic sequestration, and vaso-occlusive crises in childhood. Severe cases of vaso-occlusive pain crises can result in acute chest syndrome or ischemic central nervous system events. Bacterial sepsis can manifest as fever and may rapidly progress to uncompensated shock and death due to functional asplenia.

- *Diagnosis:* newborn screening is available in 44 states and the District of Columbia to identify sickle cell disease. This allows for early identification and intervention. In states where newborn screening is not available, physicians must rely on family history and clinical judgment when deciding who to screen. In patients with known disease, acute chest syndrome should be ruled out with serial chest X-rays when patients present with pain in the chest, abdomen or back.

- *Treatment:* patients should be monitored closely for signs of shock and respiratory failure. Fever is treated as an emergency in sickle cell anemia due to the high risk of sepsis from encapsulated organisms. Blood cultures should be obtained and empiric broad spectrum antibiotics should be given immediately to cover *Streptococcus pneumoniae*. IV fluid resuscitation is necessary to prevent shock and reduce sickle deformation of red blood cells. Pain should be addressed, typically by morphine boluses and then by patient controlled analgesia, and oxygen should be given as needed to further prevent sickling. When treating acute chest syndrome, atypical bacteria including *Mycoplasma* should be covered with macrolide antibiotics. Exchange transfusion may be necessary if signs of end-organ damage do not improve after initial resuscitative efforts. Hospital admission is required in most cases when a child with sickle cell disease presents with fever.

- *Definitive therapy:* hematopoietic stem cell transplant from an HLA-matched donor sibling is the only existing curative treatment for sickle cell disease; however, very few patients have such donors available to them. Median survival for homozygous SS disease is approximately 45 years with current therapy. All children with sickle cell anemia should be followed by a pediatric hematologist, and families should be educated on how to manage vaso-occlusive crises and fever in their children. The mainstay of treatment is in preventative therapies, such as penicillin prophylaxis until age 5, folic acid supplementation, hydoxyurea and frequent red blood cell transfusions. Long-term morbidity related to iron overload can result from chronic transfusions, and chelation therapy is often required.

Clinical course

The keys to this patient's diagnosis are recognition of the patient's underlying illness in the context of the patient's acute pain and fever. This led the provider to perform the appropriate ancillary studies to make the diagnosis.

Historical clues	Physical findings	Ancillary studies
• Known sickle cell disease	• Fever	• Elevated reticulocyte count
• Fever	• Hypoxia	• Anemia
• Back and abdominal pain	• Respiratory distress	• Chest X-ray with infiltrate
	• Tachycardia	

In this patient, the correct diagnosis was made very quickly. He was hydrated in the ED with a 20 mL/kg bolus of normal saline and given morphine analgesia. He was given a dose of cefuroxime to cover for infection with encapsulated organisms, as well as azithromycin for community-acquired pneumonia. He was admitted to the general pediatrics floor and placed on a sickle cell protocol that included IV fluid hydration, oxygen to keep his oxygen saturations greater than 97%, incentive spirometry every 2 hours, and morphine via patient-controlled analgesia for pain control. Despite these measures, his clinical course declined with increasing pain and worsening serial chest X-rays consistent with a right-sided pleural effusion, requiring transfer to the intensive care unit (ICU). In the ICU, a chest tube was placed to relieve the pleural effusion, and his antibiotics were changed to piperacillin/tazobactam with azithromycin. He also underwent a partial exchange transfusion as a means to treat the acute chest syndrome. He soon stabilized and was transferred back to the general pediatric floor, where he gradually improved. He was discharged home with a plan to complete a total of 3 weeks of antibiotics for his pneumonia.

Further reading

Driscoll, MC. Sickle cell disease. *Pediatr Rev J* 2007;**28**:243–79.

Vichinsky EP, et al. Causes and outcomes of the acute chest syndrome in sickle cell disease. *N Engl J Med* 2000;**342**:1855–65.

Behrman R, Kliegman R, Jenson H, eds. *Nelson Textbook of Pediatrics*, 17th edition. Elsevier, 2004, pp. 1624–8.

Case #7

History

This 69-year-old woman, status post a cadaveric renal transplant 2 weeks ago, presents to the ED with a fever. The patient has had 10 days of worsening dry, non-productive cough, chills, mild shortness of breath, and a fever up to 38.7°C. She reports that the dry cough has been present for 2 months, but has become worse over the last several days. She also reports feeling increasing fatigue and wheezing. She denies dysuria or frequency, diarrhea, nausea, or vomiting. Her review of systems is otherwise negative.

Past medical history

The patient has a history of end-stage renal disease secondary to polycystic kidney disease. She also has a history of supraventricular tachycardia, asthma, hypertension, hyperlipidemia, hypothyroidism, and total abdominal hysterectomy. The patient denies alcohol, tobacco, or recreational drug use. She is an avid gardener. She has a family history of polycystic kidney disease in both her mother and her sister.

Medications

The patient takes sirolimus, tacrolimus, mycophenolate mofetil, iron, fluticasone, atenolol, estradiol, calcium, flecainide, folic acid, atorvastatin, ezetimibe, docusate, and aspirin.

Allergies

The patient has no known drug allergies.

Physical exam and ancillary studies

- *Vital signs:* the patient's current temperature is 37.0°C. Her blood pressure is 125/66 mmHg, her pulse is 86 bpm, her respiratory rate is 18, and her oxygen saturation is 98% on room air.
- *General:* the patient is awake, alert, and oriented. She is in no apparent distress.
- *HEENT:* she has no conjunctivitis or scleritis. Her oral mucosa is moist without lesions. She has no pharyngeal erythema or exudates. There is no cervical, supraclavicular, or axillary lymphadenopathy.
- *Lungs:* the patient's lungs are clear to auscultation bilaterally, without wheezes, rales, or rhonchi. Her chest is resonant to percussion. There is no change in tactile fremitus.
- *Cardiovascular:* the patient's heart is regular. She has a soft systolic murmur.
- *Abdomen:* the patient's abdomen is soft, non-tender, and non-distended. Her right flank incision is intact without drainage or erythema.
- *Extremity:* her extremities have no clubbing, cyanosis, or edema.

- *Neurologic:* the patient has a normal neurologic exam.
- *Pertinent labs:* all of the patient's lab values are within normal limits except for a creatinine of 1.9.
- *Radiographs:* the patient's chest X-ray shows no abnormalities.

Questions for thought

- What is causing this patient's symptoms?
- Does a recent history of a kidney transplant make a difference in the diagnostic approach?
- What workup should you initiate for this patient in the ED?
- What can be done for the patient in the ED while waiting for the workup to be completed?

Diagnosis

Aspergillus pneumonia.

Discussion

- *Epidemiology: Aspergillus* is a ubiquitous fungal organism found frequently in soil and decaying organic matter. The most common pathogenic species include *A. fumigatus* (most common), *A. niger, A. flavus,* and *A. glaucus.* Aspergillosis is the second most common opportunistic fungal infection (after candidiasis) in the immunocompromised patient and occurs almost exclusively through inhalation of spores. Invasive aspergillosis is extremely uncommon in the immunocompetent population, but affects 5–25% of immunocompromised individuals.
- *Pathophysiology:* pulmonary aspergillosis generally begins after inhalation of spores. Alveolar macrophages, which usually kill *Aspergillus* species, are unable to eradicate the spores if macrophage dysfunction exists, or the immune system is suppressed by cytotoxic medications (immunosuppressants) or another underlying infection (HIV, leukemia). The spores germinate, producing hyphae, which then manage to evade host defenses via numerous secreted proteases and other immunosuppressive metabolites.
- *Presentation: Aspergillus* most often causes pulmonary disease, but has been shown to cause endocarditis, sinus infection, disseminated disease, or cutaneous infection after direct implantation during trauma. Pulmonary aspergillus infection generally occurs in three forms: allergic bronchopulmonary aspergillosis, invasive aspergillosis, and aspergilloma. Allergic bronchopulmonary aspergillosis generally affects asthmatics or cystic fibrosis patients who present with elevated IgE levels and complain of upper respiratory infection (URI) symptoms (cough, fever, wheezing, dyspnea, pleuritic pain) with hemoptysis. Invasive aspergillosis frequently affects leukemia patients who present with URI symptoms, unremitting fevers not responding to standard antibiotic regimen and have radiographic evidence of pulmonary cavitations or bronchopneumonia. Aspergilloma (mycetoma or "fungus ball") most often presents as a round density in the upper lobes and 50–80% of patients present with hemoptysis (30% subsequently have massive bleeding). Most serious infections occur several months after the

transplant; however, earlier infections may occur if the patient experiences an unusual epidemiological exposure (for example, travel, construction, gardening). Early diagnosis combined with aggressive and specific therapy is vital to the patient's well-being and survival. Despite a reduced inflammatory response, a fever in these patients will often be the first sign of infection.

- *Definitive therapy:* a febrile transplant patient should be hospitalized and receive broadspectrum antibiotics soon after appropriate initial fever workup labs are obtained. Once a specific infectious agent has been identified, the antibiotics should be tailored accordingly. Invasive aspergillosis carries a mortality of 93–100% in a bone marrow transplant patient, and 38% in a kidney transplant patient. Traditionally, amphotericin has been the standard antifungal therapy. Recently, new antifungal agents with fewer side-effects such as caspofungin and voriconazole have been used with good results. Surgery is reserved for *Aspergillus* infection complication or hemoptysis associated with invasive pulmonary disease. Generally a lobectomy is required for complete eradication.

Clinical course

Aspergillosis is not a diagnosis that is made definitively in the ED. However, appropriate ED evaluation provides the necessary framework to obtain the diagnosis. The transplant patient with a fever requires a comprehensive evaluation, the specifics of which are as follows:

Critical history	Physical findings	Ancillary studies
• Transplant date	• Vital signs	• Complete blood count
• Reason for organ failure	• Thorough cardiovascular exam	• Comprehensive chemistry panel
• Cadaveric, living, or living related donor	• Skin and mucosal findings	• Cultures of all potential sources
• Recent medication changes	• Assessment of wound	• Chest X-ray
• History of rejection episodes	• Even minor physical findings can represent serious infection	• CT of chest if high index of suspicion
• History of opportunistic infections		
• Even minor symptoms can represent serious infection		

This patient was identified to be at high risk for opportunistic infection, as she was a recent transplant recipient on maximal immunosuppression. Although her chest X-ray showed no specific acute disease, her symptoms pointed to a likely pulmonary process. Therefore, the patient underwent a CT of her chest, which is shown below. While awaiting this study, she received broad-spectrum antibiotics, and the transplant service was contacted for the patient to be admitted.

After admission, the patient underwent bronchoscopy and bronchoalveolar lavage based on the abnormalities on her chest CT. This is the diagnostic study of choice for pulmonary aspergillosis. These studies identified an ulcerating lesion in the trachea with copious secretions. Cultures of the lesion and a trans-bronchial biopsy were positive for *Aspergillus* and the patient was started on voriconazole. She quickly improved once appropriate therapy was instituted, and was discharged home with a 2 month course of voriconazole.

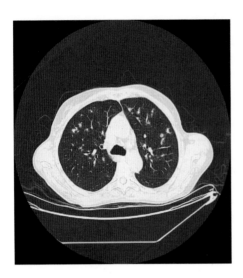

Figure 2.3. This chest CT shows bilateral upper lobe nodules concerning for an atypical pneumonia.

Further reading

Doherty GM, Way LW. Chapter 18. *Current Surgical Diagnosis and Treatment*, 12th edition. New York: McGraw-Hill, 2005.

Chirch L, Roche P, Fuhrer J. Successful treatment of invasive Aspergillus sinusitis with caspofungin and voriconazole. *Ear Nose Throat J* 2008;**87**(1): 30–3.

Makawka L. *The Handbook of Transplantation Management*. Austin: R.G. Landes, 1991.

Fishman JA. Approach to the immunocompromised patient with fever and pulmonary infiltrates. Retrieved from www.UpTodate.com. May 24, 2006.

Sugar AM. Clinical features and diagnosis of invasive aspergillosis. www.UpTodate.com. November 6, 2007.

Case #8

History

The patient is a 19-year-old female who presents to the ED stating "I always feel hot." The sensation has been worsening over the past few months and she has been sweating frequently. These symptoms have been associated with frequent watery bowel movements and generalized fatigue. She was originally told by her primary care doctor that this was "probably a stomach bug" but her symptoms have continued for many weeks without improvement. She also had noticed that she has missed her last two periods and, although she is sexually active, three home pregnancy tests have all been negative. When home from college recently, her parents became quite concerned by a noticeable weight loss and asked her whether she had an eating disorder or drug use. She insistently denied this to her parents, but has been feeling anxious, jittery, and today says that her heart is racing. Her review of systems is otherwise negative.

Past medical history

She states she has no significant past medical history.

Medications

The patient takes an oral contraceptive pill daily.

Allergies

She has allergies to penicillin and sulfa.

Physical exam and ancillary studies

- *Vital signs:* the patient's temperature is 38.3°C. Her blood pressure is 135/68 and her heart rate is 112 bpm. She is breathing at 22 breaths per minute with an oxygen saturation of 99% on room air.
- *General:* she is a thin female who appears quite agitated, with darting glances around the room and a fine resting tremor.
- *Head and neck:* the mucous membranes are mildly dry. The thyroid gland is diffusely and symmetrically enlarged and a thyroid bruit can be auscultated. The thyroid is also mildly tender to palpation. The remainder of the exam shows no abnormalities.
- *Cardiovascular:* S1 and S2 are auscultated with a regular rate and rhythm. There are no appreciable clicks, rubs, or murmurs, but she is mildly tachycardic.
- *Lungs:* her lungs are clear to auscultation bilaterally without wheezes, rhonchi, or rales.
- *Abdomen:* the patient's abdomen is soft, non-tender, non-distended but remarkable for hyperactive bowel sounds.
- *Extremities and skin:* her extremities show no clubbing, cyanosis, or edema. The skin is warm and diaphoretic with decreased turgor. She has brittle hair.

- *Neurological:* the patient has no focal deficits, although her strength is only 4/5 in both upper and lower extremities bilaterally.
- *Pertinent labs:* her complete blood count is remarkable for a white blood cell count of 13.2 with elevated granulocytes and lymphocytes, a hemoglobin of 10.8, and a hematocrit of 33%. The patient's AST is 84, her ALT is 76, the alkaline phosphatase level is 234, and her calcium is 10.1. The patient's thyroid stimulating hormone (TSH) level is 0.1. The remainder of her laboratory data are within normal limits.
- *EKG:* her EKG shows a sinus tachycardia.

Questions for thought

- What is the differential diagnosis for this patient?
- How does one treat this condition urgently in the emergency department?
- What is the definitive treatment for this condition?
- Does this patient need to be admitted to the hospital?

Diagnosis

Thyrotoxicosis.

Discussion

- *Epidemiology:* the prevalence of hyperthyroidism in community-based studies has been estimated at 2% for women and 0.2% for men, for an overall prevalence around 1.2%. Overall, Grave's disease is the most common cause of thyrotoxicosis. However, older patients are more likely to have toxic nodular goiters, and may have blunted symptoms labeled "apathetic thyrotoxicosis."
- *Pathophysiology:* the thyroid produces T4 hormone, and a smaller amount of T3 hormone. Circulating T4 is converted into the active T3 form in the periphery. The hormone has many effects, including its influences on metabolism, protein synthesis, and sensitivity to catecholamines. Thyrotoxicosis is the hypermetabolic syndrome that is a consequence of excessive thyroid hormone. Often this may be due to hyperthyroidism, where the gland over-produces its hormones. Such overproduction represents a failure of the homeostatic negative-feedback loop. In other cases, inflammation of the thyroid gland induces the release of stored thyroid hormone, rather than an overproduction of hormone per se. Finally, some patient's ingest exogenous thyroid hormone, which is termed thyrotoxicosis factitia.
- *Presentation:* patients present with symptoms referable to their hypermetabolic state and catecholamine sensitivity. Tachycardia, anxiety, and tremor are common. In addition, in patients in whom the disease has been undiagnosed for some time, weight loss is common, as is amenorrhea. Vomiting, diarrhea, and hyperactive bowel sounds are common findings on gastrointestinal exam. Patients may have dry or brittle hair, diaphoresis, and sensitivity to heat. Proptosis is common in Graves disease. In severe cases, patients may present with high output heart failure and psychosis.

Measurement of the TSH level is the primary test in initially diagnosing hyperthyroidism in most cases. Generally, TSH levels are low because an excess of thyroid hormone suppresses TSH release. With suppressed TSH, an elevated free T4 level suggests primary hyperthyroidism. Radioactive iodine uptake may indicate Graves disease, toxic adenoma, or toxic multinodular goiter, where the uptake is high. These are distinguished by the uptake pattern. A diffuse uptake pattern is seen in Graves disease, whereas a single nodule represents a toxic adenoma and multiple areas are seen in toxic multinodular goiter. In contrast, low uptake of radioactive iodine may suggest thyroiditis, extraglandular production, iodide exposure, or thyrotoxicosis factitia. Thyroglobulin levels are low in the case of exogenous thyroid hormone, but higher in the other cases. Antithyroid antibodies are seen in Graves disease or lymphocytic thyroiditis.

In rarer cases, hyperthyroidism is due to a pituitary abnormality. In these cases, an excess of TSH stimulates an excess of thyroid hormone production. This is confirmed by documenting a high free T4 and would necessitate further imaging of the pituitary gland.

Nonspecific findings in the diagnostic workup may include anemia, elevated granulocytes and lymphocytes, elevated transaminase and alkaline phosphatase levels, and hypercalcemia.

- *Treatment:* symptomatic treatment of thyrotoxicosis is obtained via beta-blockade for control of hypersympathetic activity, including tachycardia and tremors. Propranolol is commonly used both due to familiarity with it, and due to its inhibition of peripheral conversion to T4 to T3. Esmolol is an alternative. When beta-blockers are contraindicated, including asthmatics or CHF, calcium-channel blockers can be used for the same purposes. Fever is treated with antipyretics. Salicylates are not used, however, because they may exacerbate the thyrotoxicosis by decreasing thyroid protein binding and increasing free thyroid hormone. Nonpharmacologic options include ice packs and cooling blankets, but shivering should be avoided. Oral rehydration, if tolerated, can be used to treat the fluid loss through diaphoresis and GI losses. Fluid requirements may be as much as 3 to 5 L/day and, if intravenous fluids is needed, a fluid dextrose and electrolyte solution can replace depleted stores. Symptomatic thyrotoxicosis may necessitate hospitalization. In most patients with mild or moderate hyperthyroidism, outpatient care is appropriate.
- *Definitive therapy:* treatment depends on the cause of thyrotoxicosis. Thyrotoxicosis factitia is treated by discontinuation of the exogenous thyroid hormone. For endogenous hyperthyroidism, the main treatment strategies are antithyroid drugs, radioactive iodine, and thyroid surgery. Antithyroid drugs used most commonly are methimazole or propylthiouracil (PTU). These medications inhibit organification of tyrosine to block T4 synthesis. PTU also blocks peripheral conversion of T4 to T3. Alternatively, ablation by radioactive iodine is a common option for Graves disease but leads to hypothyroidism within 4 to 12 months. Lifelong thyroid hormone therapy is routine. Surgery is less common, requires the patient be euthyroid before surgery, and may also cause permanent hypothyroidism.

Clinical course

The keys to this patient's diagnosis are careful attention to her history, physical exam, and ancillary studies.

Historical clues	Physical findings	Ancillary studies
• Feeling hot	• Febrile	• Low TSH level
• Diaphoresis	• Tachycardia	• Sinus tachycardia on EKG
• Vomiting	• Enlarged, tender thyroid	• Elevated LFTs
• Amenorrhea	• Tremor	• Elevated alkaline phosphatase
• Weight loss	• Hyperactive bowel sounds	
• Racing heart	• Diaphoresis	
• Anxious	• Brittle hair	

After the patient was suspected of being hyperthyroid based on her presentation, she was given propranolol for symptom control in the ED, and was given acetaminophen for her fever with good relief. Her symptoms were relieved over the course of an hour, and she was admitted to the hospital, where she was transitioned to an oral beta-blocker.

As an inpatient the workup included a radioactive iodine uptake study which revealed diffuse uptake. Laboratory data also identified the presence of immune autoantibodies. With the low TSH level and an elevated free T4, these findings suggested the diagnosis of Graves disease.

The patient was initiated on propylthiouracil 300 mg daily initially. She responded well to therapy. She soon noted an improvement in her diaphoresis, resolution of her palpitations and agitation, and more regularity with her bowel movements. Over the course of a number of months, her menses returned and she was able to put on the weight she had lost. Given the improvement in her symptoms and good response to therapy, her daily medication dose of propylthiouracil was eventually reduced to 150 mg daily.

Further reading

Schraga E. Hyperthyroidism, thyroid storm, and Graves disease. Retrieved from eMedicine.com on December 1, 2008.

McKeown NJ, Tews MC, Gossain VV, Shah SM. Hyperthyroidism, *Emerg Medicine Clin North Am* 2005;**23**:669–85.

Ross DS. Overview of the clinical manifestations of hyperthyroidism in adults. Retrievd from Uptodate.com on December 1, 2008.

Nayak D, Burman K. Thyrotoxicosis and thyroid storm. *Endocrinol Metab Clin North Am* 2006;**35**:663–86.

Case# 9

History

A 14-day-old girl presents to the ED with a 1 day history of fever, vomiting, and decreasing oral intake. She felt warm, so her mother took a rectal temperature, which was 38.6°C. The patient was immediately taken to the hospital by her parents. Her mother notes that the patient appears to be irritable, and is not taking her "normal" amount of formula. She usually ingests approximately 5 ounces of formula every 3 hours, but overnight had only taken in 5 ounces total, 3 ounces of which were plain water. The infant had a couple of episodes of vomiting which were non-projectile and non-bilious. She has not had diarrhea, and she has had her usual number of wet diapers.

Past medical history

The child is a full-term infant, a product of a normal spontaneous vaginal delivery, without any obstetrical complications.

Medications

The patient is not on any medications.

Allergies

She has no known drug allergies.

Physical exam and ancillary studies

- *Vital signs:* the patient's temperature is 38.0°C, her pulse is 148 bpm, her blood pressure is 80/40 mmHg, her respiratory rate is 40 per minute, and her oxygen saturation is 100% on room air.
- *General:* she is sleeping in her mother's arms, in no acute distress.
- *HEENT:* the patient's anterior fontanelle is open and flat. Her red reflex is present bilaterally. Her pupils are equally round and reactive to light. She has slightly dry mucus membranes. Her neck is supple.
- *Cardiovascular:* the patient's heart sounds are regular with no murmur. Her capillary refill is approximately 3 seconds, and she has equal pulses in all four extremities.
- *Respiratory:* her lungs are clear to auscultation bilaterally.
- *Abdomen:* the patient's abdomen is soft, non-tender to palpation, and non-distended. She has no hepatosplenomegaly or masses. Her bowel sounds are normal.
- *Extremities:* her hips are stable without clicks or clunks, and the patient is able to move all four extremities.
- *Neurologic:* the patient's deep tendon reflexes are present bilaterally, and her grasp/suck/Moro reflexes are present and normal.

- *Pertinent labs:* the patient's complete blood cell count is normal for her age. Her white blood cell differential shows segmented neutrophils of 64 (17–22)%, band neutrophils of 18 (0–17)%, lymphocytes of 15 (10–63)%, and monocytes of 3 (0–18)%. Her electrolytes and renal function are normal, as is her glucose. Her cerebrospinal fluid studies are shown in the table below.

Tube number	1	4
Fluid color	Hazy	Hazy
Fluid WBC Tho/CMM (none)	2.863	1.890
Fluid RBC (none) Tho/CMM	0.048	0.035
Crenated RBC %	10	15
Fresh RBC %	90	85
Fluid neutrophils %	47	65
Fluid lymphocytes %	8	4
Fluid monocytes %	45	31
Fluid eosinophils %	0	0
Fluid blasts %	0	0
Other cell lines %	0	0

In addition, the patient's CSF glucose was 20 mg/dL (40–75), her protein was 190 mg/dL (15–100), and her CSF smear showed 4+ polymorphonuclear cells.
- *Radiographs:* the patients' chest X-ray is unremarkable.

Questions for thought

- How does the patient's history fit in with her laboratory values?
- Does the patient's age affect how you would approach her workup?
- What are some of the organisms that may cause a similar presentation in this age group?

Diagnoses

Listeria meningitis.

Discussion

- *Epidemiology:* bacterial meningitis in the United States is thought to have an incidence of 0.3 per 1000 live births. Common organisms for meningitis in the neonate (< 1 month old) are group B *Streptococcus* (most common), enterobacteriaceae (e.g. *E. coli*), and *Listeria monocytogenes*. Viruses may also be a cause of meningitis, including the more common HSV, and the less common varicella virus.
- *Pathophysiology:* bacterial meningitis is inflammation of the leptomeninges caused by bacteria. The route of spread is typically respiratory. In the neonate, transmission typically

occurs during the birthing process, and the spectrum of pathogens reflect this mode of transmission.

- *Presentation:* the neonate may or may not present with symptoms suggestive of meningitis, which may include a bulging anterior fontanelle and/or nuchal rigidity, seizures, hemiparesis, or cranial nerve palsies. More commonly, infants will present with symptoms such as fever or hypothermia, apnea, irritability, feeding intolerance, or lethargy. Any child with these symptoms and any febrile child less than 28 days of age requires admission to the hospital for a full septic workup, including blood culture, urine culture, lumbar puncture, and empiric broad-spectrum antibiotics until an organism or source of infection is identified.
- *Treatment:* empiric broad-spectrum antibiotics must be started immediately in a neonate when infection is suspected. One possible choice may be meningitic doses of ampicillin and cefotaxime; alternatively, one may also choose ampicillin and gentamicin.
- *Definitive therapy:* again, broad-spectrum antibiotics must be initiated until a culprit organism is identified. Antibiotic therapy may then be tailored to a specific organism or cause, or discontinued altogether if the diagnostic workup is negative for any infectious cause of fever.

Clinical course

The keys to this patient's diagnosis are the recognition of the significance of a fever in this age group. A neonate with a fever should lead to a full septic workup.

Historical clues	Physical findings	Ancillary studies
• Fever	• Fever • Dehydration	• White blood cell differential with elevated bands
• Vomiting		• CSF with elevated protein
• Irritability		• CSF with low glucose
• Feeding intolerance		• CSF with elevated white cells

Given the patient's age and presence of a fever, a lumbar puncture and complete septic workup was performed, although her physical exam findings showed little except for fever and dehydration. This patient had the classic CSF findings of meningitis, including an elevated CSF protein, and a decreased CSF glucose. In addition to the CSF glucose and protein, the CSF cell counts and color were consistent with meningitis. The patient was started on empiric broad-spectrum antibiotics at meningitic doses, and later was maintained on ampicillin for a full 14 day course after her CSF culture became positive for *Listeria*. The patient completed her full course of antibiotics without any side effects. She was also given IV hydration therapy for dehydration, until she was able to tolerate all oral intake without difficulty. The patient also had a full neurologic evaluation upon admission and throughout her stay, in addition to daily head circumferences for surveillance of post-meningitis hydrocephalus. Audiology testing was performed to ensure that the patient did not have any hearing loss secondary to the meningitis. The patient made a full recovery.

Further reading

Barnett S. Neonatal meningitis. www.Emedicine.com. 2006.

Garges HP, et al. Neonatal meningitis: what is the correlation among cerebrospinal fluid cultures, blood cultures, and cerebrospinal fluid parameters? *Pediatrics* 2006;**117**(4):1094–100.

Pickering LK, et al. *Red Book: 2006 Report of the Committee on Infectious Disease*, 27th edition. American Academy of Pediatrics, 2006.

Robertson J, Shilkofsky N. *The Harriet Lane Handbook. Microbiology and Infectious Disease*. Elsevier Mosby, 2005, pp. 415–19.

Case #10

History

A 76-year-old female patient arrives from an acute rehabilitation facility where she has been recovering from a total hip replacement 3 weeks ago. She is normally awake, alert, and until her hip fracture had been independent in all activities of daily living. Over the past 2 days the patient has had a low-grade fever which has been treated with acetaminophen. This morning, facility staff found the patient "unresponsive" in bed and were unable to rouse her.

Past medical history

The patient has a history of hypertension, hypercholesterolemia, overactive bladder, and osteoporosis.

Medications

The patient's medications include atenolol, lisinopril, calcium supplement with vitamin D, low-dose aspirin, multivitamin, tolterodine, acetaminophen, percocet, and a bowel regimen.

Allergies

The patient has no known drug allergies.

Physical exam and ancillary studies

- *Vital signs:* the patient's temperature is 39.1°C rectally, her heart rate is 134 bpm, her blood pressure is 76/38, her respiratory rate is 26 and shallow, and her room air oxygen saturation is 87%.
- *General:* she is pale, thin, unresponsive, and ill-appearing.
- *Head and neck:* the patient's pupils are equally round and sluggishly reactive to light; her cranial nerves are unable to be meaningfully assessed as she is non-participatory in the exam, but no focal deficits are noted. The patient's mucous membranes are extremely dry. Her neck is supple with a midline trachea. Her neck veins are flat.
- *Cardiovascular:* she has a regular tachycardic rhythm, with non-palpable peripheral pulses.
- *Lungs:* the patient's breath sounds are decreased throughout with shallow respirations, no wheezes, rales, or rhonchi.
- *Extremities and skin:* the patient has no edema or clubbing. She has poor capillary refill throughout with cool and mottled extremities.
- *Pertinent abnormal labs:* the patient's complete blood count is remarkable for a white blood cell count of 18.6 (neutrophils 60%, bands18%), a hematocrit of 31.4%, a blood

urea nitrogen of 96, a creatinine of 2.1 (0.9 one month ago). The patient's urinalysis shows positive leukocyte esterase, positive nitrites, 50–100 white blood cells per high-powered field, 5–10 red blood cells per high-powered field, and many bacteria. Her serum lactic acid is 4.67.

Questions for thought

- What are the appropriate initial actions to take to stabilize this patient?
- What studies and labs are critical in the initial workup of this patient?
- How does one urgently treat this condition in the emergency department?
- What is definitive treatment of this condition?

Diagnosis

Septic shock as a result of urosepsis.

Discussion

- *Epidemiology*: approximately 750 000 cases of sepsis are diagnosed in the United States each year. The incidence of sepsis increases yearly. Reasons for this are speculated to include an aging population, increased incidence of drug-resistant pathogens, and increased frequency of high-risk surgeries. With shorter lengths of stay in the hospital and more aggressive at-home and out-of-hospital care, particularly among the elderly, the emergency department is increasingly where septic patients initially present and are diagnosed. Sepsis has a high mortality: in Rivers' study in 2001, he found 59% in-hospital mortality among septic patients undergoing standard care at the time.
- *Definitions*: the systemic inflammatory response syndrome, or SIRS, is an inflammatory response, which may or may not be a response to infection. Criteria by which SIRS is defined include two or more of the following: (1) a body temperature greater than 38°C or less than 36°C; (2) a heart rate greater than 90 bpm; (3) tachypnea, with a respiratory rate of greater than 20 breaths per minute, or hyperventilation, as indicated by a $paCO_2$ of less than 32 mmHg; and (4) an alteration in the white blood cell count, either greater than 12 000 mm³, less than 4000 mm³, or more than 10% bandemia. Sepsis is the inflammatory response to an infection, and exists when a patient meets the criteria for SIRS, and an infectious etiology is the underlying cause. Severe sepsis is defined as sepsis associated with organ dysfunction, hypoperfusion, or hypotension. Hypoperfusion may present as altered mental status, oliguria, or lactic acidosis. Septic shock exists in the worst cases of severe sepsis, and is said to exist when sepsis-induced hypotension persists despite adequate fluid resuscitation, along with the presence of hypoperfusion abnormalities or organ dysfunction.
- *Pathophysiology*: the pathophysiology of sepsis represents a complex interaction between characteristics of the infecting organism and the host response to infection. Complex cytokine-mediated inflammatory cascades bring about nitric-oxide-induced vasodilatation, macrophage activation, increased endothelial cell adhesion and resultant

small vessel damage, and alteration of the procoagulant–anticoagulant balance. The end result is widespread vasodilatation, a dramatic increase in endothelial permeability (leaky capillaries), a decrease in available clotting factors, and microvascular thrombosis.

- *Presentation:* this patient is typical of an elderly patient with septic shock, presenting with altered mental status as a result of profound hypoperfusion. Other septic patients may present with shortness of breath as a result of an underlying pneumonia, acute renal failure due to pre-renal azotemia, pain associated with a cellulitis, weakness and fatigue, or simply with a complaint of "fever." The astute clinician is aware that the natural course of sepsis is to progress rapidly from sepsis, to severe sepsis, to septic shock, and then to multiple organ dysfunction. Early diagnosis is essential to prevent progression of the disease state. The presence of SIRS criteria, along with a suspicion of an infectious etiology, even when an infectious source is not immediately identifiable, should prompt the diagnosis of sepsis and the initiation of appropriate treatment.

- *Treatment:* treatment of the septic patient needs to be multi-factorial and implemented promptly. Cultures of blood, urine, sputum if available, and any possible wound source should be obtained immediately and ideally before antibiotic therapy is started. Broad-spectrum antibiotics should be started within an hour of the diagnosis of sepsis. Antibiotics should be tailored to the source of the infection when one is apparent. If no clear source is available, a broad range of antibiotics to cover Gram-negative, Gram-positive, anerobic, pseudomonas, and methicillin-resistant *S. aureus* should be started. Immune-suppressed patients should be covered for yeast and fungal infections as well.

- *Early goal-directed therapy:* early goal-directed therapy (EGDT) is a combination of measureable goal-oriented interventions which when successfully executed in the first 6 hours of treatment have been shown to significantly decrease mortality from sepsis. EGDT begins with identifying patients who meet SIRS criteria despite an initial fluid bolus. Oxygen (100%) is administered, and intubation performed if required. A central line allowing central venous pressure (CVP) monitoring and an arterial line allowing continuous arterial blood pressure monitoring should be placed. Initial resuscitation should be with crystalloid fluid resuscitation to achieve central venous pressures of 8–12 mmHg. Once volume is restored and a normal CVP is achieved, either dopamine or norepinephrine should be started as needed to maintain mean arterial pressures (MAP) between 65 mmHg and 90 mmHg. Once the CVP and MAP goals are met, a central venous oxygen saturation ($ScvO_2$) should be obtained. This can be performed with a special catheter designed to measure pulse oximetry at the catheter tip, or by sending a central venous blood gas. If the $ScvO_2$ returns less than 70%, then transfusion with packed red blood cells should be performed as needed to establish a hematocrit of at least 30%. If the $ScvO_2$ remains below 70% despite a normalized hematocrit, then inotropic agents should be started or increased until the $ScvO_2$ exceeds 70%. EGDT is completed when the patient has a normal CVP of 8–12 mmHg, a normal MAP of 65–90 mmHg, and $ScvO_2$ of greater than 70%.

- *Definitive therapy:* unless initial resuscitation measures are overwhelmingly successful, septic patients require management in an intensive care unit. Ongoing management should consist of low-pressure ventilator management to minimize lung injury, narrowing the antibiotic spectrum rapidly in response to culture and Gram stain results, and ongoing hemodynamic monitoring to ensure that the goals achieved during EGDT are maintained.

Clinical course

The keys to this patient's diagnosis are recognition of SIRS criteria along with a suspicion for infection. A non-astute clinician might waste much time getting head CTs, neurology consults, and other not useful ancillary studies to work up this patient's altered mental status while grossly under-resuscitating her.

Historical clues	Physical findings	Ancillary studies
• Recent low-grade temperature	• Tachycardia	• Elevated WBC with bandemia
• Skilled nursing facility patient at increased risk for infection.	• Hypotension	• Elevated lactic acid
	• Altered mental status	• UA findings consistent with infection
	• Obvious hypoperfusion on exam	• New-onset renal insufficiency

This patient was recognized to have septic shock by her provider. Two peripheral IVs were established and volume resuscitation was immediately started with normal saline. Two separate blood cultures and a urine culture were obtained. Due to her altered mental status, the patient was intubated and sedated. Deep endotracheal tube aspirate samples were obtained for sputum culture. Low ventilator volumes were used to minimize lung damage.

Antibiotics were initiated. While every institution will have a slightly different antibiotic resistance profile, the provider here elected to start pipercillin-tazobactam, which will provide good Gram-negative coverage as well as anti-pseudomonal coverage, vancomycin to cover methicillin-resistant *Staphylococcus aureus*, and amikacin to cover additional Gram-positives and to double cover pseudomonal infection.

An internal jugular central line was placed, and initial CVP readings of 2–3 mmHg were obtained. Massive crystalloid resuscitation ensued, and after 7 liters of normal saline, the patient had CVP readings consistently between 9 and 10 mmHg. A radial arterial catheter was inserted to allow continuous blood pressure monitoring. Initial MAPs after CVP normalization were only 50 mmHg. A norepinephrine infusion was started and titrated up until the patient's MAP exceeded 65 mmHg.

A central venous blood gas was sent to obtain an $ScvO_2$, which returned 63%, reflecting a lack of adequate oxygen delivery. The patient's hematocrit was redrawn (to account for hemodilution following volume resuscitation), and returned 25%. A transfusion of two units of packed red blood cells was initiated.

After 5 hours of overall resuscitation, the patient had a CVP of 11 mmHg, a mean arterial pressure of 68 mmHg, and an $ScvO_2$ of 76%. She had received a total of 7.5 liters of crystalloid fluid, two units of packed red blood cells, and was able to be weaned down on her norepinephrine drip. Urine output significantly improved and she was producing in excess of 70 mL of urine an hour by the time she was transferred to the intensive care unit.

She was extubated on hospital day 2 and remained hemodynamically stable. Urine and blood cultures grew out pan-sensitive *E. coli*, and her antibiotic regimen was immediately narrowed to a second-generation cephalosporin. She was transitioned to oral antibiotics, and discharged back to her rehabilitation facility on hospital day 5.

Further reading

Martin GS, Mannino DM, Eaton S, Mass M. The epidemiology of sepsis in the United States from 1979 through 2000. *N Engl J Med* 2003;**348**:1546–54.

Rivers E, Nguyen B, Havstad S, et al. Early goal directed therapy in the treatment of severe sepsis and septic shock. *N Engl J Med* 2001;**345**:1368–77.

Bone RC, Balk RA, Cerra FB, et al. Definitions for sepsis and organ failure and guidelines for the use of innovative therapies in sepsis. The ACCP/SCCM Consensus Conference Committee. American College of Chest Physicians/Society of Critical Care Medicine. *Chest* 1992;**101**:1644–55.

Dellinger RP, Levy MM, Carlet JM, et al., for the Surviving Sepsis Campaign guidelines committee. Surviving Sepsis Campaign: international guidelines for management of severe sepsis and septic shock: 2008. *Crit Care Med* 2008;**36**:296–327.

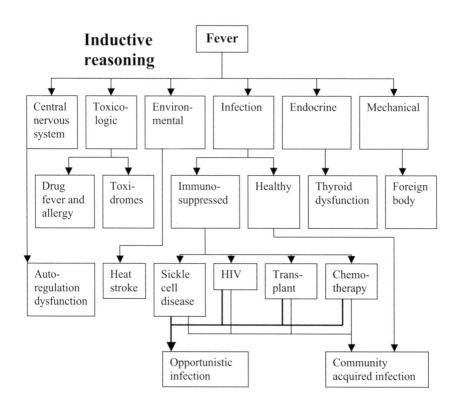

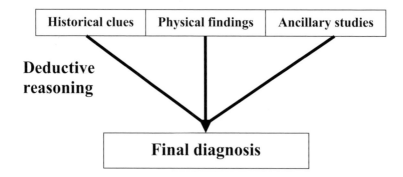

Chapter

3

Chief complaint: chest pain

Mara McErlean, Wendy DeMartino, Damian Compa, Dan Mayer, Lorraine Thibodeau, Jennifer E. Pelesz, Tammy Adamson, Nitza Alvarez

Case #1

History

A 63-year-old woman presents to the ED at 2:00 a.m. complaining of nausea that began 3 hours ago. She denies any prodromal symptoms and has not had any vomiting, pain, or diarrhea. She states she and her husband had the same meal last night and that he is feeling well. She offers no other complaints. She is brought by EMS, who started an IV of normal saline. Three hundred milliliters of crystalloid have been given for an initial blood pressure of 92/60. On arrival to the ED, she began vomiting.

Past medical history

The patient has a 10-year history of diabetes, which is treated with oral hypoglycemic medication. In addition, she has a history of hypertension and elevated cholesterol. She quit smoking 5 years ago and drinks alcohol occasionally.

Medications

The patient's medications include glypizide, lisinopril, and atorvastatin.

Allergies

The patient has no known drug allergies.

Physical exam and ancillary studies

- *Vital signs:* temperature 36.2°C, heart rate 55 bpm, blood pressure 102/71, respiratory rate 24, room air saturation 98%.
- *General:* awake and alert, diaphoretic and with dry heaves.

Case Studies in Emergency Medicine, ed. R. Jeanmonod, M. Tomassi and D. Mayer.
Published by Cambridge University Press © Cambridge University Press 2010.

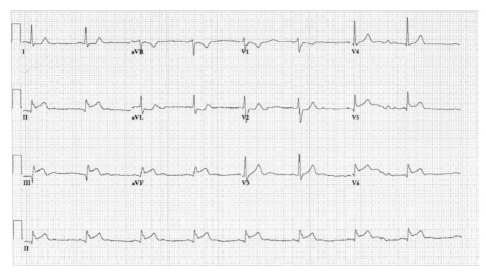

Figure 3.1 ST segment elevation acute myocardial infarction (STEMI). ST elevations in leads II, III, aVF, V5 and V6.

- *Head and neck:* pupils are equally round and reactive to light, cranial nerves intact. The patient's mucous membranes are moist. Her neck is supple with a midline trachea. There is no jugular venous distension.
- *Cardiovascular:* regular bradycardia without murmurs or rubs, no third or fourth heart sounds, peripheral pulses present throughout.
- *Lungs:* clear.
- *Extremities and skin:* trace bilateral edema, no clubbing, no calf tenderness. Her skin is cool and clammy.
- *CXR:* no acute changes.
- *EKG:* see Figure 3.1.

Questions for thought

- What are the appropriate initial actions to take to stabilize this patient?
- What other diagnostic modalities are appropriate in the ED?
- What therapeutic interventions are appropriate?
- How does ED treatment differ based on the abilities of the institution?
- What are indications for transfer?
- What is optimal EMS care?

Diagnosis

Acute inferior wall ST elevation myocardial infarction.

Discussion

- *Epidemiology:* ST elevation MI (STEMI) is one form of acute coronary syndrome (ACS). ACS includes unstable angina, non-STEMI and STEMI. Although the exact incidence of ACS is unknown, there were 1.68 million hospitalizations for ACS in 2007 in the USA. In patients younger than 70, men have a higher incidence than women. In patients over the age of 70, the incidence is equal.

- *Pathophysiology:* myocardial ischemia is most often the result of atheromatous deposits in the lumen of the coronary arteries, which compromise the supply of oxygenated blood to the myocardium. When increased demand is placed on the heart, symptoms result, typically occurring gradually over time with worsening symptoms associated with lesser degrees of exertion. Plaques can rupture, causing acute blockage of the coronary artery from thrombosis. Infrequently, myocardial ischemia can result from arterial emboli or from significant spasm of a coronary artery sometimes secondary to the use of cocaine or amphetamines. Finally, occlusion of a coronary artery can occur as the result of aortic dissection. Risk factors include: age, male gender, a family history of premature coronary artery disease, tobacco use, hypertension, diabetes, hypercholesterolemia, and hyperlipidemia.

- *Presentation:* the classic symptom of crushing substernal chest pain radiating to the left arm is not frequently seen. Patients younger than 40 and older than 70 are more likely to present with atypical symptoms such as dyspnea, nausea, weakness, or dizziness without pain. The autonomic nervous system dysfunction caused by protracted hyperglycemia will often make the presentation atypical in diabetics.

- *Diagnosis:* the diagnosis of acute coronary syndrome is based largely on the patient's history. The physical exam is often normal or demonstrates nonspecific abnormalities of the blood pressure or pulse. Patients with complications of ACS can have signs of congestive heart failure or cardiogenic shock. Patients should have an EKG performed as soon as the diagnosis is suspected and interpreted by the ED provider within 10 minutes of arrival. A negative EKG or cardiac enzymes are not sufficiently sensitive to exclude a diagnosis of acute coronary syndrome and a single normal measurement should never be used to determine that a patient may be discharged from the ED. A chest X-ray should always be done to look for signs of congestive heart failure or thoracic aortic aneurysm.

- *Treatment:* initial treatment of acute coronary syndrome and STEMI is directed at decreasing myocardial oxygen demand and establishing optimal flow through the coronary arteries. Sublingual nitroglycerin by pill or spray is still the mainstay of chest pain treatment and should be given if the blood pressure is reasonably elevated. Beta-blockers should be given to patients who present with an elevated pulse or blood pressure. Supplemental oxygen improves oxygen delivery to ischemic myocardial tissue. Anxiolytics and morphine can be used to decrease anxiety and pain, thereby decreasing myocardial oxygen demand. Aspirin should be given to all patients unless there is a specific contraindication. Patients may benefit from heparin, either standard or low molecular weight, and from other antiplatelet agents. Patients with evidence of STEMI are at greatest risk of complication if the blockage is not immediately relieved. These patients must be urgently evaluated for definitive therapy.

- *Definitive therapy:* thrombolytic therapy or primary angioplasty is the primary therapy for patients who present with STEMI. Current studies demonstrate that angioplasty is preferred when available. Patients with other forms of ACS are treated with medical management when possible and may require additional diagnostic procedures such as stress testing, chest CT or diagnostic angiography. Coronary artery bypass grafting is reserved for lesions that are not amenable to angioplasty and when symptoms are not controlled with medical management. All patients with ACS require hospitalization with telemetry monitoring for observation and additional testing.

Clinical course

The keys to this patient's diagnosis are careful attention to her history, physical exam, and ancillary studies.

Historical clues	Physical findings	Ancillary studies
• Nausea without concomitant GI symptoms	• Bradycardia	• EKG with STEMI
• History of diabetes	• Initial hypotension responsive to fluids	• Normal chest X-ray
• Multiple risk factors for coronary artery disease	• Otherwise unremarkable exam	

This woman was recognized as having acute coronary syndrome, specifically an ST elevation myocardial infarction. Because the ED had access to urgent heart catheterization services, the catheterization lab was activated and responded within 30 minutes. The patient underwent diagnostic heart catheterization, which revealed a 99% blockage of the right coronary artery. This blockage was successfully ballooned and a stent was placed to maintain vessel patency. The patient was transferred to the CCU in good condition.

Further reading

Gandhi MM, Lampe FC, Wood DA. Incidence, clinical characteristics, and short-term prognosis of angina pectoris. *Br Heart J* 1995;**73**(2):193–8.

ACC/AHA 2002 guideline update for the management of patients with unstable angina and non-ST-segment elevation myocardial infarction–summary article: a report of the American College of Cardiology/American Heart Association task force on practice guidelines (Committee on the Management of Patients With Unstable Angina). *J Am Coll Cardiol* 2002;**40**(7):1366–74.

Fesmire FM, Hughes AD, Fody EP, et al. The Erlanger chest pain evaluation protocol: a one-year experience with serial 12-lead ECG monitoring, two-hour delta serum marker measurements, and selective nuclear stress testing to identify and exclude acute coronary syndromes. *Ann Emerg Med* 2002;**40**(6):584–94.

Hollander Judd E, Chapter 50. Acute coronary syndromes: acute myocardial infarction and unstable angina. In Tintinalli JE, Kelen GD, Stapczynski JS, Ma OJ, Cline DM, eds., *Tintinalli's Emergency Medicine: A Comprehensive Study Guide*, 6th edition. New York: McGraw-Hill, 2004.

Case #2

History

A 27-year-old male with a history of Down's syndrome presents with shortness of breath and chest pain that have been increasing over the last 5 days. At baseline he is on oxygen at home at a rate of 2 liters by nasal cannula. His mother increased this to 5 liters to help with his shortness of breath. He appears short of breath at rest and most notably when speaking. He has not had any fevers, cough, or cold. He has no known sick contacts. Two weeks ago he had nausea and vomiting for several days, which has since resolved, and he has been tolerating oral intake. His mother is most concerned about the patient's chest pain. His pain is diffuse and vague in nature, but worse when he breathes. He has an umbilical hernia and a ventral hernia, which are unchanged in size according to his mother. He has also been a little constipated, which is normal for him and was treated at home with over-the-counter medications. His last bowel movement was yesterday.

Past medical history

The patient has a history of chronic obstructive pulmonary disease, congestive heart failure, Down's syndrome, and mild mental retardation. He has a surgical history including inguinal hernia repair as well as coronary artery bypass grafting as a child.

Medications

The patient takes albuterol, budesonide, and furosemide.

Allergies

He has no known drug allergies.

Physical exam and ancillary studies

- *Vital signs:* at triage, the patient's oxygen saturation was 84% on 2 L of oxygen. Upon arrival to his ED room and on 3 L of oxygen by nasal cannula, his saturation ranges from 90% to 100%. His temperature is 37.2°C, his blood pressure is 128/82 mmHg, his heart rate is 90 bpm, and his respiratory rate is 20.
- *General:* the patient is awake and alert, and is non-toxic-appearing. He has no respiratory distress at this time.
- *Head and neck:* there are no signs of trauma. His pupils are equal, round, and reactive to light. The patient has moist oral mucosa. His neck is supple with a midline trachea.
- *Cardiovascular:* his heart has a regular rate and rhythm, with normal S1 and S2. He has no murmurs, rubs, or gallops.
- *Lungs:* there are decreased breath sounds in the patient's right lower lobe, otherwise no wheezes, rales, or rhonchi.

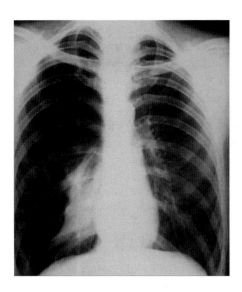

Figure 3.2. Right side pneumothorax of almost the entire right lung. There is a slight shift in the mediastinum to the left, suggesting that this is going to progress to a tension pneumothorax leading to cardiovascular compromise.

- *Abdomen:* a large ventral hernia is noted. An umbilical hernia is also present. Both are soft and easily reducible. He has normoactive bowel sounds with no organomegaly and no peritoneal signs.
- *Extremities and skin:* he has no pedal edema or calf tenderness. There are no petechiae or skin lesions.
- *Labs:* the patient's complete blood count, electrolytes, liver function tests, and lipase are all within normal limits.
- *Radiographs:* see Figure 3.2: chest X-ray.

Questions for thought

- What are the appropriate initial actions to take to stabilize this patient?
- What is the appropriate emergency therapy for this patient?
- What constitutes definitive therapy for this patient?
- What is the risk of recurrence?

Diagnosis

Spontaneous right pneumothorax.

Discussion

- *Epidemiology:* there are two types of spontaneous pneumothorax; primary and secondary. Primary pneumothorax develops in healthy individuals without underlying lung disease. Secondary pneumothorax occurs in patients with underlying lung disease, most commonly COPD. Other causes of secondary pneumothorax include cystic fibrosis, asthma, collagen vascular disease, pulmonary infection, interstitial lung disease, tuberculosis, AIDs, cancer, and drug use. Secondary pneumothorax is usually seen in patients over

40 years of age. The incidence of spontaneous pneumothorax is increasing. There are 20 000 new cases of spontaneous pneumothorax each year in the United States. The incidence of secondary pneumothorax is greater in men, with a 3.2:1 predominance, and has a recurrence rate of 40–50%.

- *Pathophysiology:* pneumothorax can be due to trauma, iatrogenic, or spontaneous. A pneumothorax results from a break in the pleura and air entering the potential space between the visceral and parietal pleura of the lung. This occurs because of damaged alveoli or rupture of an apical bleb or bulla and in the setting of increased intrathoracic pressure, such as with vomiting or exhaling against a closed glottis. Air travels down a pressure gradient into the intrapleural space until pressure equilibrium is achieved resulting in partial lung collapse. Complete lung collapse is rare with secondary spontaneous pneumothorax. As the pneumothorax increases, the lung becomes smaller. This alters the ventilation perfusion ratio, causing a decrease in vital capacity leading to dyspnea and hypoxemia.

- *Presentation:* symptoms are related to the size of the pneumothorax, rate of development, and underlying clinical status of the patient. Common symptoms include acute pleuritic pain (usually on the side of the pneumothorax), dyspnea, cough, and generalized malaise. Decreased breath sounds, decreased chest excursion, hyper-resonant percussion, subcutaneous emphysema, increased heart rate, and increased respiratory rate may be noted on physical exam. On EKG, nonspecific ST changes and T-wave inversions may be present. Tension pneumothorax is rarely seen with spontaneous pneumothorax and is diagnosed in a patient with pleuritic chest pain, dyspnea, hypotension, tachycardia, and unilaterally absent breath sounds.

- *Treatment:* there are multiple treatment options. All patients should receive oxygen at 3–4 L via nasal cannula, which increases pleural resorption of air by 3–4 fold. If the pneumothorax is small and the patient's clinical condition stable, observation or needle decompression may be appropriate. However, a chest tube is eventually required in up to 40% of observed patients. The majority of patients with secondary pneumothorax will require a chest tube and admission. Short-term complications include tension pneumothorax, failure of the lung to re-expand, persistent air leak, infection, and re-expansion pulmonary edema.

Clinical course

The keys to obtaining this patient's diagnosis are careful attention to history, physical exam, and chest X-ray.

Historical clues	Physical findings	Ancillary studies
• History of COPD	• Increased oxygen requirement	• Chest X-ray demonstrating pneumothorax
• Pleuritic chest pain	• Elevated respiratory rate	
• History of forceful vomiting	• Decreased breath sounds on the right	
• Complaint of dyspnea		

This patient was suspected to have intrapulmonary pathology based on his increased oxygen requirement, dyspnea, and history of chronic obstructive pulmonary disease. This prompted the clinician to order an X-ray, which showed a visceral pleural line on an upright

PA chest film. This line is the interface of the lung and pleural air and is 83% sensitive. Based on this finding, the patient underwent therapy in the emergency department with right-sided chest tube placement. His right lung was re-expanded, with immediate symptomatic improvement. He was admitted to the cardiothoracic surgery service, his chest tube was removed after a few days, and he was discharged home in good condition.

Further reading

Chang A. Pneumothorax, iatrogenic, spontaneous and pneumomediastinum. Emedicine. Topic 469. Nov 14, 2007.

Light R. Secondary spontaneous pneumothorax in adults. Up-To-Date. Sept 21, 2007.

Olsen C. Spontaneous pneumothorax treatment guidelines previewed. Pulmonary Reviews.com. Jan 2000.

Young WF, Humphries R. Spontaneous and iatrogenic pneumothorax. In Tintinalli JE, et al., eds., *Tintinalli's Emergency Medicine: A Comprehensive Study Guide*, 6th edition. New York: McGraw-Hill, 2004, pp. 513–16.

Case #3

History

A 63-year-old woman presents with chest pain after vomiting. She has a history of ovarian carcinoma and is currently receiving chemotherapy. Her course has been complicated by persistent nausea and frequent emesis, poorly controlled by anti-emetics. She reports that she vomits most mornings after eating. In addition, she is being treated for known gastroesophageal reflux. She states the onset of chest pain was sudden and that the pain is severe. She states it is different from her prior discomfort with reflux. She denies other shortness of breath, cough, fever, and diarrhea.

Past medical history

Ovarian carcinoma, GERD, Type II DM and HTN.

Medications

Chemotherapy weekly. Ranitidine, glucophage, lisinopril.

Allergies

None.

Physical exam and ancillary studies

- *Vital signs:* heart rate 123 bpm, blood pressure 100/58, respiratory rate 26, temperature 37.8°C, room air saturation 95%.
- *General:* ill-appearing woman, complaining of 10/10 pain.
- *Head and neck:* dry oral mucosa, otherwise normal.
- *Cardiovascular:* regular tachycardia, thready pulses, otherwise normal.
- *Lungs:* normal.
- *Extremities and skin:* cool, clammy skin, delayed capillary refill.
- *Pertinent abnormal labs:* WBC 18 000, CO_2 18, BUN 26, Cr 0.9.
- *EKG:* sinus tachycardia with no acute ischemic changes.
- *Chest X-ray:* see Figure 3.3.

Questions for thought

- What are the appropriate initial actions to take to stabilize this patient?
- Once stable, what are other diagnostic tools you can use to make a diagnosis?
- What medications should be avoided in this patient?
- How does one urgently treat this condition in the emergency department?
- What is definitive treatment of this condition?

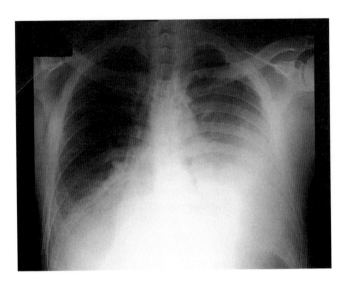

Figure 3.3. Bilateral pleural effusions from esophageal rupture.

Diagnosis

Esophageal rupture (Boerhaave's syndrome).

Discussion

- *Epidemiology:* Boerhaave's syndrome originally was described as esophageal rupture following forceful emesis. Due to the increased use of endoscopy for diagnosis and treatment, iatrogenic esophageal perforation is now the most common etiology. Other etiologies include foreign body ingestion, trauma (both penetrating and blunt), and erosion by neoplasm. Men are more likely to suffer esophageal perforation than women.
- *Pathophysiology:* esophageal rupture occurs either from direct trauma, due to instrumentation, penetrating injury, or neoplasm, or from increased pressure within the esophageal lumen. The esophagus is a thin-walled organ without an outer serosal layer. The location of rupture is either at the site of direct injury, as in the case of iatrogenic or penetrating trauma, or just above the gastroesophageal (GE) junction in the case of spontaneous rupture. Esophageal rupture results in leakage of saliva and ingested materials into the mediastinal space, causing necrosis and infection within the mediastinum. Often, this progresses to include the pleural space as well. With diagnosis and treatment within 24 hours, mortality is 10%. Delays in diagnosis and treatment are associated with increased morbidity and mortality.
- *Presentation:* patients may present following esophageal instrumentation or trauma. Patients with spontaneous rupture will present after forceful emesis. Spontaneous rupture has also been described following weight-lifting and childbirth. Patients present initially with pain. Unrecognized perforation that progresses to mediastinitis will present with fever and generalized symptoms. Patients may present in shock.
- *Diagnosis:* diagnosis is suspected on the basis of history and presentation. Chest X-ray (CXR) may show pneumomediastinum, pneumothorax, or pleural effusion. However, early studies may be normal. Diagnosis is confirmed by gastrograffin swallow, which has a 10% false negative rate. Barium has a greater density and may identify more leaks in patients with high clinical suspicion. CT may be useful.

- *Treatment:* all patients should be maintained with an NPO status and all should have IV fluid treatment as necessary for shock and to maintain adequate hydration. Antibiotics are used to treat infection as the mediastinal contamination contains polymicrobial organisms. Steroids are of no proven benefit.
- *Definitive therapy:* definitive treatment depends on the site of injury and the time delay between injury and identification. Therapeutic options include primary repair, debridement, expectant management with tube thoracostomies, and diversions of the esophagus. Although there is no gold standard currently, it is clear that delays in diagnosis are associated with longer ICU and inpatient stays and increased mortality.

Clinical course

The keys to this diagnosis were the history, clinical presentation, and pneumomediastinum apparent on plain film.

Historical clues	Physical findings	Ancillary studies
• Chest pain following emesis	• Ill appearance	• Plain radiographs with effusions and mediastinal air
• Increased risk with history of GE reflux	• Abnormal vital signs on presentation	
	• Presence of shock on presentation	• Gastrograffin swallow

Summary

The potential diagnosis of esophageal rupture was recognized in this patient who presented with excruciating chest pain following forceful emesis. The patient was initially treated with crystalloid to normalize vital signs and reverse the clinical signs of shock, as well as antibiotics to cover oral flora. A CXR was obtained and the presence of mediastinal emphysema further supported this presumptive diagnosis, which was confirmed by gastrograffin swallow. Thoracic surgery was consulted and the patient was taken immediately to the OR for primary repair.

Further reading

Henderson JA, Peloquin AJ. Boerhaave revisited: spontaneous esophageal perforation as a diagnostic masquerader. *Am J Med* 1989;**86**(5):559–67.

Justicz AG, Symbas PN. Spontaneous rupture of the esophagus: immediate and late results. *Am Surg* 1991;**57**(1):4–7.

Tong BC, Yang SC, Harmon J. Esophageal perforation. In *Principles of Surgery*, 8th edition. New York: McGraw-Hill, 2004, pp. 10–14.

Case #4

History

A 77-year-old woman presents to the ED complaining of sudden onset of severe chest pain and dizziness starting about 1 hour prior to arrival. Her pain is described as a tearing sensation mid-substernal, radiating to her mid upper back. She also notes that she has been lightheaded, worse when standing up, and she almost passed out when the pain initially started. She denies any previous history of similar events. She had some mild nausea but has had no active vomiting, fever, chills, shortness of breath, diaphoresis, abdominal pain, or any recent changes in her bowel or urinary habits. She states she has had a dry cough for about 5 days for which she did not seek treatment. On arrival in the ED the patient appears to be in severe pain and is agitated. After 5 minutes, the patient becomes less responsive with a GCS of 7 and is intubated.

Past medical history

The patient on arrival is able to give a partial history of hypertension, hypercholesterolemia, and hypothyroidism, but denies any cardiac history. Patient is a 50 pack-year smoker.

Medications

Patient states that she is on a blood pressure medication and thyroid medication, but cannot recall the names.

Allergies

The patient has no known drug allergies.

Physical exam and ancillary studies

- *Vital signs:* temperature 37.3°C, heart rate 83 bpm, blood pressure 124/68, but drops to 95/35, respiratory rate 15, room air saturation 96%.
- *General:* awake and alert, diaphoretic and pale, is able to answer questions initially, but soon becomes unresponsive.
- *Head and neck:* pupils are equally round and reactive to light, cranial nerves intact. The patient's mucous membranes are moist. Her neck is supple with a midline trachea. Her jugular veins are distended when the stretcher is flat.
- *Cardiovascular:* heart sounds are muffled. Regular rate and rhythm with a diastolic murmur, peripheral pulses decreased throughout. Left radial pulse cannot be appreciated.
- *Lungs:* clear to auscultation bilaterally, no wheezes, rales, or rhonchi.
- *Extremities and skin:* no edema, clubbing, or calf tenderness. There is poor capillary refill throughout and her skin is pale.

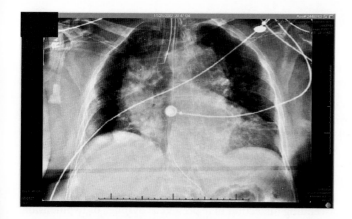

Figure 3.4 Chest X-ray demonstrating widened mediastinum.

- *Pertinent abnormal labs:* WBC 10.5, HCT 34.6%. The rest of her chemistries including cardiac enzymes were within normal limits or negative.
- *EKG:* low-voltage and minimal nonspecific ST-T wave changes consistent with mild left ventricular hypertrophy
- *Chest X-ray:* see Figure 3.4.

Questions for thought

- What are the appropriate initial actions to take to stabilize this patient?
- Once stable, what are other diagnostic tools you can use to make a diagnosis?
- What medications should be avoided in this patient?
- How does one urgently treat this condition in the emergency department?
- What is definitive treatment of this condition?
- Why is this patient short of breath?

Diagnosis

Aortic dissection, Stanford type A.

Discussion

- *Epidemiology:* aortic dissection is the most common catastrophe of the aorta. Thoracic aortic dissections are classified by two methods, with the more common being the Stanford classification, which divides dissections into 2 types based on treatment. Type A involves the ascending aorta and type B the descending aorta. The DeBakey classification system divides dissections into three types. Untreated dissections lead to a mortality rate of 33% within 24 hours and 50% within 48 hours of onset of symptoms.
- *Pathophysiology:* the aorta is composed of three layers: the intima, media, and adventitia. In aortic dissection, a tear develops in the intimal layer, creating and propagating a sub-intimal hematoma. The resulting false lumen can occasionally surround the entire aorta, reducing blood flow to arteries branching off the aorta. The most common site

95

of aortic dissection is the first few centimeters of the ascending aorta followed by the area just distal to the left subclavian artery. Diseases that weaken the aortic wall include Marfan, Ehlers-Danlos, and Turner syndrome, bicuspid aortic valve, syphilis, and coarctation of the aorta. Incidence is also increased in pregnancy, secondary to crack cocaine use, after cardiac catheterization, and because of shearing forces secondary to blunt trauma.

- *Presentation:* aortic dissection should be considered in all patients reporting acute, sudden, and severe chest pain that is maximal at onset and often characterized as ripping or tearing. This chest pain may be located in the anterior chest and can mimic or cause an AMI. Mid-thoracic or intrascapular pain may represent a dissection involving the descending aorta. Neurologic symptoms such as syncope, mental status changes, and limb paresthesias or pain may represent dissection of the aortic arch. Tamponade from an ascending dissection may present as dyspnea or hypotension. Flank pain may indicate renal artery involvement. Additional clues may include bruits, asymmetrical pulses, asymmetrical blood pressure measurements, and a new diastolic murmur.

- *Diagnosis:* blood work may indicate compromised blood flow and ischemia to organs such as the heart or kidneys. Chest X-ray findings may include a widened mediastinum, abnormal aortic knob, a displaced aorta greater than 5 mm, a left apical cap, and tracheal or esophageal deviation. The sensitivity of these findings is about 80%. Spiral CT and CT angiography have a sensitivity of 83–94% and a specificity of 87–100% for dissection and are replacing angiography as the diagnostic test of choice. Drawbacks are transportation of the emergency patient out of the ED and need for contrast material. Transesophageal echocardiography (TEE) is most useful in identifying ascending aortic dissections, cardiac tamponade, and aortic regurgitation. Transthoracic echocardiography may be used as a non-invasive bedside screening test, recognizing that ascending dissections are more likely to be diagnosed correctly.

- *Treatment:* the mortality rate of patients with aortic dissection is 1–2% per hour for the first 24–48 hours. Once diagnosis is suspected, the patient should have IV access, oxygen, and cardiac and respiratory monitoring. Beta-blockers should be given initially for a target heart rate of 60–80 bpm and target systolic blood pressure of 100–120 mmHg. Emergency surgical intervention is required for type A dissections. Uncomplicated type B dissections are generally treated medically with control of blood pressure. Surgery may be used for distal dissections that are complicated and are leaking, ruptured, or compromising blood flow to a vital organ. Surgery for type A dissections is typically resection and replacement with a Dacron graft. The operative mortality rate is usually less than 10%, and serious complications are rare with ascending aortic dissections. Inability to control hypertension with medication is also an indication for surgery in those with type B dissections. Long-term medical therapy involves a beta-adrenergic blocker combined with other antihypertensive medications.

Clinical course

The keys to this patient's diagnosis are careful attention to her history, physical exam, and ancillary studies. This woman was recognized to probably have aortic dissection based on her presentation and chest X-ray. It was elected to intubate the patient after she became less responsive, had altered mental status, and was unable to protect her own airway.

Historical clues	Physical findings	Ancillary studies
• Mid-sternal chest pain radiating to the back	• Beck's triad; hypotension, jugular venous distension, and muffled heart sounds	• Widened mediastinum on the chest X-ray with loss of normal mediastinal contours and rightward tracheal shift
• Tearing nature of chest pain	• Diastolic murmur	
• Gradual loss of consciousness with need to intubate	• Asymmetric peripheral pulses	
• Neurological symptoms	• Pallor	
	• Poor peripheral perfusion	

BP stabilized, and the patient was sent off for CT, which showed a type A aortic dissection, with hemopericardium indicating a tear at root of aorta. The dissection extended from aortic root to left common iliac artery. The cardiothoracic surgery department was contacted but they determined that the patient was not a candidate for surgery and she was subsequently designated DNR and given comfort care.

Further reading

Menon V, Sengupta J, Unzek S. Optimal management of acute aortic dissection. *Curr Treat Options Cardiovasc Med* 2009;**11**(2):146–55.

Lin PH, Huynh TT, Kougias P, et al. Descending thoracic aortic dissection: evaluation and management in the era of endovascular technology. *Vasc Endovascular Surg* 2009;**43**(1):5–24.

Golledge J, Eagle KA. Acute aortic dissection. () *Lancet* 2008;**372**(9632):55–66.

Prince LA, Johnson GA, Chapter 58. Aortic dissection and aneurysms. In Tintinalli JE, Kelen GD, Stapczynski JS, Ma OJ, Cline DM, eds., *Tintinalli's Emergency Medicine: A Comprehensive Study Guide*, 6th edition. New York: McGraw-Hill, 2004.

Case #5

History

A 45-year-old white male comes to the ED complaining of chest pain and shortness of breath which has worsened over the past 4 days. The chest pain is in his right lateral chest, and he describes it as dull and non-radiating. The pain is worse with inspiration. The dyspnea is worse with exertion and associated with a mildly productive cough. There is no associated post-nasal drip, sore throat, ear pain, rash, or heartburn symptoms. He has a mild frontal headache and his girlfriend feels that he is a bit confused. He had some mild non-bloody diarrhea the night prior to presentation. He has had no recent travel or sick contacts. He denies having pets or recent construction to his home, but does recall recently placing an air conditioner in his apartment window which he had purchased from a local garage sale.

Past medical history

The patient's history is remarkable for hypertension, celiac sprue, and gastroesophageal reflux disease. He smokes one pack of cigarettes per day, but denies alcohol or illicit drug use.

Medications

The patient's medications include atenolol, ranitidine, and a daily multivitamin.

Allergies

The patient is allergic to sulfa-containing medications.

Physical exam and ancillary studies

- *Vital signs:* the patient's temperature is 39.3°C, his heart rate is 120 bpm, his blood pressure is 95/50, his respiratory rate is 32, and his room air oxygen saturation is 90%.
- *General:* the patient is awake and alert, with three-word dyspnea.
- *Head and neck:* his pupils are equally round and reactive to light. His cranial nerves are intact. The patient has dry mucous membranes. His neck is supple and non-tender. His trachea is midline and he has no jugular venous distension.
- *Cardiovascular:* the patient's heart has a regular tachycardia, without gallops, rubs or murmurs. His pulses are slightly diminished throughout.
- *Lungs:* his lungs have normal excursion. They are resonant to percussion throughout except for dullness at the right base. He also has decreased breath sounds at the right base with egophony and an increase in tactile fremitus.
- *Abdomen:* the patient's abdomen is non-tender and non-distended. His bowel sounds are normal.
- *Extremities and skin:* the patient has no edema, clubbing, or calf tenderness. There is no evidence of jaundice, ecchymosis, or petechiae.

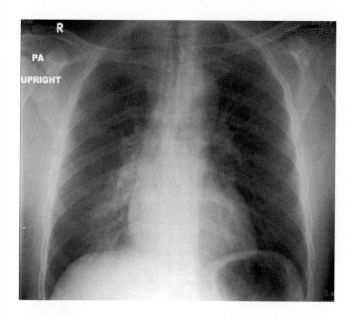

Figure 3.5. Chest X-ray showing right lower lobe infiltrate. You can still see the right heart border and diaphragm, suggesting that the consolidation is in the right lower lobe.

- *Neurological:* the patient is alert and oriented times three. He cannot remember three objects at 5 minutes.
- *Pertinent labs:* the patient's complete blood count is remarkable for a white blood cell count of 18.1 with 18% bands. His hematocrit is 45%, and his platelet count is 125. The patient's chemistries are remarkable for a sodium of 129, a creatinine of 1.8, a creatine kinase of 801 (3% CKMB), an AST of 201, and an ALT of 210. His troponin is 0.04. His remaining labs are normal or negative.
- *Chest radiographs:* see Figure 3.5.

Questions for thought

- What initial measures should be taken to stabilize this patient?
- What historical and ancillary information is helpful in establishing a likely etiology for this patient's pneumonia?
- How can the diagnosis be confirmed?
- What is the definitive therapy for this patient?

Diagnosis

Legionella pneumonia.

Discussion

- *Epidemiology: Legionella* pneumonia is reported to be among the top causes of community-acquired pneumonia in immunocompetent persons and is the second most frequent cause of severe pneumonia requiring intensive care unit admission. In general,

Legionella colonizes up to 70% of hospital water supplies and is virtually impossible to eradicate. Hospital-acquired *Legionella* pneumonia is a well-described entity with considerable morbidity and mortality.

- *Pathophysiology: Legionella* is not part of the normal human flora. The organism has been isolated in freshwater streams and lakes, water reservoirs and artificial sources such as cooling towers and potable water distribution systems. The usual mode of transmission of *Legionella* is inhalation. Despite considerable colonization in water supplies in residential and commercial facilities, most people do not contract *Legionella* infection. Smoking, chronic lung disease, diabetes mellitus, and immunosuppression are risk factors for infection. Transmission occurs by means of aerosolization or aspiration of water contaminated with *Legionella* organisms. Wounds may become infected after contact with contaminated water. Person-to person transmission has never been demonstrated. Once infection has occurred, *Legionella* replicates within alveolar macrophages.

- *Presentation: Legionella* pneumonia usually presents with a mild productive cough, dyspnea, and abdominal symptoms. Chest pain is quite common and usually reflects associated pleuritis or rarely a complicated effusion. A fever greater than 39.7°C occurs in the majority of cases. Bradycardia relative to the elevated temperature may be present but is neither sensitive nor specific for the diagnosis. There may be associated neurologic sequelae such as headache and confusion. Many patients will have gastrointestinal complaints, such as diarrhea. There is often an impressive leukocytosis with mild thrombocytopenia, hyponatremia, and mild renal and hepatic dysfunction. The chest exam usually shows changes typical of consolidation with egophony and an increase in tactile fremitus.

- *Treatment:* the intracellular location of the pathogen is relevant to the efficacy of the chosen antibiotic. Antibiotics capable of achieving adequate intracellular concentrations are the standard of care and include macrolides, quinolones, tetracyclines, and rifampin. In general, either azithromycin or a respiratory fluoroquinolone are chosen at doses sufficient to treat pneumonia. The exact duration of therapy is unclear, but depending on the severity of illness a course of 14–21 days is reasonable. In addition to specific therapy for the etiologic agent, patients with *Legionella* pneumonia often require aggressive cardiorespiratory support. These patients are often critically ill and mandate admission, frequently to a critical care bed.

Clinical course

The keys to this patient's diagnosis are careful attention to his history, physical exam, and ancillary studies.

Historical clues	Physical findings	Ancillary studies
• Pleuritic chest pain	• Fever	• Elevated WBC
• Dyspnea	• Hypoxia	• Elevated liver function tests
• Mild confusion	• Tachypnea	• Low sodium
• Diarrhea	• Focal lung exam	• Elevated creatinine
• Smoking history		• Radiograph consistent with pneumonia
• Recent exposure to a new air-conditioning unit		

The provider caring for this patient recognized the critical nature of his illness and the patient was intubated for respiratory support in light of his low oxygenation and elevated respiratory rate. He was given 3 liters of normal saline for hypotension, with improvement in his hemodynamics, and was empirically started on ceftriaxone and azithromycin to cover likely community-acquired lung pathogens. Blood and sputum were sent for routine culture. In addition, the provider recognized the possibility that this patient might have *Legionella*, and sent a *Legionella* urinary antigen as well as a respiratory specimen for *Legionella* culture. This requires a special medium. The patient was admitted to the intensive care unit. His status initially worsened, and he briefly required vasopressors, but after 5 days he began to improve and was weaned from the ventilator on hospital day 8. His laboratory and hemodynamic parameters improved over the following week, and he was discharged home with no sequelae. He has since quit smoking.

Further reading

Cunha BA. Atypical pneumonias: current clinical concepts focusing on Legionnaires' disease. *Curr Opin Pulm Med* 2008;**14**(3):183–94.

Mandell LA, Wunderink R. Chapter 251. Pneumonia. In Fauci AS, Braunwald E, Kasper DL, et al., eds., *Harrison's Principles of Internal Medicine*, 17th edition. New York: McGraw-Hill, 2008.

Moffa DA, Emerman CL. Chapter 63. Bronchitis, pneumonia, and pleural emphysema. In Tintinalli JE, Kelen GD, Stapczynski JS, et al., eds. *Tintinalli's Emergency Medicine: A Comprehensive Study Guide*, 6th edition. New York: McGraw-Hill, 2003.

Case #6

History

A 34-year-old man arrived at the emergency department about 10:00 a.m. He had been making himself some breakfast with some leftover fish and while eating he felt a sudden sharp pain in his throat. He feels that the pain is still there and is sure there is a fishbone stuck in his throat. The neck pain radiates to his upper chest. He initially was able to swallow without any difficulty but now is gagging on his own saliva. Otherwise the patient has no complaints.

Past medical history

He has been in good health all of his life, he has no medical problems and never had any difficulty swallowing before. There is no history of reflux or other symptoms relating to swallowing.

Physical exam and ancillary studies

- *Vital signs:* all normal.
- *General:* awake and alert, appears to be uncomfortable but is sitting quietly on the stretcher in no acute distress.
- *Head and neck:* completely normal, there is no scleral icterus and the conjunctivae are normal color. No foreign body is visible in the hypopharynx and his tongue and uvula are both normal. Normal ear and nose examination. Neck examination essentially normal with a little bit of increased pain when his trachea is moved from side to side.
- *Lungs:* clear bilaterally with no rales, rhonchi, or wheezes.
- *Cardiovascular:* regular heartbeat without rubs, murmurs, or gallops. Peripheral pulses normal.
- *Extremities and skin:* normal without edema, clubbing, or calf tenderness. Good capillary refill throughout.
- *Abdomen:* bowel sounds are normal. The abdomen is soft with no tenderness.
- *Pertinent labs:* none are ordered.

Questions for thought

- What would make you think of an esophageal foreign body?
- What symptoms are typical of esophageal foreign body?
- Which foreign body needs to be removed urgently?
- What is the best way to remove esophageal foreign bodies?
- What other diseases might predispose to esophageal foreign body?

Diagnosis

Fishbone esophageal foreign body.

Discussion

- *Epidemiology:* meat impaction is the most common esophageal foreign body in adults. These food boluses are more common in patients with dentures and who have had some alcoholic beverages with a meal. Common ingestions in children include coins, magnets, and button battery ingestion. The latter is becoming a more common clinical event as these batteries are put into more objects. They are easily ingested and have a certain attractiveness to children.
- *Pathophysiology:* most ingested foreign bodies will pass through the gastrointestinal tract without difficulty. The "tight" parts of the GI tract are the esophagus at the level of the cricopharyngeus muscle and the gastroesophageal junction. Once the object has passed through to the stomach, treatment in most cases is expectant only. Objects that may get stuck are sharp objects such as needles and fish bones, button batteries, magnets, and large coins. If a foreign body obstructs the esophagus, aspiration or perforation may occur and this requires mechanical removal of the foreign body. Swallowed magnets may attract each other in the intestine, producing an area of ischemia and leading to perforation. Sharp and pointed objects should be considered for removal because of the potential for perforation.
- *Presentation:* esophageal foreign objects typically cause retrosternal pain and anxiety. The patient will have a painful sensation on swallowing, if they are able to swallow at all. Choking, coughing, and aspiration are potential problems if the patient tries to eat or drink anything. Inability to swallow their own secretions is a common presentation in adults and this history is usually all the information needed to make the diagnosis and initiate treatment. In children 16 years and younger, symptoms may be more vague and also include nonspecific vomiting, refusal to eat, gagging, choking, stridor, neck or throat pain, inability to swallow, and increased salivation.
- *Diagnosis:* the presence of an esophageal foreign body requires a high degree of suspicion in patients with characteristic signs and symptoms. Potential diagnostic methods available to locate foreign bodies include CT scans and ultrasound, neither of which is as reliable as endoscopy.
- *Follow-up care:* subsequent progress of the object through the gastrointestinal tract should be monitored with frequent abdominal examinations and radiographs where indicated. Foreign objects stuck high up in the esophagus should have emergency esophagoscopy to remove the object. Button batteries and magnets may be followed clinically with repeat radiographs if they have clearly passed into the stomach. Any patient with foreign body ingestion who returns with abdominal pain should be considered to have a perforation or obstruction until proved otherwise. Meat bolus impaction can be observed and delayed endoscopy done if the patient has no difficulty with their secretions. Swallowing meat tenderizer was recommended in the past but should not be used because of the increased likelihood of perforation. Intravenous glucagon was thought to relax esophageal smooth muscle, but has not been shown to be beneficial in well-controlled studies. Other spasmolytic drugs have been equally ineffective although there is some evidence that nifedipine reduces lower esophageal sphincter pressure and may assist in the

passage of food boluses caught at the gastroesophageal junction. Button battery ingestion is a true emergency because burns to the esophagus have occurred in as little as 4 hours and perforation after 6 hours of ingestion. Blood and urine mercury levels should be measured if a mercury-containing cell breaks open while in the gastrointestinal tract. Once the battery passes through the pylorus, watchful waiting is considered the treatment of choice.

Clinical course

The keys to this patient's diagnosis are careful attention to his history, and physical exam.

Historical clues	Physical findings	Ancillary studies
• Pain after eating fish	• Tenderness of the larynx	
• Difficulty swallowing		
• Persistent vomiting, especially of saliva		

Clinical course

Based on his history a soft tissue lateral X-ray of his neck was taken. This was felt to show something that could have been his hyoid bone but might also have been a foreign body. Because of this question the ear, nose, and throat resident was called in to consult. The resident examined him with a fiberoptic nasopharyngoscope and found a fishbone in his soft tissue just above the vallecula. It was removed without difficulty and the patient was observed for an hour and then was discharged home with a liquid diet for 24 hours.

Further reading

Schwartz GF, Polsky HS. Ingested foreign bodies of the gastrointestinal tract. *Am Surg* 1976;**42**:236.

Mosca S, Manes G, Martino R, et al. Endoscopic management of foreign bodies in the upper gastrointestinal tract: report on a series of 414 adult patients. *Endoscopy* 2001;**33**:692.

Tibbling L, Bjorkhoel A, Jansson E, Stenkvist M. Effect of spasmolytic drugs on esophageal foreign bodies. *Dysphagia* 1995;**10**:126.

Litovitz T, Schmitz BF. Ingestion of cylindrical and button batteries: an analysis of 2382 cases. *Pediatrics* 1992;**89**:747.

Case #7

History

A 36-year-old female presents to the ED complaining of chest and back pain associated with mild shortness of breath. She was in her usual state of health this morning, dropped her 5-month-old at day care as usual and then went to work. Just before lunch, she felt a sudden cramp in her chest "like someone kicked her." While at work she felt the chest pain and was somewhat short of breath but thought that it was secondary to the pain. She has never had anything like this before and there is no family history of early cardiac disease. Her pain has been constant since its onset and does not have alleviating or exacerbating factors, except that it hurts more when she takes a deep breath. She has been in good health since the birth of her child, and just went back to work last month. The patient denies nausea, vomiting, diaphoresis, or fever.

Past medical history

She has no past medical problems. She smokes one pack of cigarettes a day and denies alcohol or any recreational drugs use. She was breast feeding until she went back to work last month.

Medications

She just started back on oral contraceptives.

Allergies

The patient has no known drug allergies.

Physical exam and ancillary studies

- *Vital signs:* temperature 36.7°C, heart rate 92 bpm, blood pressure 128/72, respiratory rate 24, room air saturation 97%.
- *General:* awake and alert, in no respiratory distress.
- *Head and neck:* pupils are equally round and reactive to light, cranial nerves intact. The patient's mucous membranes are moist. Her neck is supple with a midline trachea. She has no jugular venous distension.
- *Cardiovascular:* regular rate, rhythm and tachycardic without murmurs, gallops or rubs.
- *Lungs:* clear equal breath sounds throughout without any rales, wheezes, or rhonchi. No accessory muscle use.
- *Extremities and skin:* trace bilateral edema, no clubbing. Both legs appear slightly swollen although there is no frank edema and no calf tenderness.
- *Pertinent labs:* pregnancy test is negative, WBC 10.2, HCT 38.2. The remainder of laboratory studies are normal or negative.

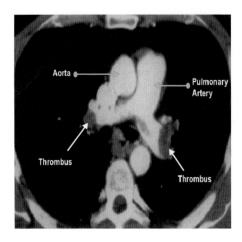

Figure 3.6. Chest CT angiogram showing two large clots in the main pulmonary arteries.

- *CXR:* normal chest.
- *EKG:* sinus tachycardia with right heart strain (S1-Q3- T3 configuration).
- *CT angiogram:* see Figure 3.6.

Questions for thought

- What are the standard diagnostic tests used in most patients with chest pain?
- What are other diagnostic tools you can use to make a diagnosis?
- How does one treat this condition in the emergency department?
- Why is this patient short of breath?

Diagnosis

Acute pulmonary embolism.

Discussion

- *Epidemiology:* pulmonary embolus (PE) is a relatively common phenomenon and should always be considered in the differential in any patient presenting with chest or back pain, or shortness of breath. Most patients who present with PEs have predisposing factors that promote clot formation or a hypercoagulable state. Key underlying risk factors include pregnancy, oral contraceptive use, protein C or S deficiency, Factor V Leiden, smoking, prolonged bed rest or travel, recent surgery, and trauma.
- *Pathophysiology:* patients with PE have a clot in their pulmonary blood vessels that limits perfusion of the lungs. The clot has formed elsewhere (commonly the leg as a deep vein thrombosis or DVT) and has traveled to the lungs via the blood stream.
- *Presentation:* this presentation is typical for PE from any cause. Most patients will present with relatively sudden onset of symptoms, which may include chest or back pain and shortness of breath. Severity of symptoms is based on total size of the embolus and

location of the vessel in which it is lodged. If the PE is small, it may not compromise respiratory function to a significant degree and the patient may not exhibit any hypoxia or tachycardia. Therefore, it may go undiagnosed. This presents a problem in that this small PE is not itself harmful, but the next one (from the initial source) could be life-threatening or lethal. If the PE is large and obstructs major pulmonary vessels, the patient will present with significant hypoxia and sometimes hypotension.

- Clinicians must assign a pretest probability to help determine how likely it is that the patient has had a PE. For instance, if the patient has many risk factors and/or has signs such as pleuritic chest pain associated with hypoxia, then the pretest probability would be high. Otherwise-healthy patients without any risk factors who present with less clear symptoms and no signs have a low pretest probability.

- *Diagnosis:* if the diagnosis of pulmonary embolus is in question, the most definitive study to obtain is a CT angiogram of the chest. This study is both sensitive and specific, and shows the size and location of the clot. The down side is that there is both a dye and a radiation load to the patient. In addition, small peripheral clots can be missed. Nonetheless, CT angiogram has replaced others as the test of choice when evaluating a patient for a PE.

- There are a number of other testing modalities available as well. Ventilation-perfusion scans have been performed for years, and can be helpful in select patients. This modality is particularly helpful in patients without any underlying lung disease in whom the pretest probability is very low. It is helpful if the read is "negative" or "high probability," but a reading of low probability does not clear the patient from the concern for PE. In some institutions, D-dimer assays are utilized to help place the patient into a risk category. Each institution should evaluate their own assays to determine whether they are the correct type to use in this setting. Only the enzyme-linked immunosorbent assay (ELISA) D-dimer test can be used to help differentiate patients when pulmonary embolus is suspected. Echocardiogram can also be useful, but is not often readily available for routine cases. While the EKG may be normal, a tracing showing right-sided heart strain should be considered a strong clue to the presence of a PE.

- *Treatment:* initial treatment of the patient with pulmonary embolus is oxygen and fluid resuscitation. Increasing the patient's preload or venous pressure helps to temporarily overcome the increased intrathoracic pressure, improving perfusion and oxygenation. The patient should be anticoagulated with heparin. If the patient is very unstable and does not improve with fluids, urgent thrombolysis may be indicated.

- *Definitive therapy:* since pulmonary emboli come from clots elsewhere in the body, efforts are made to determine the source of the clot and the presence of any underlying disease process or hypercoagulable state. Patients are typically anticoagulated for a minimum of 6 months, started on a form of heparin then switched to Coumadin for long-term therapy.

Clinical course

The keys to this patient's diagnosis are careful attention to her history, physical exam, and ancillary studies.

This woman was recognized to have likely pulmonary embolus and was started on anticoagulants prior to confirmatory CT. Her pretest probability of PE was high, therefore therapy

Historical clues	Physical findings	Ancillary studies
• Recent pregnancy	• Tachycardia	• EKG with an S1Q3T3
• Dyspnea	• Hypoxia	• Chest X-ray normal
• Pleuritic chest pain	• Lower extremity edema	• Chest CT demonstrates PE
• Rapid onset of pain		
• Smoking		
• Oral contraceptive use		

was warranted. An IV was placed, oxygen administered, and she was placed on a monitor. When her blood pressure dropped after morphine in the CT scanner, she was given a liter of normal saline as a bolus. The patient's blood pressure and dyspnea improved with fluid resuscitation. The CT confirmed that she did indeed have a pulmonary embolus, and she was continued on her anticoagulation and admitted to the hospital.

Further reading

Kline JA. Chapter 56. Pulmonary embolism. In Tintinalli JE, Kelen GD, Stapczynski JS, et al., eds., *Tintinalli's Emergency Medicine: A Comprehensive Study Guide*, 6th edition. New York: McGraw-Hill, 2004.

Fengler BT, Brady WJ. Fibrinolytic therapy in pulmonary embolism: an evidence-based treatment algorithm. *Am J Emerg Med* 2009;**27**:84–95.

Shakoor H, Santacruz JF, Dweik RA. Venous thrombo-embolic disease. *Compr Ther* 2009;**35**:24–36.

Case #8

History

A 28-year-old female complains of chest pain, which has slowly been worsening over the last 3 days. She describes it as a constant ache that is located under her right breast and gets much worse if she coughs or takes a deep breath. She doesn't feel frankly short of breath, but states she feels like she is unable to take a full breath secondary to pain. She states she had the "flu" about a $1\frac{1}{2}$ weeks ago, with a productive cough and fever that lasted several days. She did not seek medical attention and her symptoms have improved greatly with supportive care. She denies radiation of the pain, paresthesias, palpitations, headache, dizziness, or leg or back pain. She has been eating and drinking normally, denies nausea or vomiting and has had no history of trauma or strain.

Past medical history

She is healthy. She drinks a glass or two of wine weekly, and denies tobacco or illicit drug use.

Family history

Parents are both alive and well. Her father has hypertension.

Medications

She has tried acetaminophen, and had been using an over-the-counter cough and cold medicine daily until several days ago. She takes a daily multivitamin.

Allergies

There are no known allergies.

Physical exam and ancillary studies

- *Vital signs:* temperature 36.8°C, heart rate 92 bpm, respiratory rate 20, blood pressure 116/72, pulse oximetry 99% on room air.
- *General:* she is alert, pleasant and well-dressed. She is tall and thin and appears somewhat uncomfortable sitting in the chair, but she is not in any distress.
- *HEENT:* unremarkable.
- *Chest:* there are no retractions or palpable crepitus; expansion is equal bilaterally. There is marked tenderness of the costo-sternal junction along the right side at approximately ribs 5–7. The tenderness extends to just under her right breast. There is no overlying edema, erythema, or warmth. There is no palpable step off or depression of the ribs. She states that palpation reproduces the pain she feels with inspiration.
- *Heart:* regular rate and rhythm with no murmurs or rubs audible.

- *Lungs:* clear bilaterally, although her breaths are somewhat shallow and with diffusely decreased breath sounds.
- *Abdomen:* flat with normal bowel sounds; there is no guarding, tenderness, or masses. There is no Murphy's sign or organomegaly palpable. There is no costovertebral angle (CVA) tenderness.
- *Back/extremities:* there is no tenderness of her spine or paravertebral muscles. She ambulates normally. There is full range of motion in all four extremities; there is no edema, clubbing, or cyanosis noted. There are no cords or calf tenderness. Pulses are strong and regular bilaterally. She does note some pain in her right chest wall with strength testing of her right arm, in particular when using her pectoral muscles on that side.
- *Skin:* warm and dry. There is no rash noted. There are no petechiae, ecchymoses, or bruising noted.
- *CXR:* no acute process, specifically, no visible rib fracture or pneumothorax.

Questions for thought

- What are the potentially life-threatening causes of chest pain in this patient?
- How can they be quickly and efficiently ruled out?
- How is this patient's pain best treated in the ED? At home?
- Are additional studies necessary?

Diagnosis

Costochondritis.

Discussion

- *Introduction:* chest pain is one of the most common symptoms that patients will seek medical attention for in the outpatient setting. While the initial evaluation may focus on potentially life-threatening cardiac and pulmonary causes, conditions affecting the musculoskeletal structures of the chest wall are the most common category of non-cardiac chest pain presenting to the emergency department. The initial evaluation of the patient with chest pain should consider the context of age, sex, family history, cardiopulmonary risk factors, and the patient's general health. Middle-aged or elderly patients or those with comorbid conditions and/or other risk factors will require more ancillary studies to rule out more serious conditions.
- *Presentation:* musculoskeletal chest pain is often insidious and persistent. It may last for days. It is frequently sharp and localizes to a specific area of the chest wall. It is usually positional and can be exacerbated with deep breathing or certain arm movements. There is often a history of repetitive or unusual physical activity involving the upper trunk or arms. Patients may report a recent history of respiratory illness or describe feeling "short of breath" because of the pain involved with inspiration. Restriction of breathing due to pain with breathing (inspiration) must be distinguished from true dyspnea.
- *Differential diagnosis:* the differential for patients with chest pain is large. Many conditions are obviously life-threatening and need to be immediately addressed. In this particular

patient, with young age and no comorbid conditions or risk factors, a cardiac condition is extremely unlikely. As she had a recent history of a febrile respiratory illness, pneumonia is still a possibility. Also her tall and thin stature makes spontaneous pneumothorax a consideration as well. A pleuritic source of pain in this patient is also possible given the nature of the pain such as in this case. A chest film was adequate to rule out these more serious diagnoses. Pulmonary embolism is almost definitely not the cause of her pain as she lacks any risk factors and has good room air oxygen saturation. Thoracic aortic aneurysm is also extremely unlikely since she lacks any of the usual risk factors and it would be effectively ruled out with a negative chest X-ray. Other causes of chest pain such as gastroesophageal reflux disease (GERD) or other musculoskeletal causes should be sought with clues from the history and physical. At age 28, coronary artery disease is extremely unlikely, especially with pleuritic chest pain that has been constant for 3 days.

- *Diagnosis:* costochondritis is associated with palpable tenderness of the chest wall that can occur anywhere over the chest wall at any of the costochondral joints. Patients will often say it reproduces their pain exactly. This finding has been noted in myocardial infarction as well and therefore a diagnosis of costochondritis or musculoskeletal chest pain should not be made until other causes have been thoughtfully excluded. In this case, a chest film was the only ancillary study needed. However, in older patients, or those with other comorbidities, EKG, chest CT, and lab work, including cardiac enzymes, brain natriuretic peptide (BNP) or D-dimer, may be necessary.

- *Treatment:* therapeutic interventions for musculoskeletal pain in the chest are generally the same as those for musculoskeletal pain elsewhere in the body. Patient education is an important component of care as chest pain is associated with a level of anxiety regarding its etiology. Patients need reassurance that their pain is real, but benign in nature. If there is an exertional or over-use component of the pain, patients need to be instructed to stop the offending behavior at least temporarily. Nonsteroidal anti-inflammatory drugs (NSAIDs) are generally considered the standard treatment and should be given in the ED. Patients can then be discharged on ibuprofen or an equivalent medication. Muscle relaxants may occasionally be helpful and narcotics should be used in patients for whom NSAIDs are contraindicated (peptic ulcer disease, GI bleed, or renal insufficiency) or have not provided adequate relief.

Clinical course

The keys to this patient's diagnosis are careful attention to her history and examination. Ancillary studies support the diagnosis by excluding other etiologies.

Historical clues	Physical findings	Ancillary studies
• Increasing pain with cough and deep breath	• Normal vital signs	• Chest X-ray normal
• Recent respiratory illness with coughing	• Tenderness of chest wall at the costochondral-sternal junction exactly duplicate the pain	• EKG normal
• Constant pain for 3 days	• Normal heart and lungs	

Given her reproducible pain and otherwise benign exam, the diagnosis of costochondritis was made relatively easily in this patient. A negative chest X-ray confirmed the diagnosis.

She was treated in the ED with oral ibuprofen. This adequately relieved her pain and she was discharged with instructions to continue taking 600 mg of ibuprofen every 6–8 hours. In this particular case, there were no strain or overuse issues that needed to be addressed. The cause was probably coughing during her recent URI. She was instructed to follow up with her primary doctor in 7–10 days.

Case #9

History

A 34-year-old HIV-positive male presents to the ED complaining of fever, odynophagia, substernal burning chest pain, and nausea for 1 day. His chest pain does not radiate, is 10/10 in severity, worsened with food intake, and constant. He has not been compliant with Highly Active Anti-Retroviral Therapy (HAART) medications in the past year and has not recently started any new medications. His last CD4 count, 1 year ago, was 100 cells/mm^3. He denies recent travel, sick contacts, vomiting, diarrhea, bloody stools, dysuria, hematuria, cough, and weight loss.

Past medical history

HIV-positive, hepatitis C, tobacco dependence (30 pack-year history).

Medication

None.

Allergies

No known allergies.

Physical exam and ancillary studies

- *Vital signs:* temperature 38.4°C, heart rate 90 bpm, blood pressure 112/78, respiratory rate 14, room air saturation 97%.
- *General:* awake and alert, appears to be in pain.
- *Head and neck:* pupils are equally round and reactive to light, no scleral icterus or injection, tympanic membranes clear bilaterally, oral mucosa dry with no intraoral lesions noted, oropharynx benign with no exudates or erythema, no cervical lymphadenopathy, no JVD, neck is supple, trachea is midline.
- *Cardiovascular:* regular rate and rhythm, no murmurs, rubs, or gallops. Good peripheral pulses.
- *Respiratory:* lungs clear to auscultation bilaterally.
- *Extremities:* no clubbing, cyanosis, edema, or asterixis. No calf tenderness.
- *Skin:* warm and well-perfused, no lesions or rashes.
- *Pertinent abnormal labs:* WBC 11 000, HCT 40%, BUN 20, Cr 1.4; otherwise chemistries including cardiac enzymes are negative, blood cultures pending.
- *EKG:* rate 88, normal sinus rhythm.
- *Upper endoscopy:* multiple well-circumscribed "volcano"-like lesions in the mid-esophagus, biopsy revealed multinucleated giant cells with ground-glass nuclei and eosinophilic inclusions (Cowdry type A inclusion bodies).

Questions for thought

- What are other causes of esophagitis?
- What other tests/procedures can be done to obtain a diagnosis?
- What are the possible complications of herpetic esophagitis?

Diagnosis

Herpes simplex virus (HSV) type 1 esophagitis.

Discussion

- *Epidemiology:* when the CD4 cell count is less than 100/mm^3, HIV-positive patients are at a much higher risk of HSV esophagitis. In addition to HSV, when an HIV-positive patient presents with odynophagia or dysphagia, other infectious etiologies must also be considered, most notably CMV, candida, and fungal and mycobacterium tuberculosis esophagitis. Other causes of esophagitis include gastroesophageal reflux disease, medications (doxycycline, aspirin (ASA), ibuprofen, potassium, Fosamax), esophageal adenocarcinoma, food impaction from Schatzki's ring, and foreign body.
- *Pathophysiology:* in the earliest stage, vesicles form on the squamous mucosa. Well-circumscribed ulcers form as the vesicles coalesce. Irritation of the mucosa causes the symptoms of odynophagia, dysphagia, and substernal chest pain.
- *Presentation:* the most common presenting symptom is odynophagia. Nausea, vomiting, fever, hematemesis, and dyspepsia are less common symptoms. Nineteen to 38% of patients have oral, labial, or cutaneous HSV as well.
- *Diagnosis:* the most effective way to diagnose HSV-1 esophagitis is by upper endoscopy to visualize the mucosa and obtain biopsies. The lesions appear endoscopically as multiple, small (less than 1.5 cm), superficial ulcers with raised margins creating the "volcano"-like appearance and are typically located in the mid to distal third of the esophagus. The esophagitis may be diffuse and erosive. Histology reveals multinucleated giant cells and intranuclear Cowdrey type A inclusion bodies, but cytoplasmic inclusions are usually absent. Barium swallow may show aphthous ulcers, which are difficult to differentiate from other types of ulcers. Viral culture is more sensitive than histology.
- *Treatment:* for patients able to take oral medications, acyclovir 400 mg five times a day for 14–21 days is recommended. For patients unable to tolerate oral medications, intravenous acyclovir 5 mg/kg is given every 8 hours for 7–14 days and they may also need parenteral nutrition during their treatment.
- *Definitive therapy:* compliance with HAART therapy to keep CD4 counts above 100/mm^3 has been shown to decrease HSV-1 esophagitis. Primary prophylaxis to prevent HSV disease is not currently recommended.
- *Complications:* these include hemorrhage, esophageal perforation, tracheoesophageal fistula, and visceral dissemination.

Clinical course

The keys to this patient's diagnosis are careful attention to his history, physical and ancillary studies.

Historical clues	Physical findings	Ancillary studies
• Pain on swallowing (odynophagia)	• Pain	• Ulcerations seen on esophageal endoscopy
• Chest pain	• Fever	
• Fever		
• Presence of HIV with low CD-4 count		

The patient was admitted for IV acyclovir due to his inability to tolerate adequate oral intake. After 5 days of therapy he was able to tolerate adequate oral intake and his therapy was changed to PO acyclovir at that time. He was also restarted on his HAART therapy.

Further reading

Zaidi SA, Cervia JS. Diagnosis and management of infectious esophagitis associated with human immunodeficiency virus infection. *J Int Assoc Physicians AIDS Care* 2002;**1**:40–56.

Case #10

History

A 35-year-old Hispanic male patient presented to emergency department for evaluation of chest pain that he described as retrosternal pressure, radiating to his left arm. He described his symptoms as constant for the past 3 days. Other associated symptoms include shortness of breath. No aggravating or alleviating factors. He denies exertional angina, palpitations, paroxysmal nocturnal dyspnea (PND), or orthopnea. The patient denies any prior history of similar symptoms but reported that he has been generally sick for the last 7 days with symptoms suggestive of upper respiratory tract infection (runny nose, fever, chills, cough, sore throat, skin rash on the face), and generalized muscular weakness that is most pronounced in his lower extremities. He was recently diagnosed with presumptive polymyositis or dermatomyositis and received treatment with methotrexate, prednisone, and folic acid without significant improvement in his symptoms. He denies palpitations, lightheadedness, dizziness, diaphoresis, nausea, vomiting, dark urine, or hematuria.

Past medical history

Osteoarthritis.

Medications

Methotrexate, folic acid and prednisone.

Allergies

The patient has no known drug allergies.

Social history

Married. The patient denies smoking, alcohol or recreational drug use.

Family History

No history of premature coronary artery disease.

Physical exam and ancillary studies

- *Vital signs:* temperature 36.8°C, respiratory rate 14, blood pressure 138/96, pulse 115 bpm.
- *General:* active, alert and oriented. He was in no acute distress. Able to speak in full sentences.
- *Head and neck:* periorbital hyperpigmented erythema. No carotid bruits, no jugular venous distention.
- *Heart:* regular rate and rhythm. Tachycardic. Normal S1 and S2. No murmurs, gallops, or rubs.

- *Chest:* no evidence of trauma, no reproducible chest pain.
- *Lungs:* clear to auscultation, no rales, rhonchi, or wheezes.
- *Abdomen:* obese. Not tender or distended. No bruits.
- *Extremities:* significant muscle weakness in proximal and distal upper and lower extremities. No edema.
- *Pertinent labs:* Complete blood count (CBC) is within normal limits. Complete metabolic profile is normal except AST 382, ALT 260, Tbil 1.0, ALK-P 61. Cardiac enzymes: CPK 10 525, CK-MB 1390, %MB 13.2 and troponin 0.46.
- *EKG:* Sinus tachycardia at 111 with early repolarization pattern and left axis deviation.
- *Radiographs:* no abnormalities.
- *2D echocardiogram:* normal LV systolic function with an EF > 55%.

Questions for thought

- What are the non-ischemic causes of chest pain?
- Can the emergency physician reliably diagnose non-ischemic causes of chest pain?
- What systemic illness can directly affect the myocardium?

Diagnosis

Myocarditis.

Discussion

- *Epidemiology:* although several non-infectious causes are known, the majority of cases of myocarditis are considered to be of infectious origin. There is solid evidence to suggest that the microbial pathogenesis may be complex. Viral infection of the heart is relatively common, most often from enteroviruses.
- *Pathophysiology:* myocarditis is an inflammatory disease of the cardiac muscle that is caused by intramyocardial infiltration of immunocompetent cells and direct viral cytotoxic effect on myocardial tissue. Etiologically, the relevant factors are the direct or indirect influence of infectious pathogens, toxic, chemical, or physical agents, allergic-hyperallergic reactions and myocardial inflammatory events in the context of systemic diseases.
- *Presentation:* inflammatory cardiomyopathy may have a variety of clinical presentations, including (a) acute onset of symptoms mimicking those of myocardial infarction; (b) cardiac insufficiency of acute or insidious onset that may develop into dilated cardiomyopathy; and (c) sudden unexpected cardiac death. The severity of symptoms is highly variable and subclinical myocarditis is common. Rarely viral-induced myocarditis develops over a few days and leads to life-threatening arrhythmias or rapid progression of myocardial dysfunction. The majority of patients have a clinically inapparent course with minimal cardiovascular symptoms. Frequently, only transient EKG changes or minimal echocardiographic signs of ventricular wall motion dysfunction are present. Pathologic findings may recede completely in a few days or weeks. Wall motion abnormalities or clinical complaints such as fatigue, angina, dyspnea, or arrhythmias persisting over a period of several

weeks or months without improvement suggest a chronic inflammatory process or a persistent viral infection. Tachypnea and tachycardia are the most common signs. A chronic cough is suggestive of pulmonary venous congestion. Neck vein distension may be prominent, together with hepatomegaly secondary to elevated systemic venous pressure, and the symptoms and signs are not distinguishable from those of dilated cardiomyopathy.

- *Diagnosis:* blood tests that should be done are: erythrocyte sedimentation rate (ESR), CBC, C-reactive protein (CRP), and cardiac enzymes. An EKG should be done and may show nonspecific findings, sinus tachycardia, diffuse ST-T wave abnormalities, prolonged QT interval, bundle branch block (left bundle branch block (LBBB) found in 20%), myocardial infarction pattern, complete heart block, supraventricular tachyarrhythmias, or ventricular tachyarrhythmias.
- *Definitive diagnosis:* diagnosis requires endomyocardial biopsy (EMB). The 1987 Dallas criteria require: lymphocytic infiltration associated with myocyte injury in the absence of ischemia. This finding is highly specific but only 10% to 22% sensitive. The lack of precision of the Dallas criteria arise from sampling error and high interobserver variability in interpretation.
- *Non-invasive evaluation:* this includes 2D echocardiogram and gallium-67 scan. Cardiac magnetic resonance (CMR) imaging is currently the most accurate diagnostic method for both guiding biopsy and following up disease activity over time. CMR is likely to become the standard diagnostic test in suspected myocarditis.
- *Treatment:* the treatment of the patient with myocarditis is supportive. If rhabdomyolysis is present, aggressive fluid hydration should be initiated. While small studies suggest a role for immunosuppressants, there is no evidence to support routine use of immunosuppressive agents in acute myocarditis. Immunoglobulin may be useful. The rest of the treatment depends on the presentation. If the patient presents with heart failure due to cardiomyopathy, the treatment of heart failure should follow conventional lines.

Clinical course

It is very important to recognize that chest pain syndrome doesn't always mean acute coronary syndrome. History, physical findings, and laboratory report play a significant role in appropriate diagnosis and management of patients with this presentation. This patient is unlikely to have myocardial ischemia or infarction since he is young and has had continuous chest pain for 3 days without any ischemic changes on his EKG.

Historical clues	Physical findings	Ancillary studies
• Prior viral upper respiratory infection	• Tachycardia	• EKG
• Chest pain	• Signs of heart failure	• Elevated CPK and troponin
• Shortness of breath		• 2D echocardiogram

This patient underwent left heart catheterization, revealing normal coronary arteries. He received supportive treatment with normal saline for adequate hydration and a small dose of beta-blockers to control his persistent sinus tachycardia, in an attempt to prevent tachycardia-mediated cardiomyopathy. He was subsequently evaluated by the rheumatology department and they recommended high-dose steroids and muscle biopsy for further evaluation of his myopathy. After being on high-dose steroid therapy the patient's symptoms started to improve.

Further reading

Mann DL. Determinants of myocardial recovery in myocarditis: has the time come for molecular fingerprinting? *J Am Coll Cardiol* 2005;**46**;1043–4.

Sarda L, Colin P, Boccara F, et al. Myocarditis in patients with clinical presentation of myocardial infarction and normal coronary angiograms. *J Am Coll Cardiol* 2001;**37**;786–92.

Skouri HN, Dec GW, Friedrich MG, et al. Noninvasive imaging in myocarditis. *J Am Coll Cardiol* 2006;**48**;2085–93.

McNamara DM, Rosenblum WD, Janosko KM, et al. Intravenous immune globulin in the therapy of myocarditis and acute cardiomyopathy. *Circulation* 1997;**95**:2476–8.

Mahrholdt H, Wagner A, Deluigi CC, et al. Presentation, patterns of myocardial damage, and clinical course of viral myocarditis. *Circulation* 2006;**114**:1581–90.

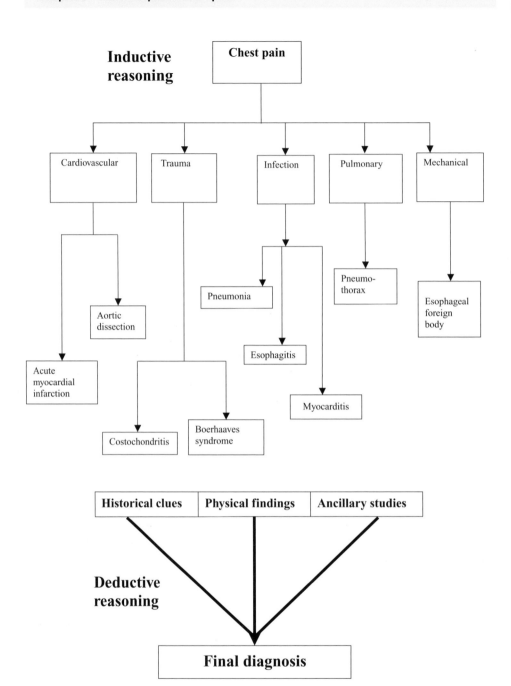

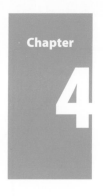

Chief complaint: shortness of breath

Shellie Asher, Wendy DeMartino, Donald Jeanmonod, Rebecca Jeanmonod, Kevin Jones, Mikhail Kirnus, Chad S. Lewis, Mara McErlean

Case #1

History

A 63-year-old woman presents to the ED complaining of severe shortness of breath which has become progressively worse over the past several days. Her dyspnea is much worse with exertion, but not when she lies down. She states she is "breathing like a fish," and that she is "retaining water in my stomach and legs." She has gained several pounds over the last week. The patient denies chest pain, nausea, vomiting, diaphoresis, or fever. She states she has a dry cough. She called her primary care physician 3 days ago because of her symptoms, and he increased her furosemide dose over the phone. However, since that time, the patient feels like she has become worse.

Past medical history

The patient had a pacemaker placed 10 days ago for "problems with my heart." She has a history of congestive heart failure, chronic obstructive pulmonary disease, a massive heart attack 15 years ago, hypertension, hypercholesterolemia, frequent pneumonias, and hypothyroidism. The patient quit smoking 15 years ago, and has a 40 pack-year history.

Medications

The patient's medications include atenolol, losartan potassium, furosemide, aspirin, lovastatin, levothyroxine, Albuterol, and estrogen replacement.

Allergies

The patient has no known drug allergies.

Case Studies in Emergency Medicine, ed. R. Jeanmonod, M. Tomassi and D. Mayer.
Published by Cambridge University Press © Cambridge University Press 2010.

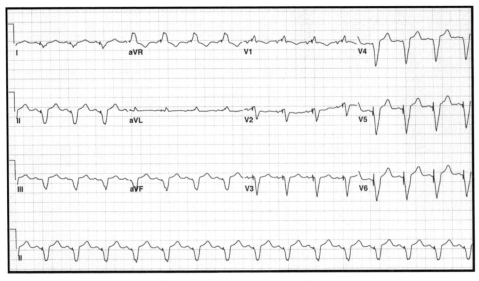

Figure 4.1. This EKG shows sinus tachycardia with a ventricular pacemaker.

Physical exam and ancillary studies

- *Vital signs:* the patient's temperature is 36.2°C, her heart rate is 120 bpm, her blood pressure is 108/51 mmHg, her respiratory rate is 24, and her room air oxygen saturation is 94%.
- *General:* she is awake and alert, somewhat pale, and speaking in three-word sentences.
- *Head and neck:* the patient's pupils are equally round and reactive to light, and her cranial nerves are intact. The patient's mucous membranes are dry. Her neck is supple with a midline trachea. She has jugular venous distension.
- *Cardiovascular:* the patient's heart is regularly tachycardic without rubs. Her peripheral pulses are decreased throughout.
- *Lungs:* her lungs are decreased throughout, with bibasilar rales and scattered wheezes.
- *Extremities and skin:* the patient has trace bilateral edema, with no clubbing or calf tenderness. She has poor capillary refill throughout with pale skin.
- *Pertinent labs:* the patient's complete blood count reveals a white blood cell count of 12.8 and a hematocrit of 28.6% (it had been 39% one month prior to this ED visit). The remainder of her chemistries including cardiac enzymes are normal or negative.
- *EKG:* see Figure 4.1.
- *Radiographs:* the patient's chest X-ray is shown in Figure 4.2.

Questions for thought

- What are the appropriate initial actions to take to stabilize this patient?
- Once stable, what are other diagnostic tools you can use to make a diagnosis?
- What medications should be avoided in this patient?

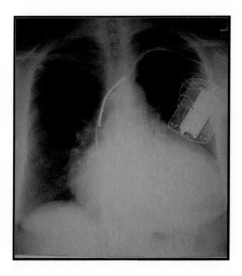

Figure 4.2. Chest X-ray showing clear lung fields. The patient has an enlarged cardiac silhouette (water-bottle heart) on PA study, and the lateral shows a displaced epicardial fat pad (lucency just anterior to the tip of the pacer) consistent with pericardial effusion.

- How does one urgently treat this condition in the emer~
- What is definitive treatment of this condition?
- Why is this patient short of breath?

missed Tamponade
list emergency heart
causes by heart

Diagnosis

Cardiac tamponade as a complication of pacemaker placement.

Discussion

- *Epidemiology:* tamponade is a rare but fatal cause of dyspnea. The most common cause of tamponade in the United States is malignancy, but trauma and infectious and iatrogenic causes are also frequently seen. In endemic areas, tuberculosis is a common cause.
- *Pathophysiology:* patients with cardiac tamponade have fluid (blood, exudative, or trans-udative fluid) in their pericardial sacs which compromises the pump function of their hearts. As tamponade progresses, the pressure from the pericardial fluid inhibits the heart's ability to fill and decreases venous return from the systemic circulation. This leads to overall decreased perfusion secondary to decreased stroke volume and eventual shock.
- *Presentation:* this presentation is typical for tamponade from any cause. Rapidity and severity of symptoms are based on total volume of pericardial fluid and rate of accumu-lation over time. Patients typically present with shortness of breath or weakness because they are not perfusing; their problem is not one of oxygenation, as their lungs are func-tioning normally, but one of not getting oxygen to where it is needed. Many patients will have one or two of the findings of Beck's triad (hypotension, distant heart sounds, and jugular venous distension), but most will not have all three elements. This patient had hypotension and JVD, and was clearly hypoperfused.
- *Treatment:* initial treatment of the patient with cardiac tamponade is fluid resuscita-tion. Increasing the patient's preload or venous pressure helps to temporarily overcome

[handwritten note: furo makes it worse !! clue]

the _____ pericardial effusion, improving perfusion and oxygenation. Conversely, medications that decrease preload, such as furosemide, narcotics, and nitroglycerin, should be avoided. If the patient is very unstable and does not improve with fluids, urgent bedside pericardiocentesis should be performed. Even removal of a small amount of pericardial fluid can cause dramatic improvement in a patient's hemodynamic status, and this can be done either as a blind procedure or under ultrasound guidance. Even without a definitive echocardiographic diagnosis, if tamponade is suspected, treatment should be initiated, as it may be life-saving.

- *Definitive therapy:* since many of the underlying causes of pericardial effusion are persistent and patients run the risk of re-accumulating fluid, definitive therapy usually involves placement of a catheter for ongoing pericardial fluid drainage under ultrasound or CT guidance. Another common definitive treatment is surgical windowing of the pericardial sac to allow for continued drainage.

Clinical course

The keys to this patient's diagnosis are careful attention to her history, physical exam, and ancillary studies.

Historical clues	Physical findings	Ancillary studies
• Recent pacemaker placement	• Tachycardia	• Falling hematocrit after a minor procedure
• Dyspnea on exertion	• Hypotension	• Chest X-ray with water-bottle heart and clear lung fields
• Peripheral edema and weight gain	• Jugular venous distension	• Lateral CXR with lucency anterior to pacemaker lead, diagnostic of effusion
• Worsening symptoms with treatment with diuretics	• Pallor	
	• Poor peripheral perfusion	
	• Lower extremity edema	

[handwritten note: ↓ Ht. clue → blood loss happening somewhere]

This woman was recognized to have likely cardiac tamponade based on her presentation and chest X-ray. Therefore, after IV placement, oxygen administration, and placement on a monitor, the patient was given a liter of normal saline as a bolus. The patient's blood pressure and dyspnea improved with fluid resuscitation. An urgent bedside echocardiogram was performed, which is the diagnostic study of choice in tamponade. Although CT can delineate the size of a pericardial effusion, a patient can have a large effusion without tamponade. Tamponade is defined by physiologic compromise of pump function, and this is manifested by collapse of the right ventricle during diastole, which can be seen on bedside echo. The patient then underwent CT guided placement of a drainage catheter in her pericardial sac. Seven hundred milliliters of blood were removed, and the patient had a full recovery.

Case #2

History

A 59-year-old gentleman presents to the emergency department complaining of difficulty breathing. The patient states that he has been progressively short of breath with exertion for the last several months. His dyspnea improves with rest. The patient also reports that he has been coughing up copious amounts of thick white sputum. He denies chest pain, orthopnea, or paroxysmal nocturnal dyspnea.

Past medical history

The patient has a past medical history of hypertension.

Medications

The patient takes atenolol daily.

Allergies

The patient has no known drug allergies.

Social history

The patient has smoked two packs of cigarettes per day for the last 45 years.

Physical exam and ancillary studies

- *Vital signs:* the patient has a temperature of 36.9°C, a heart rate of 96 bpm, a blood pressure of 165/92 mmHg, a respiratory rate of 18, and a room air oxygen saturation of 95%.
- *General:* the patient appears older than his stated age. He is in no acute respiratory distress.
- *Head and neck:* the patient's mucous membranes are moist. His sclerae are non-icteric. His neck is supple without jugular venous distension or carotid bruit.
- *Cardiovascular:* his heart has a regular rate and rhythm without murmur, rub, or gallop. The patient's distal pulses are normal in all four extremities.
- *Lungs:* the patient's chest wall is non-tender with equal expansion. He is somewhat barrel-chested. His lung sounds are symmetrical with scattered expiratory wheezes throughout. There are no rales or rhonchi. He is able to speak in full sentences at rest. With exertion, the patient becomes short of breath, is only able to speak in two- or three-word phrases, and his oxygen saturation decreases to 88%.
- *Abdomen:* his abdomen is soft and non-tender. There are no masses. There are normal active bowel sounds.
- *Extremities and skin:* the patient's extremities are warm and well perfused. He has no edema, with normal capillary refill.

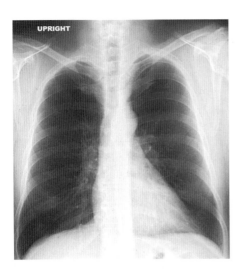

Figure 4.3. His chest X-ray demonstrates hyperinflation and flattened diaphragms.

- *Pertinent labs:* no labs are performed.
- *EKG:* his EKG reveals normal sinus rhythm with no ischemic changes, hypertrophy, or axis deviations.
- *Radiographs:* The patient's chest X-ray is shown in Figure 4.3.

Questions for thought

- What are the appropriate initial actions to take for this patient?
- What are other diagnostic tools you can use to make a diagnosis?
- How does one urgently treat this condition in the emergency department?
- What is the definitive treatment of this condition?
- What is the appropriate disposition for this patient?

Diagnosis

Dyspnea secondary to chronic obstructive pulmonary disease (COPD).

Discussion

- *Epidemiology:* COPD, which includes chronic bronchitis and emphysema, affects up to 32 million people in the United States, and is the fourth leading cause of death. Most cases are associated with smoking, but other etiologies include cystic fibrosis, alpha-1 antitrypsin deficiency, bronchiectasis, and bullous lung disease.
- *Pathophysiology:* three distinct diseases in combination result in clinical COPD. They are chronic bronchitis, emphysema, and asthma. The hallmark of chronic bronchitis is excessive mucous production which overwhelms the ciliary clearance mechanisms with concomitant airway obstruction. Emphysema is characterized by destruction of the small

airways and pulmonary capillary beds. In addition, many patients have some component of reactive airways contributing to deficiencies in oxygenation and ventilation.

- *Presentation:* most patients present with shortness of breath, especially with exertion. In patients with primary chronic bronchitis, predominant symptoms are productive cough, frequent pulmonary infections, and associated cardiac failure. Patients with predominant emphysema tend to present with a steady decline in pulmonary function, with cachexia and eventual respiratory failure. Physical examination varies depending on the underlying pathology, but is commonly characterized by wheezing on pulmonary exam and use of accessory muscles.
- *Treatment:* first-line therapies include oxygen, bronchodilators, and corticosteroids. Oxygen supplementation should be titrated to maintain oxygen saturations of at least 90%. Monitor mental status carefully, as hypercarbia and respiratory acidosis will lead to altered mentation and may require endotracheal intubation for adequate oxygenation and ventilation. Non-invasive ventilation may be attempted in the patient with an appropriate mental status and the ability to cooperate. Inhaled bronchodilators and anticholinergics in the acute setting may have a synergistic effect in dilating airways, improving mucous clearance, and reducing inflammation. Corticosteroids act to decrease inflammation and may be given orally, intravenously, or inhaled. Adjunctive therapies include helium-oxygen, methylxanthines, and magnesium.
- *Definitive therapy:* all patients should be strongly counseled to stop smoking, and resources to promote success should be provided. Patients who return to their previous baseline can be discharged with outpatient pulmonary follow-up. You should prescribe a short course of corticosteroids as well as short-term increases in dosing frequency of inhaled rescue medications. Maintenance medications include long-acting bronchodilators, anticholinergics and inhaled corticosteroids.

Clinical course

The keys to this patient's diagnosis are careful attention to history, physical exam, and ancillary studies.

Historical clues	Physical findings	Ancillary studies
• Smoking history	• Barrel chest	• Chest X-ray with mild hyperinflation and flattening of the diaphragm
• Productive cough	• Wheezing	• Workup negative for other etiologies of dyspnea
• Progressive dyspnea	• Hypoxia with exertion	

This patient was suspected of having an acute COPD exacerbation for a variety of reasons. He had a substantial smoking history, which is the most common cause of COPD. In addition, he was wheezing on exam. This typically reveals limitation of airflow during forced expiration due to decreased airway compliance or increased resistance secondary to mucous obstruction, and this is usually irreversible, even with bronchodilators. The degree of limited airflow on expiration can be measured using pulmonary function testing, which typically reveals a decrease in forced expiratory volume in 1 second (FEV1) and decreased FEV1 to forced vital capacity (FVC) ratio. These tests, however, are usually not performed in the ED. Finally, the patient's X-ray revealed hyperinflation with flattening of the diaphragms, which is common in COPD.

This gentleman was treated in the emergency department for chronic obstructive pulmonary disease with inhaled bronchodilators, ipratroprium, and oral steroids. His dyspnea with exertion improved dramatically. His lung exam cleared and his hypoxia with exertion resolved. He was counseled to stop smoking, and discharged to follow-up with his primary care physician. Discharge medications included inhaled bronchodilators, anticholinergics, and a short course of oral steroids. A referral was made for pulmonary function testing and pulmonary specialist follow-up.

Case #3

History

A 91-year-old female presents with obvious shortness of breath. According to the prehospital providers, the patient had been breathing rapidly since their initial contact. The patient has a recent history of frequent falls, with the initial fall being almost 1 month ago. Her family states that she had a cough and shortness of breath at that time. An evaluation by her primary care physician revealed a negative chest X-ray, and the patient was placed on antibiotics. She had a follow-up with her primary physician 10 days after the initial fall. Since that time, 2 weeks ago, she has continued to fall. Her daughter recently moved in with her due to the number of falls. The family does not believe she has passed out after any of these falls. She had been eating normally until today. She had some breakfast this morning and developed nausea that caused her to refrain from eating for the rest of the day. The patient was alert and active earlier today. This evening she was sewing, looked up at her daughter, had a blank look on her face, and started twitching her right hand. This lasted 5 to 6 minutes. Although awake, the patient was not responsive to questioning during this episode. This prompted her daughter to call EMS. At this time, the patient does not have any complaints. Her primary language is German. She does speak English well, as she has been in this country for 16 years; however, she is speaking and responding to primarily German this evening. She states she feels fine and could go home. She denies any pain. She has had no fever. She does have some nausea, but no vomiting.

During evaluation, the patient has two episodes of vomiting. She then complains of some abdominal pain. Her family recalls that she did complain of abdominal pain earlier in the day, but had not mentioned it since that time. She continues to be short of breath.

Past medical history

The patient has a history of breast cancer, diabetes, hypertension, atrial fibrillation, and cervical cancer. She has had a total mastectomy and a total hysterectomy.

Medications

The patient takes folic acid, atenolol, aspirin, vitamin B6, and diltiazem.

Allergies

She has no known drug allergies.

Physical exam and ancillary studies

- *Vital signs:* the patient's temperature is 36.1°C, her heart rate is 76 bpm, her respiratory rate is 26, her blood pressure is 78/42 mmHg, and her oxygen saturation is 96% on room air.

- *General:* she is awake and non-toxic in appearance. She is breathing fast, but does not appear to be in distress.
- *Head and neck:* the patient's head is normocephalic. She has two healing bruises beneath her eye from the initial fall 1 month ago. She has a large hematoma on the front portion of her right forehead as well as a hematoma over her chin. The patient's pupils are equal and minimally reactive to light. Her extraocular muscles are intact. Her conjunctivae are pale. She has dry oral mucosa. Her neck is non-tender and supple with full range of motion. Her trachea is midline. There is no evidence of hemotympanum.
- *Cardiovascular:* the patient's heart has a regular rate and rhythm, with no murmurs, rubs, or gallops.
- *Lungs:* the patient has coarse breath sounds with faint crackles throughout. She has decreased breath sounds in her left lower lobe.
- *Abdomen:* the patient is initially examined at 17:00. Her abdomen is soft, non-tender, and non-distended. She has normoactive bowel sounds. There are no masses or abdominal wall bruising. On repeat examination at 21:30, the patient has minimal upper abdominal tenderness with some guarding.
- *Extremities and skin:* she is able to move her arms and legs, and has no extremity tenderness. She has swelling in her lower extremities, the left greater than the right. Her skin is cool and her face is slightly diaphoretic.
- *Neurologic:* she is awake and alert. Her cranial nerves are intact. She intermittently has some twitching-like activity of her upper extremities, which lasts 1 to 2 minutes. She has 5/5 distal strength and 4/5 proximal strength. Her gait is not assessed at this time. Her sensation is intact.
- *Pertinent labs:* the patient's initial labs are drawn at 17:20. They are remarkable for a hematocrit of 37%, an INR of 1.1, a potassium of 5.2, a bicarbonate of 27, a blood urea nitrogen of 30, and a creatinine of 1.5. Her venous blood gas shows a pH of 7.27, a pCO_2 of 54, a pO_2 of 16, and a bicarbonate of 24. All her other labs are normal. At 19:50, the patient has a lactic acid level drawn, which is 2.2. At 21:45, the patient has repeat blood work drawn, which shows a hematocrit of 26%. She has an arterial blood gas drawn, which shows a pH of 7.17, a pCO_2 of 50, a pO_2 of 137, a bicarbonate of 18, and an oxygen saturation of 98%.
- *Radiographs:* the patient's chest X-ray shows minimal atelectasis in her left lung base, but otherwise no abnormalities. Her head CT shows mild soft tissue swelling involving the right frontal scalp. The brain parenchyma is normal. A representative cut of the patient's abdominal CT is shown in Figure 4.4.

Questions for thought

- What are the appropriate initial actions to take to stabilize this patient?
- What is the differential diagnosis for this patient?
- What are other diagnostic tools you can use to make a diagnosis?
- What is the definitive treatment of this condition?

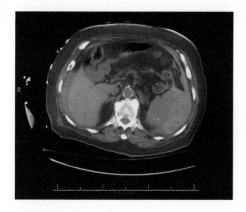

Figure 4.4. This CT shows massive left intraperitoneal hematoma, probably originating from the shattered spleen. There is a prominent subcapsular perihepatic hematoma.

Diagnosis

Dyspnea from hemorrhagic shock secondary to ruptured spleen.

Discussion

- *Epidemiology:* although difficult to quantify, it is estimated that 25% of hospital trauma admissions involve blunt splenic injury. The spleen is the most commonly injured organ in blunt abdominal trauma, and geriatric patients with splenic injury have a higher mortality and require more resources than younger patients.
- *Pathophysiology:* three mechanisms of splenic injury include: blunt, penetrating, and explosive injuries. Of these, blunt injuries are the most common. The spleen is normally protected by the ribcage. However, there are many diseases that lead to enlargement of the spleen and increase the likelihood of injury. With injury to the spleen shock is likely. Hemorrhagic shock can result in dyspnea by causing decreased tissue oxygenation secondary to decreased oxygen carrying capacity. It is important to remember that anything that decreases perfusion, be it lung disease, inability to bind oxygen (such as with carbon monoxide poisoning), low hematocrit, or poor cardiac pump function, can result in dyspnea.
- *Presentation:* patients with splenic injury can present with abdominal pain or left shoulder pain. Shoulder pain, known as Kehr sign, is referred pain from the irritation of the subdiaphragmatic nerve root. Diffuse abdominal pain and peritoneal irritation are likely with free intraperitoneal blood. If intraabdominal bleeding results in the loss of 5–10% of the blood volume, shock may be detected. Signs of shock include tachycardia, tachypnea, hypotension, restlessness, anxiety, decreased capillary refill, and decreased urine output. Elderly patients have a decreased physiologic reserve that impairs their ability to compensate for blood loss. In addition they are often on medications that will blunt normal physiologic response to shock.
- *Treatment:* treatment of patients with known splenic injury is directed by the stability of their vital signs. Unstable patients will proceed to the OR for staging, repair, and possible splenectomy. Stable patients may undergo angiography and embolization or may be

observed depending on the degree of damage to the spleen. All patients in shock should be treated by starting with the ABCs. Most importantly, the airway must be protected. Intubation and mechanical respirations will help decrease the work of breathing and consumption of oxygen. Circulation should be optimized by fluid resuscitation and possible transfusion. If fluid resuscitation is adequate but the patient is still hypotensive, one can consider adding vasopressor agents.

- *Definitive therapy:* the definitive therapy for hypovolemic shock is to stop the cause of bleeding and correct associated abnormalities. When it is caused by a splenic injury, splenectomy is the definitive therapy. Other modalities of stabilization, such as embolization, are often attempted to preserve spleen function, since immunosuppression results from splenectomy.

Clinical course

The keys to this patient's diagnosis are careful attention to her history, exam, and ancillary studies. In this case, it is critical to pay close attention to how the patient's exam and labs changed over time, as well.

Historical clues	Physical findings	Ancillary studies
• Recent frequent falls	• Hypotension	• Renal insufficiency suggesting hypovolemia
• Vomiting	• Pale conjunctivae	• Chest X-ray ruling out other causes of dyspnea
• Abdominal pain	• Abdominal tenderness on re-exam	• Falling hematocrit
• Dyspnea without lung abnormalities on previous X-ray		• CT with shattered spleen
		• Worsening acidosis secondary to global hypoperfusion

The patient's diagnosis was not obvious on initial evaluation, so abnormal vital signs were aggressively treated while seeking a cause. The patient's history, although notable for falls, did not initially highlight abdominal injury as the main cause for concern. Physical exam signs of persistent hypotension despite fluid boluses, dyspnea without hypoxia or X-ray abnormalities, and lack of fever to suggest infectious source of dyspnea added to diagnostic deduction. Finally, the ancillary studies including a normal chest X-ray with shortness of breath, acidosis on labs, and a positive abdominal CT led to the correct diagnosis. Bedside ultrasound FAST exam would have been an appropriate alternative to CT scan in this patient, as she was persistently hypotensive. In a stable patient, angiography may further delineate the extent of splenic injury and may be therapeutic if embolization is performed. This was not appropriate in this patient.

This patient took several hours to diagnose. Once it was known that she had a splenic injury, she was transferred urgently to the operating room for exploratory laparotomy. She was found to have a substantial amount of blood in her peritoneal cavity and a shattered spleen. The patient underwent urgent splenectomy and repair of two enterotomies that were made during previous abdominal operations. She had approximately 2.5 liters of blood loss. She was brought to the surgical ICU. She continued to deteriorate clinically. She was given

IV fluids and chemical resuscitation, but no CPR was performed, as was her family's wishes. The patient was declared deceased shortly thereafter.

Further reading

Huijnen L, Van Der Horst F, van Amelsvoort L, et al. Dyspnea in elderly family practice patients. Occurrence, severity, quality of life and mortality over an 8-year period. *Fam Pract* 2006;**23**:34–9.

Case #4

History

This 13-month-old male toddler is brought to the ED by his mother for evaluation of wheezing. This morning, she heard wheezing while dressing him. Since he has never been known to wheeze before, this concerned her and she brought him to the ED for evaluation.

She states that he has a history of placing things in his mouth. Yesterday, she noted the child chewing on a red crayon. When she attempted to remove it, he gagged and coughed but appeared to expel all fragments of the crayon. He ate and behaved normally through the remainder of the day, and slept well last night. He has had no fever, cough or respiratory distress.

Past medical history

The patient is a healthy term infant with up-to-date immunizations.

Medications

He takes no medications.

Allergies

The child has no allergies.

Physical exam and ancillary studies

- *Vital signs:* the patient is afebrile. His heart rate is 123 bpm, his respiratory rate is 26, his blood pressure is 96/66 mmHg, and his room air oxygen saturation is 93%.
- *General:* he is cheerful, interactive, and appropriate.
- *Head and neck:* the patient's head and neck exam are normal.
- *Cardiovascular:* his heart is regular with no murmurs or rubs. He has good perfusion.
- *Lungs:* the patient has diminished breath sounds on the right. He has wheezing in his right upper lung fields.
- *Extremities and skin:* the patient's extremities are warm and well-perfused. He has no rashes or skin lesions.
- *Pertinent labs:* the patient has no indication for lab work.
- *Radiographs:* the patient's chest X-ray shows no abnormalities.

Questions for thought

- What are the appropriate initial actions to take to stabilize this patient?
- Once stable, what are other diagnostic tools you can use to make a diagnosis?

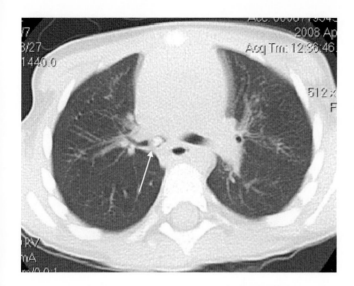

Figure 4.5. This CT scan shows a foreign body in the patient's right main stem bronchus.

- What medications should be avoided in this patient?
- How does one urgently treat this condition in the emergency department?
- What is definitive treatment of this condition?

Diagnosis

The patient underwent CT of the chest, which is shown in Figure 4.5. He was diagnosed with aspirated foreign body.

Discussion

- *Epidemiology:* foreign body aspiration is a potentially fatal cause of upper airway obstruction. It is most common in young children and the elderly. In young children, it occurs because of the tendency to place foreign objects into the mouth, and because mastication is incomplete due to lack of dentition. In the elderly, it is associated with dentures, neuromuscular disorders and intoxication. Although foreign body aspiration can lead to immediate airway obstruction and death, partial airway obstruction can present at a time remote from the aspiration itself.
- *Pathophysiology:* aspirated foreign bodies can be lodged in the upper airway, but are more commonly found in the bronchi. Foreign body blockages of the upper airway that are complete are not compatible with survival to hospital presentation. Bronchial foreign bodies are more common on the right due to the more linear orientation of the right main stem bronchus relative to the trachea.
- *Presentation:* patients with complete obstruction of the upper airway will not survive to hospital presentation unless the obstruction is removed immediately. The majority of patients with partial obstruction will present within 1 week, but presentation may be delayed far longer. Most patients present with respiratory complaints, including cough, wheeze, dyspnea, fever, or hemoptysis.

- *Treatment:* complete airway obstruction of the upper airway must be treated immediately. Cricothyrotomy may be necessary to establish an airway below the larynx if direct visualization and removal of the foreign body is not possible by laryngoscopy. Patients without complete airway obstruction should proceed to bronchoscopy as soon as safely feasible. Supplemental oxygen may be necessary.
- *Definitive therapy:* removal by bronchoscopy under controlled conditions is possible for the majority of patients. Rarely, patients will require an open procedure to remove a deep foreign body not accessible by bronchoscopy. Many patients will require admission for observation post-bronchoscopy as airway edema is possible. In addition, patients with post-obstructive pneumonia may require admission for antibiotic therapy and respiratory care.

Clinical course

The keys to this presentation are the history of potential aspiration and new wheezing in this otherwise well toddler.

Historical clues	Physical findings	Ancillary studies
• Known oral foreign body	• Wheezing	• CT scan showing foreign body
• Subsequent coughing and gagging	• Mild hypoxia	
• New complaint of wheezing		

The most important step in this case is to consider the diagnosis. Radio-opaque foreign bodies will be readily apparent on plain chest films, but in cases like this one involving a non-radio-opaque foreign body, a high index of suspicion is critical. To exclude high, partial obstructions, films of the neck may also be necessary. Non-radio-opaque foreign bodies may be inferred by plain-film findings, which include atelectasis, air trapping on the affected side, pneumonia and abscess. Comparison of inspiratory and expiratory films may demonstrate air trapping. However, 20% of films are entirely normal, as in this case. In these cases, CT may be useful. Based on history, it may be appropriate to proceed directly to bronchoscopy for direct visualization of the airway.

The potential for airway foreign body was recognized in this toddler who presented with new respiratory symptoms following an episode of choking on a crayon. When the plain film was normal, a CT scan was obtained, which confirmed the clinical suspicion. The child was taken to the OR for bronchoscopy and a green crayon was successfully removed. He was discharged the following day without need for further therapy.

Case #5

History

This is a 6-year-old male brought in by his mother with the chief complaint of breathing difficulties. The patient had been sick for the last 2 days with cough, clear rhinorrhea and low-grade fever. Tonight the child went to bed at his normal time, but awoke with a hoarse cough and difficulty breathing with audible wheezes during both inspiration and expiration. He improved slightly when he was going from the house to the car, but has become worse upon arrival to the emergency department. There were no episodes of cyanosis at home. He has not complained of headache, neck stiffness, photophobia, or acute otic complaints. He has not had any nausea, vomiting, diarrhea, or abdominal pain. He was eating and drinking appropriately earlier today.

Past medical history

The patient has no significant past medical history, and his immunizations are up to date.

Medications

He takes no medications.

Allergies

The patient has no known drug allergies.

Physical exam and ancillary studies

- *Vital signs:* the patient's temperature is 38.3°C, his heart rate is 150 BPM, his blood pressure is 123/87 mmHg, his respiratory rate is 40, and his room air oxygen saturation is 88%.
- *General:* he is awake and alert, nodding his head to yes or no questions. He is in severe respiratory distress, and is unable to speak in full sentences.
- *Head and neck:* the patient has inspiratory and expiratory stridor on anterior cervical auscultation. His pupils are equally round and reactive to light, and his cranial nerves are intact. The patient's mucous membranes are moist. His neck is supple with a midline trachea. He has no jugular venous distension.
- *Cardiovascular:* the patient's heart is regularly tachycardic at 150. He has no murmurs, rubs, or gallops. His radial pulses are 2+ bilaterally.
- *Lungs:* intercostal, suprasternal notch, and sternal retractions are present. The patient has bilateral inspiratory and expiratory wheezes present in all lung fields, with the inspiratory component louder than the expiratory component.
- *Abdomen:* his abdomen is soft, non-tender, and non-distended with positive bowel sounds. He has no peritoneal signs.

137

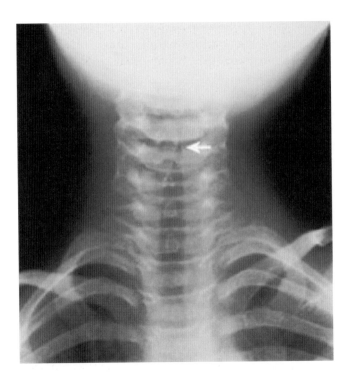

Figure 4.6. Neck X-ray demonstrating symmetric subglottic airway narrowing, known as a steeple sign.

- *Extremities and skin:* the patient has no edema, clubbing or cyanosis. His capillary refill is 2 seconds.
- *Radiographs:* the patient's chest X-ray was unremarkable. His neck X-ray is shown in Figure 4.6.

Questions for thought

- What are the appropriate initial actions to take to stabilize this patient?
- Once stable, what are other diagnostic tools you can use to make a diagnosis?
- What medications should be used in this patient?
- How does one urgently treat this condition in the emergency department?
- Why is this patient short of breath?

Diagnosis

Croup.

Discussion

- *Epidemiology:* croup or laryngotracheitis is a respiratory illness characterized by stridor, barking cough, and hoarseness. It usually occurs in children 6 months to 3 years of age, peaking at 1–2 years. The cause is almost always viral, with the most common type being parainfluenza. Respiratory syncytial virus, adenovirus, rhinovirus and influenza are also known viral sources of croup. Croup is relatively uncommon after age 6 although it can be seen in patients with recurrent croup. It has a higher incidence in patients with anatomic defects such as tracheomalacia and laryngomalacia. In children older than 5, *Mycoplasma pneumoniae* can cause a croup-like syndrome.

- *Pathophysiology:* inflammation and edema of the subglottic larynx and trachea, especially near the cricoid cartilage, lead to the stridor, barking cough and hoarseness of croup. Croup is mainly a disease of young children due to inflammation of the narrowest part of the pediatric upper airway. The swelling significantly reduces the diameter of the airway, limiting airflow and leading to stridor. Laryngotracheitis is seen in older children and adults; however, the larger diameters of their airways do not manifest croup-like symptoms. Hypoxemia may occur from progressive luminal narrowing and impaired alveolar ventilation and ventilation-perfusion mismatch.

- *Presentation:* croup usually begins with nonspecific respiratory symptoms, including rhinorrhea, cough, and fever. Within 1–2 days, the hoarseness, barking cough, and inspiratory stridor develop, often suddenly, along with a variable degree of respiratory distress. ED visits mostly occur from 10 p.m. to 4 a.m. Symptoms typically resolve within 3–7 days. Severe disease consists of frequent cough, prominent inspiratory and expiratory stridor, noticeable suprasternal, intercostal, and/or subcostal retractions, and decreased air entry with significant distress and agitation.

- *Treatment:* when the diagnosis of croup is suspected, humidified oxygen should be initially given. Most patients do not present in extremis, but intubation should be considered for those who do. Racemic epinephrine is used initially for patients with moderate to severe respiratory distress, with effects seen within minutes of therapy. Racemic epinephrine acts directly on mucosal edema by acting as a vasoconstrictor and reducing the amount of swelling. The other mainstay of treatment for croup is steroids, mainly dexamethasone. The medication has the same absorption rate regardless of route of administration. Most literature shows benefit at 0.3–0.6 mg/kg, not to exceed 10 mg per dose. The steroids act by reducing inflammation of the upper airway, but it usually takes 3–4 hours before positive results are seen. Heliox is a controversial therapy modality in croup. It acts by increasing laminar flow due to its decreased density. The drawback comes in that most Heliox preparations have helium:oxygen concentrations of 70:30. Patients with poor oxygen saturation should not receive this, as the oxygen in the heliox is equivalent to 3 L of oxygen by nasal cannula.

Clinical course

The keys to this patient's diagnosis are careful attention to his history, physical exam, and ancillary studies.

Historical clues	Physical findings	Ancillary studies
• Recent upper respiratory tract infection symptoms	• Stridor on auscultation	• Steeple sign on X-ray
• Sudden-onset barking cough	• Tachypnea	
• Inspiratory stridor	• Barking cough	
• Transient improvement when exposed to the cold	• Intercostal and suprasternal retractions	

The diagnosis of croup is a clinical one, based on history and exam. This patient was diagnosed with croup based on his findings, and his neck X-ray ruled out other causes of respiratory distress, such as foreign body or epiglottitis. In this case, the patient had a steeple sign, which is a classic finding in croup, but is not necessary to make the diagnosis.

This patient's croup was severe, based on his level of respiratory distress and degree of retractions. Initial humidified oxygen and racemic epinephrine caused mild improvement in his respiratory rate and reduced his stridor. Dexamethasone (10 mg) was given immediately. Heliox was given when the patient showed improving signs, and after a 4 hour observation period the patient had no stridor and was deemed stable to be discharged home.

Case #6

History

A 78-year-old man presents to the ED with complaints of severe shortness of breath. He admits to having this difficulty breathing for quite a while, but not this severe. About a week ago, it started progressing. Initially it was worse with exertion, and over the past several days he has had dyspnea at rest. His dyspnea is much worse when he lies down. During the two previous nights, he woke up short of breath and had to sit up in bed to make himself more comfortable. He has gained a few pounds over the last month. He denies any chest pain, nausea, vomiting, diaphoresis, or fever. He states he has had a cough for a while, and this cough has become worse over the last several days.

Past medical history

He has a history of anterior wall myocardial infarction many years ago. He also has a history of hypertension, diabetes, and hypercholesterolemia.

Social history

The patient does not drink alcohol or use illicit drugs. He quit smoking 15 years ago, and has a 40 pack-year history. It is Thanksgiving weekend, and he has been off his cardiac diet in honor of the holiday.

Medications

The patient's medications include atenolol, lisinopril, aspirin, lovastatin, and metformin.

Allergies

The patient has no known drug allergies.

Physical exam and ancillary studies

- *Vital signs:* the patient's temperature is 36.8°C, his heart rate is 60 bpm, his blood pressure is 128/59 mmHg, his respiratory rate is 26, and his room air oxygen saturation is 90%.
- *General:* he is an awake and alert, somewhat pale man, speaking in three-word sentences.
- *Head and neck:* the patient's pupils are equally round and reactive to light, and his cranial nerves are intact. The patient's mucous membranes are dry. His neck is supple with a midline trachea. He has appreciable jugular venous distension.
- *Cardiovascular:* the patient's heart has a regular rate and rhythm. He has an S3 gallop appreciated over the anterior precordium. He has no murmurs or rubs. His peripheral pulses are somewhat decreased.
- *Lungs:* he has decreased breath sounds throughout, with crackles bilaterally in the lower third of his lungs.

141

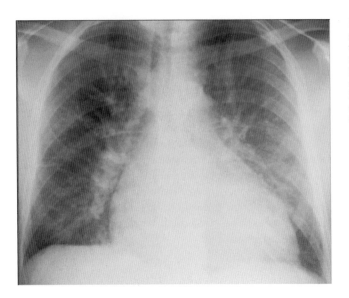

Figure 4.7. This chest X-ray shows cardiomegaly. There is vascular redistribution, with upper lobe blood diversion (cephalization), Kerley B lines, cuffing around the bronchi, and interstitial edema. This is consistent with congestive heart failure.

- *Abdomen:* the patient's liver protrudes approximately 3 cm from under his rib cage.
- *Extremities and skin:* he has 1+ bilateral lower extremity edema. He has no clubbing. He has poor capillary refill throughout with pale skin.
- *Pertinent labs:* the patient's complete blood count is remarkable for a hematocrit of 32%. His BNP level is > 3000. The remainder of his chemistries including cardiac enzymes are normal or negative.
- *EKG:* the patient's EKG shows no evidence of ischemia or arrhythmia.
- *Radiographs:* the patient's chest X-ray is shown in Figure 4.7.

Questions for thought

- What are the appropriate initial actions to take to stabilize this patient?
- Once stable, what are other diagnostic tools you can use to make a diagnosis?
- What medications can be administered in this patient?
- How does one urgently treat this condition in the emergency department?
- What is definitive treatment of this condition?
- Why is this patient short of breath?

Diagnosis

Acute on chronic congestive heart failure (CHF).

Discussion

- *Epidemiology:* more than 3 million people in the United States have CHF, and more than 400 000 new patients present yearly. Approximately 30–40% of patients with CHF are hospitalized every year. The most common cause of death in these patients is progressive heart failure, but sudden death may account for up to 45% of all deaths. Patients with coexisting insulin-dependent diabetes mellitus have a significantly increased mortality rate.

- *Pathophysiology:* patients with heart failure have an imbalance in cardiac pump function in which the heart fails to adequately maintain the circulation of blood. The most severe manifestation of CHF, pulmonary edema, develops when this imbalance causes an increase in lung fluid secondary to leakage from pulmonary capillaries into the interstitium and alveoli of the lung.

- *Presentation:* heart failure may be left-sided or right-sided. Left-sided heart failure most commonly presents with symptoms that are respiratory in nature. Pumping failure of the left ventricle causes backward congestion of the pulmonary veins, and, consequently, capillaries. The patient will have dyspnea on exertion and, in more severe cases, at rest. Easy fatigueability is also a common, although nonspecific, complaint. Orthopnea, increasing breathlessness while lying down, occurs. It is often measured by the number of pillows required to lie comfortably, and in severe cases the patient may sleep while sitting up. Another symptom of heart failure is paroxysmal nocturnal dyspnea, which is a sudden severe breathlessness at night. Signs of the poor peripheral perfusion, such as dizziness and confusion, or cool extremities at rest, may be present in advanced cases.

  Right-sided failure presents with systemic venous congestion, manifesting as peripheral edema or nocturia (frequent nighttime urination when the fluid from the legs is going back to the bloodstream). Ascites (transudate in the peritoneal cavity) and painful hepatomegaly (enlargement of the liver) may develop in more advanced cases. Passive hepatic congestion can impair liver function, too.

  Chronic heart failure may exacerbate easily. The most common causes of this are dietary indiscretions, noncompliance with medications, increased metabolic needs from concomitant illnesses of any kind, atrial fibrillation, anemia, and poorly controlled hypertension.

- *Treatment:* initial treatment of the patient with CHF exacerbation consists of nitroglycerin to reduce afterload and improve cardiac pump function. This can be administered sublingually or intravenously. Diuretics are given to relieve congestive symptoms. ACE inhibitors improve symptoms, decrease mortality, and reduce left ventricular hypertrophy. Beta-blockers are indicated for patients with systolic heart failure due to left ventricular systolic dysfunction only after stabilization with diuretic and ACE inhibitor therapy. Digoxin (a positive inotrope and negative chronotrope) is reserved for control of ventricular rhythm in patients with atrial fibrillation, or where adequate CHF control is not achieved with an ACE inhibitor, a beta-blocker, and a loop diuretic. There is no evidence that digoxin reduces mortality in CHF. Phosphodiesterase inhibitors (milrinone) are utilized in severe cardiomyopathy. Their mechanism of action is through inhibition of the adenosine receptors, resulting in inotropic effects and modest diuretic effects. The addition of spironolactone can improve mortality, particularly in severe cardiomyopathy (ejection fraction less than 25%).

  In patients with New York Heart Association (NYHA) class II-III, left ventricular ejection fraction of 35% or less and a QRS interval of 120 ms or more may benefit from cardiac resynchronization therapy with pacing from both the left and right ventricles, through implantation of a bi-ventricular pacemaker. Surgical remodeling of the heart may also be undertaken. These treatment modalities may make the patient symptomatically better, and in some trials have been proven to reduce mortality.

- *Definitive therapy:* for end-stage heart failure, the only definitive treatment is heart transplantation. If heart failure develops after a myocardial infarction due to scarring and aneurysm formation, reconstructive surgery may be an option.

Clinical course

The keys to the patient's diagnosis are careful attention to his history, physical exam, and ancillary studies.

Historical clues	Physical findings	Ancillary studies
• History of the MI	• Tachycardia	• Chest X-ray with congestive heart failure
• Dyspnea on exertion	• Crackles in the lungs	• Elevated BNP level
• Peripheral edema and weight gain	• Jugular venous distension	
• Orthopnea	• S3 gallop	
• Paroxysmal nocturnal dyspnea	• Liver enlargement	
• Cough	• Poor peripheral perfusion	
	• Lower extremity edema	

This patient was believed to have CHF because of his underlying risk factors and physical findings. An EKG was done which showed no evidence of a precipitating arrhythmia or ischemia, and his chest X-ray confirmed the exam findings of pulmonary edema. In addition, the patient had a high BNP level. Although a mid-range value for BNP is not terribly specific for heart failure, a level as high as this patient's is very specific for the diagnosis of heart failure.

An IV was placed and the patient was given oxygen. He was given IV nitroglycerin and furosemide with improvement in his symptoms and was admitted to the hospital for 2 days. His symptoms resolved and he was discharged home on a low-salt diet. Furosemide was added to his medical regimen.

Further reading

Davis RC, Davies MK. *ABC of Heart Failure*. Malden, MA: Blackwell, 2006.

Abraham WT, Krum H. *Heart Failure*. New York: McGraw-Hill, 2007.

Case #7

History

A 38-year-old woman presents to the ED complaining of severe shortness of breath. She is unable to give any further history secondary to severe dyspnea. Her boyfriend states that they were arguing and she became very short of breath and has since been clutching her chest and gasping for air. This occurred less than 5 minutes ago. The patient has had intermittent shortness of breath over the last several days, which she has been treating with her albuterol inhaler.

Past medical history

The patient has a lifelong history of asthma for which she has been hospitalized several times a year, most recently 2 months ago. She has been intubated once before. She also has a history of seasonal allergies, anxiety, and depression. She has smoked a half pack of cigarettes per day for the last 25 years.

Medications

The patient's medications include albuterol, fluticasone salmeterol, loratadine, and sertraline. She completed a course of oral steroids 7 weeks ago.

Allergies

The patient has no known drug allergies.

Physical exam and ancillary studies

- *Vital signs:* the patient's temperature is 36.9°C, her heart rate is 135 bpm, her blood pressure is 150/78 mmHg, her respiratory rate is 40, and her room air oxygen saturation is 100%.
- *General:* she is awake and alert, anxious-appearing, and not able to speak. She is sitting leaning forward on the stretcher and is trembling.
- *Head and neck:* the patient's pupils are equally round and reactive to light, and her cranial nerves are intact. Her mucous membranes are moist. Her neck is supple with a midline trachea. She has no jugular venous distension.
- *Cardiovascular:* the patient is regularly tachycardic without murmurs or rubs. Her peripheral pulses are bounding, and she has good capillary refill.
- *Lungs:* the patient is breathing rapidly and deeply. There are inspiratory and expiratory wheezes. There is some stridor.
- *Extremities and skin:* she has no edema, no clubbing, and no calf tenderness. Her extremities are warm and well-perfused, but diaphoretic.
- *Pertinent labs:* the patient's arterial blood gas shows a paO_2 of 100 mmHg, a $paCO_2$ of 15 mmHg, a bicarbonate of 20, and an oxygen saturation of 100%. The remainder of her blood work was normal or negative.

- *EKG:* the EKG shows a sinus tachycardia with no evidence of other arrhythmia or ST abnormality.
- *Radiographs:* the patient's portable chest X-ray shows no evidence of pneumothorax or airspace disease.

Questions for thought

- What are the appropriate initial actions to take to stabilize this patient?
- What is the differential diagnosis for this patient?
- How can the definitive diagnosis be made?
- How does one urgently treat this condition in the emergency department?

Diagnosis

Panic attack with secondary dyspnea and hypocarbia.

Discussion

- *Epidemiology:* generalized anxiety disorder occurs in about 8% of primary care patients, with panic attacks occurring in about 5% of people during the course of their lifetimes. Panic occurs as a comorbid condition in a disproportionate number of asthmatics relative to the general population, and has a higher prevalence in those with severe asthma.
- *Pathophysiology:* a panic attack is defined by its rapidity of onset, with symptoms peaking within 10 minutes of onset. To meet criteria, the patient must have four of the following symptoms or findings: palpitations or tachycardia, sweating, trembling, shortness of breath, sensation of choking, chest pain, nausea, dizziness or faintness, derealization, fear of losing control, fear of dying, paresthesias, or chills. Many patients hyperventilate, causing them to have abnormal arterial blood gases. The decrease in carbon dioxide may in turn precipitate bronchospasm and worsen respiratory symptoms. For those with underlying asthma, the patient as well as the healthcare provider may be unable to distinguish panic symptoms from asthma symptoms, and will often treat with beta-agonist medications, which can worsen anxiety and panic. The underlying etiology of panic is unclear, and thought to be multifactorial, with both genetic and environmental contributors.
- *Presentation:* this presentation is typical for panic. The patient has rapid onset of symptoms, with palpitations, chest pain, diaphoresis, shortness of breath, and trembling. Some patients presenting with a panic attack will have no previous history of a panic attack or any other psychiatric disorder. Some will have a precipitating event, such as a personal tragedy or an argument, while others will have a panic attack with no precedent. Symptoms of panic are typically short-lived, peaking in 10 minutes and resolving rapidly. It is important to remember that a single panic attack does not mean that a patient has panic disorder.
- *Diagnosis:* it can be very difficult acutely to distinguish between an asthma exacerbation and a panic attack. Severe asthma will often manifest with lowered oxygen saturation and only minimally lowered or even elevated carbon dioxide level. Panic in the absence of

lung disease will not manifest with low oxygen but may have a very low carbon dioxide level from hyperventilation. The common coexistence of the two conditions in a single patient, however, makes the arterial blood gas unhelpful. Patients in the throes of a panic attack may develop inspiratory and expiratory stridor which sounds like wheezing on lung exam, which can further confuse the diagnosis, and hypocapnia can result in secondary bronchoconstriction. Some authors have recommended using peak flow to distinguish between asthma and panic, but this can be a challenge in the patient *in extremis*. Ultimately, the diagnosis of panic attack is clinical, based on history and exam. There are no definitive diagnostic tests.

- *Treatment:* if the diagnoses of both panic and asthma are being entertained, it is prudent to attempt treatment of asthma with a beta-agonist, as asthma can be an acutely life-threatening disease. If, however, the patient gets worse with beta-agonists or if panic seems likely, judicious use of benzodiazepines may relieve the symptoms. Benzodiazepines in the setting of an acute asthma exacerbation may depress respiratory drive, but are the treatment of choice for a panic attack. Breathing into a paper bag to increase carbon dioxide levels and decrease hyperventilation should be discouraged, as it has not been shown to reduce symptom duration and may cause hypoxia and death.
- *Definitive therapy:* the patient should be referred back to her primary care doctor for coordination of care for both her psychiatric and pulmonary illnesses.

Clinical course

Historical clues	Physical findings	Ancillary studies
• Anxiety history	• Tachycardia	• Normal chest X-ray
• Panic precipitant	• Diaphoresis	• Normal oxygen saturation
• Rapid symptom onset	• Trembling	• Marked hypocapnia
• Worsening symptoms with treatment of asthma		

This woman was erroneously believed to have status asthmaticus. After receiving oxygen, albuterol, atrovent, and magnesium sulfate with worsening symptoms, the patient was intubated. Upon sedation, the patient was easy to ventilate with bag valve mask, and she had no wheezing on exam. She was extubated within an hour, by which time her symptoms had resolved. In retrospect, careful attention to the patient's history, physical exam, and ancillary studies would have suggested the appropriate diagnosis.

The patient was discharged home from the emergency department to follow up with her primary care doctor.

Further reading

Diagnostic and Statistical Manual of Mental Disorders, 4th edition. Washington DC: American Psychiatric Association, 1994.

Weiller E, Bisserbe JC, Maier W, Lecrubier Y. Prevalence and recognition of anxiety syndromes in five European primary care settings. A report from the WHO study on Psychological Problems in General Health Care. *Br J Psychiatry* Suppl 1998;34:18–23.

Smoller JW, Pollack MH, Otto MW, Rosenbaum JF, Kradin RL. Panic anxiety, dyspnea, and respiratory disease. Theoretical and clinical considerations. *Am J Respir Crit Care Med* 1996;**154**(1):6–17.

Katon WJ, Richardson L, Lozano P, McCauley E. The relationship of asthma and anxiety disorders. *Psychosom Med* 2004;**66**:349–55.

Von Korff MR, Eaton WW, Keyl PM. The epidemiology of panic attacks and panic disorder results of three community surveys. *Am J Epidemiol* 1985;**122**(6):970–81.

Newton EJ. Hyperventilation syndrome. www.emedicine.com/emerg/topic270.htm. September 2005.

Case #8

History

A 48-year-old male presents to the emergency department via EMS after having an unresponsive episode and dyspnea. The patient had been sitting under the shade of a tree to escape the heat of the July sun. He had stood up to go into his house but had an episode of unresponsiveness upon getting to the front door. His wife described a couple "jerking" motions of his upper extremities associated with this event. The patient was unresponsive for a minute or two and quickly regained his normal level of consciousness. On EMS arrival the patient complained of difficulty breathing and was found to be in atrial fibrillation. En route the patient reverted to a normal rhythm and rate and no longer felt dyspneic. On arrival to the ED the patient denies headache, chest pain, palpitations, or shortness of breath. The patient does note some discomfort in his left lower extremity, which is in a short leg cast that was placed 3 days previously.

Past medical history

The patient has a history of intermittent atrial fibrillation in the past. His last episode was a couple of years previously. The patient had been seen in the ED 3 days previously for an injury to his left leg after falling 10 feet from a ladder. He was diagnosed with a tibia fracture and casted at that time. The patient reports smoking cigars.

Medications

The patient's medications include ibuprofen and hydrocodone/APAP.

Allergies

The patient has no known drug allergies.

Physical exam and ancillary studies

- *Vital signs:* the patient's vital signs include a temperature of 36.3°C, a heart rate of 78 bpm, a blood pressure of 110/64 mmHg, a respiratory rate of 16, and a room air oxygen saturation of 95%.
- *General:* he is awake and alert, resting comfortably on a stretcher.
- *Head and neck:* the patient's pupils are equally round and reactive to light, and his cranial nerves are intact. The patient's mucous membranes are moist. His neck is supple with a midline trachea. There is no jugular venous distension.
- *Cardiovascular:* the patient's heart has a regular rate and rhythm without murmurs or rubs. His bilateral femoral pulses are palpable.
- *Lungs:* the patient's lungs are clear to auscultation bilaterally without wheezes, rales, or rhonchi.

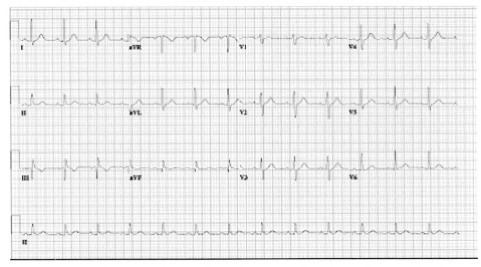

Figure 4.8. This EKG shows a normal sinus rhythm with no ischemia. The patient has the finding of an S wave in lead I, a Q wave in lead III, and an inverted T wave in lead III.

- *Extremities and skin:* he has his left lower extremity casted in a short leg cast.
- *Pertinent labs:* blood counts, chemistries, and coagulation factors are normal or negative. The patient's troponin is 0.06, which is in the indeterminate range.
- *EKG:* the patient's EKG is shown in Figure 4.8.

Radiographs: the patient's chest X-ray shows no evidence of acute airspace disease. His heart and mediastinum are normal in contour. A representative cut from the patient's CT is shown in Figure 4.9.

Questions for thought

- What is the differential diagnosis for this patient?
- What further diagnostic tools can you use to make the diagnosis?
- Why is this patient short of breath?
- What are the patient's risk factors?
- What actions should be considered in the emergency department?
- What is definitive treatment of this condition?

Diagnosis

Saddle pulmonary embolus (PE).

Discussion

- *Epidemiology:* PE is a relatively common cause of chest pain and dyspnea, effecting 0.5–1 person per 1000 per year. That said, PE frequently goes unrecognized. If untreated, PE has a mortality of 25% versus a mortality of about 5% if appropriately treated. Thirty percent

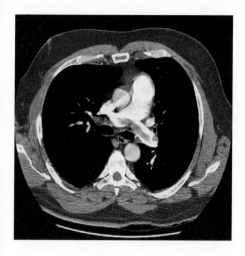

Figure 4.9. This chest CT shows evidence of a luminal filling defect in both pulmonary arteries.

of patients with PE will have a recurrence, most frequently in the first year, which carries a significantly higher mortality than the first episode.

- *Pathophysiology:* PE results from dislodgement of thrombi from the deep veins of the upper and lower extremities. When the embolus obstructs a pulmonary artery it has consequences on both the respiratory system and the cardiovascular system. Acute respiratory consequences of PE include increased alveolar dead space, ventilation-perfusion mismatch, and pulmonary infarction. The acute obstruction of the pulmonary arterial tree increases right ventricular afterload, occasionally resulting in acute right ventricular failure. Risk factors for thrombosis are numerous and were realized in the nineteenth century by Virchow as consisting of injury to the vascular intima, venous stasis, and hypercoagulability. The most prominent risk factors for PE include a previous history of deep venous thrombosis (DVT) or PE, recent surgery or immobilization, pregnancy and malignancy. Other risk factors to consider include inherited hypercoagulable states, congestive heart failure, and oral contraceptive pill use.
- *Presentation:* the most common presenting symptom of PE is dyspnea; however, this will only be present in approximately 80% of patients. About 65% of patients will have chest pain, 25–40% will have evidence of lower extremity DVT, and 8% will have circulatory collapse. Other symptoms of PE can be new-onset atrial fibrillation or multifocal atrial tachycardia or syncope from rapid increase in pulmonary intravascular pressure. Unfortunately, 5% of patients will not have dyspnea, tachypnea, chest pain, or signs of DVT.
- *Diagnosis:* the gold standard for the diagnosis of pulmonary embolus is pulmonary arteriogram, but this study has an associated morbidity in 5% of studies and a mortality of 0.5%. CT angiography (CTA) is being increasingly used for the detection of pulmonary emboli. A recent meta-analysis of 4657 patients with a negative CTA who had treatment withheld found that 1.4% of them had venous thromboembolism and the rate of fatal PE was 0.51% at 3 months. Ventilation/perfusion (V/Q) scans are rapidly becoming phased out of use because of the difficulty with interpretation, with 4% of patients with a normal V/Q having a PE and only 87% of patients with a high-probability scan having a PE. The utility of D-dimer in the diagnosis of PE is entirely dependent on the particular assay performed. Elisa-VIDAS has demonstrated sufficient sensitivity and negative predictive

value to allow it to exclude PE in those patients with low or medium pretest probability. However, other D-dimer ELISA assays have not been demonstrated to work as well.

- *Treatment:* initial treatment of the patient with PE is initiation of anti-thrombotic therapy consisting of heparin or low-molecular-weight heparin. Initial anticoagulation with heparin is usually followed by long-term anticoagulation with warfarin. Duration of treatment is dependent upon the nature of the patient's risk factors and whether they represent transient risks. For patients who cannot be anticoagulated, a vena caval filter can be placed to interrupt the passage of clot from the lower extremities to pulmonary circulation. There is some debate regarding the role of thrombolytics for the treatment of PE. Currently, thrombolytics should be reserved for those patients who are persistently hemodynamically unstable with evidence of right heart failure. Studies in patients without hemodynamic instability have failed to demonstrate significant benefits that outweigh risks of bleeding.

Clinical course

In order to make the diagnosis of pulmonary embolism, one must consider all of its subtle presentations.

Historical clues	Physical findings	Ancillary studies
• Recent fracture to lower extremity	• Relative hypoxia	• $S_I Q_{III} T_{III}$ on EKG
• Episode of syncope	• Clear lung exam	• Clear chest X-ray
• Episode of atrial fibrillation	• Lower extremity in cast	• CT scan with intraluminal filling defects (saddle embolus)
• Dyspnea		

Although the most plausible explanation for the patient's syncopal episode was an episode of atrial fibrillation with rapid ventricular response and hypotension, the clinician must not succumb to premature closure of the differential diagnosis. Given the risk factor of the recent lower extremity trauma with immobilization, PE was entertained as an explanation of the syncope, episode of atrial fibrillation, and transient dyspnea. This is why the practitioner ordered the chest CT.

The saddle embolus lodging in the right ventricular outflow tract most likely caused a transient increase in right atrial pressure and stretch resulting in the episode of atrial fibrillation. Because the pulmonary arterial blood flow was not completely obstructed the patient did not exhibit significant tachycardia or hypoxia. However, he did have an episode of syncope, which may have been from sudden decreased cardiac output from the embolus.

Although the practitioner ordered the CT early on in his ED course, an ED is a busy place, and the patient did not get his scan right away. In the interim, he was not treated prophylactically with anticoagulation because of his recent trauma. As the CT angiogram of the patient's chest was being read by radiology, the patient went into a pulseless electrical activity (PEA) cardiac arrest. Although the patient was administered epinephrine and intravenous thrombolytics, the patient expired following a prolonged resuscitative effort.

Further reading

Fields JM, Goyal M. Venothromboembolism. *Emerg Med Clin North Am* 2008;**26**:649–83.

Di Nisio M, Squizzato A, Rutjes AW, et al. Diagnostic accuracy of D-dimer test for exclusion of venous thromboembolism: a systematic review. *J Thromb Haemost* 2007;**5**:296–304.

Sinert R, Foley M. Clinical assessment of the patient with a suspected pulmonary embolism. *Ann Emerg Med* 2008;**52**:76–9.

Case # 9

History

An almost 18-year-old female patient with past medical history of a single ventricle, status post Blalock-Taussig shunt as a child, presents with shortness of breath. Her mother states that the patient normally receives chloral hydrate prior to going to bed. She was given her regular dose of medications tonight, but then as her stepfather was carrying her upstairs she became unresponsive and cyanotic. This was half an hour ago. The patient's family called EMS, who report that she required no rescue breathing en route to the hospital. She has spontaneous, shallow respirations now, but does not appear to be protecting her airway. The patient is unresponsive and somewhat pale. Her mother denies any recent fevers or chills. She has not had any nausea, vomiting, or diarrhea. There was no shortness of breath or complaints of chest pain prior to the episode. The patient has had no recent changes in her medications.

Past medical history

The patient has a past medical history of a large cerebrovascular accident with secondary left hemiparesis. She also has a history of asthma. She has congenital heart disease with a single ventricle. She has mental retardation with a 4-year-old capacity. She also has a nonfunctional cystic right kidney. Surgically, she has had an incomplete heart repair with a modified Blalock-Taussig shunt, a gastrostomy with Mickey button, a tracheostomy at 1 year of age which was removed at age 6, and a ventriculoperitoneal shunt at birth.

Medications

The patient's medications include chloral hydrate, furosemide, spironolactone, clonidine, diazepam, aspirin, and albuterol.

Allergies

The patient has an allergy to penicillins.

Physical exam and ancillary studies

- *Vital signs:* the patient's temperature is 36.7°C, her heart rate is 200 bpm, her blood pressure is 111/93 mmHg, her respiratory rate is 28, and her oxygen saturation is 88% on 100% non-rebreather (NRB).
- *General:* the patient is non-responsive to verbal and noxious stimuli, and she is in moderate to severe respiratory distress.
- *Head and neck:* the patient's head is normocephalic and atraumatic. Her pupils are equal and reactive at 3 mm down to 1 mm. The patient has moist oral mucosa. She has no nasal discharge or epistaxis. Her neck is supple, and she has no jugular venous distension.

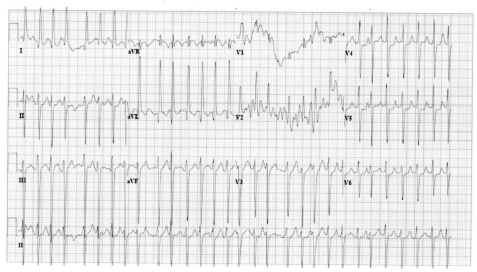

Figure 4.10. This EKG shows supraventricular tachycardia at a rate of over 200. The QRS complexes are narrow and there is no evidence of ischemia.

- *Cardiovascular:* the patient's heart is in a regular tachycardic rhythm at 200 bpm. S1 and S2 are unable to be distinguished. There are no appreciable murmurs. Her radial pulses are 1+ and thready.
- *Lungs:* the patient's lungs have equal expansion and equal breath sounds. She is using accessory muscles and is retracting.
- *Extremities and skin:* the patient has no clubbing, no calf swelling or erythema, and no tenderness. She has poor capillary refill throughout with pale, mottled skin.
- *Pertinent labs:* the patient has a glucose of 210 and a brain natriuretic peptide of 123. The remainder of her chemistries including cardiac enzymes and serum drug screen are normal or negative.
- *EKG:* the patient's EKG is shown in Figure 4.10.
- *Radiographs:* the patient's chest X-ray is shown in Figure 4.11.

Questions for thought

- What are the appropriate initial actions to take to stabilize this patient?
- Once stable, what are other diagnostic tools you can use to make a diagnosis?
- What medications should be avoided in this patient?
- How does one urgently treat this condition in the emergency department?
- What is definitive treatment of this condition?
- Why is this patient short of breath?

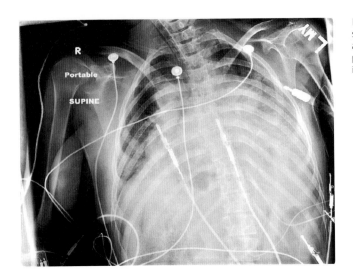

Figure 4.11. This chest X-ray shows evidence of cardiomegaly and pulmonary edema. In this picture, the patient has been intubated.

Diagnosis

Respiratory distress secondary to paroxysmal supraventricular tachycardia (SVT).

Discussion

- *Epidemiology:* respiratory distress is a common complaint for which children seek medical care. It accounts for nearly 10% of pediatric emergency department visits for all children.
- *Pathophysiology:* respiratory distress in the pediatric population is usually due to a primary respiratory disorder. These include infectious diseases such as pneumonia, bronchiolitis, croup, and tracheitis. Obstruction of the airway from foreign bodies, asthma, and reactive airway disease can also lead to respiratory distress. There are important cardiac conditions that can progress to respiratory complaints such as congestive heart failure and myocarditis. Arrhythmias, especially in congenital heart disease, can lead to respiratory distress from lack of end diastolic volume. This prevents adequate stroke volume, reduced tissue perfusion and causing acute organ dysfunction.
- *Presentation:* patients with dysrrhythmias will present as either stable or unstable. Designating an arrhythmia as stable or unstable helps guide treatment options. An unstable patient may present with severe chest pain, severe respiratory distress, pulmonary edema or altered mental status. Unstable patients are likely to decompensate and immediate electrocardioversion is indicated in most cases to help stabilize the patient. Stable patients have time for pharmacotherapy and should be treated depending on the type of arrhythmia.
- *Treatment:* electrocardioversion is indicated for the unstable patient. For patients presenting in ventricular fibrillation, unsynchronized cardioversion is indicated. For all other unstable arrhythmias, synchronized cardioversion is indicated. Output should start at 50–100 joules on a biphasic defibrillator. For unsuccessful attempts increase the output to 120, then 200 and continue at 200 joules for further attempts. The stable patient should receive pharmacotherapy for the arrhythmias. For narrow complex tachycardias, adenosine can

break paroxysmal SVT, or slow down atrial fibrillation/flutter enough to identify and allow for rate control with a beta-blocker or calcium-channel blocker. For wide complex tachydysrhythmias, amiodarone is the drug of choice as it can treat both ventricular tachycardias and supraventricular tachycardias in patients with pre-existing bundle branch blocks.

Clinical course

The keys to the diagnosis in this patient are careful attention to history, physical exam, and ancillary studies.

Historical clues	Physical findings	Ancillary studies
• History of congenital heart disease	• Regular tachycardia	• EKG with supraventricular tachycardia
• History of heart surgery	• Hypoxia	• Chest X-ray with pulmonary edema and cardiomegaly
• Sudden onset of respiratory distress	• Tachypnea	
	• Unresponsive	
	• Evidence of poor perfusion (delayed capillary refill and thready pulses)	

The diagnosis of tachyarrhythmia was considered in this patient based on her abnormal heart rate on her initial vital signs. This diagnosis was confirmed with an EKG done upon arrival.

The patient was intubated for severe respiratory distress and for protection of her airway. This only improved her oxygen saturation slightly. Synchronized cardioversion was then performed for the patient's tachycardia at 50 joules. Her rhythm was then normal sinus and the patient's oxygen saturation improved to 99%. She was admitted to the pediatric intensive care unit and extubated the next morning. She was at her baseline neurologic function. She underwent echocardiogram, which can assess for a change in her baseline cardiac structural defects or evaluate for vegetations and other abnormalities. This was unchanged from her previous echocardiograms. The patient was discharged the following day in time to enjoy her eighteenth birthday.

Further reading

Krauss, BS, Harakal, T, Fleisher, GR. The spectrum and frequency of illness presenting to a pediatric emergency department. *Pediatr Emerg Care* 1991;7:67.

Case #10

History

A 30-year-old woman presents to the ED with a 2 day history of shortness of breath. She reports that she "has been fighting a cold for the past week," but over the past 48 hours the symptoms have worsened. Currently, the dyspnea is present on both exertion and at rest and occasionally causes mild right-sided chest pain with deep inspiration. She also reports an increase in her cough with worsening sputum production, in the amount of approximately a small teacupful per day which is green and thick.

The patient reports subjective fevers and chills but has not measured her temperature at home. She has vomited twice, which was non-bloody.

She denies any recent travel. She does have several sick contacts at work and home but none with symptoms as severe.

Past medical history

The patient has a history of infectious mononucleosis at age 17. Her vaccinations are up to date. She had a splenectomy after traumatic rupture of her spleen secondary to Epstein-Barr virus splenomegaly.

Medications

The patient takes no medications.

Allergies

She has no known drug allergies.

Physical exam and ancillary studies

- *Vital signs:* the patient's temperature is 38.4°C, her pulse is 130 bpm, her respiratory rate is 26, her blood pressure is 132/89, and her oxygen saturation is 94% on room air.
- *General:* the patient is awake and alert. She is very uncomfortable-appearing, and is having a difficult time speaking because she has ongoing coughing. She is only able to speak in short sentences.
- *HEENT:* the patient has no evidence of trauma. Her eyes show mild conjuctival injection, but she has no scleral icterus. The patient has no rhinorrhea. She has significant oropharyngeal erythema. Her mucous membranes are moist.
- *Neck:* the patient's neck is supple with a midline trachea.
- *Cardiovascular:* the patient's heart is tachycardic. There are no rubs, murmurs, or gallops.
- *Lungs:* the patient has good respiratory effort, with equal chest expansion. She has crackles and rales at the base of her left lung. There are no wheezes or rhonchi. There is dullness to percussion with E to A egophony in the left base.

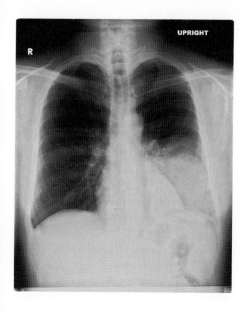

Figure 4.12. This chest X-ray demonstrates left lower lobe consolidation, consistent with pneumonia.

- *Abdominal:* the patient's abdomen is soft and without distention. There is no tenderness to palpation noted. No masses are appreciated.
- *Skin:* her capillary refill is less than 2 seconds. There are no rashes or lesions noted.
- *Extremities:* the patient has good perfusion, with no clubbing, cyanosis, or edema.
- *Neurologic:* the patient's neurologic exam is entirely normal.
- *Pertinent abnormal labs:* on complete blood count, the patient's white blood cell count is 18.3 with 60% segmented neutrophils and 9% bands. The remainder of chemistries are normal or negative.
- *Radiographs:* the patient's chest X-ray is shown in Figure 4.12.

Questions for thought

- What is the differential diagnosis?
- What are the most common pathogens for this diagnosis?
- What criteria should be used for admitting or discharging this patient?
- What is the appropriate treatment for this patient?
- What historical clues are important considerations for this patient's presentation?

Diagnosis

Community-acquired pneumonia.

Discussion

- *Epidemiology:* there are approximately 4 million cases of community-acquired pneumonia (CAP) in the United States each year. About a quarter of those will be admitted to a hospital. CAP disproportionately affects those at extremes of age, and those with pre-existing lung disease. Other host characteristics which increase the potential for infection include diseases of immunity (HIV), reduced ability to clear infections (chemotherapy treatment), or genetic characteristics limiting normal clearing of bacteria (Kartagener's syndrome causing immotile cilia). Other susceptibilities include malnutrition and unproductive or absent gag reflex.

- *Pathophysiology*: the pathogens responsible for causing CAP vary somewhat based on age and risk factors. Pathogens are divided into "typical" and "atypical." Typical pathogens include the ubiquitous *Streptococcus pneumoniae* and *Haemophilus influenzae*, among others. Those at risk for aspiration can present with anaerobic or Gram-negative pathogens. Atypical pathogens include *Mycoplasma pneumoniae*, legionella species, and *Chlamydia pneumoniae*. Empiric treatment regimens which cover both the typical and atypical pathogens are associated with decreased mortality rates. In the outpatient setting, definitive diagnosis is often not obtained prior to treatment. Therefore, most pneumonias never have a specific pathogen identified.

- *Presentation*: patients suffering from community-acquired pneumonia often present with dyspnea, a worsening and productive cough, fever, and pleuritic chest pain. Gastrointestinal complaints such as nausea, vomiting, and diarrhea are also common complaints. Fever may be absent in elderly adults or those incapable of mounting a significant immune response. An increased index of suspicion is warranted in these patients. When in question, a PA and lateral chest radiograph should always be taken.

- *Treatment*: treatment of community-acquired pneumonia consists of appropriate antibiotic coverage along with adjunctive therapy to improve ventilation, oxygenation, and patient comfort. Antibiotics should be chosen to cover both typical and atypical bacteria. In healthy patients without comorbidities and no risk factors for drug-resistant *S. pneumoniae* infection, treatment with a macrolide (azithromycin, erythromycin, clarythromycin) is usually sufficient. Doxycycline may be substituted for patients who cannot tolerate a macrolide. In high-risk patients or hospitalized patients, a β-lactam (high-dose amoxicillin, augmentin, ceftriaxone, cefuroxime, or cefpodoxime) should be combined with either a macrolide or doxycycline. A single respiratory fluoroquinolone (levofloxacin, moxifloxacin, gemifloxacin) may be used in patients who can not tolerate a β-lactam. Treatment duration should be for a minimum of 5 days, with at least 24 hours fever-free prior to the discontinuation of therapy. Tachypnea, fever, and mouth-breathing often lead to dehydration. Patients who are short of breath may have difficulty eating or drinking, as it interrupts their breathing. It should be presumed that pneumonia patients are dehydrated, and exam and lab findings usually support this. Rehydration with oral or IV fluids often improves a patient's symptoms. The use of inhaled beta-agonists such as albuterol often improves reactive bronchoconstriction and in turn ventilation. Patients may have significant improvement in shortness of breath and hypoxia with their use. Incentive spirometry improves ventilation and helps prevent atelectasis, especially in patients with pain on respiration who might be splinting and therefore under-ventilating portions of lung.

- *Definitive therapy*: the majority of patients with CAP can be managed as outpatients. Any patient with hypoxia requiring supplemental oxygen requires admission to the hospital. The Pneumonia Severity Index (PSI) was derived as a tool to help assess the risk for mortality from community-acquired pneumonia. The PSI classifies patients with CAP into one of five risk classes, from I to V. Class I patients have a 0.1% risk of mortality, whereas class V patients have a 27% risk of mortality from their pneumonia. Simple online calculators are available to help determine a patient's PSI score based upon their age, comorbidities, and some basic lab values. Patients in Class I and II are usually safe to manage as outpatients. Class III patients can be managed either with a brief inpatient observation or as outpatients with close follow-up, if reliable. Class IV and V patients almost uniformly benefit from hospitalization, with Class V patients typically requiring ICU admission.

Clinical course

The keys to obtaining this patient's diagnosis are careful attention to her history, the physical exam, and the ancillary studies.

Historical clues	Physical findings	Ancillary studies
• Respiratory distress	• Febrile	• Abnormal chest X-ray
• Sick contact	• Tachycardia	• Leukocytosis
• Splenectomy	• Tachypnea	
	• Focal findings on lung exam	
	• Benign abdominal exam	

This patient's physical exam was strongly suggestive of pneumonia. A chest X-ray was performed which revealed her left lower lobe pneumonia; however, it is important to recognize that radiographic evidence of pneumonia may not be present in patients who have not been ill for very long. Ultimately, pneumonia is a clinical diagnosis, based on the patient's history and exam. Antibiotics should not be withheld in ill patients with a clinical diagnosis of pneumonia but an unremarkable chest X-ray. In this patient in particular, antibiotics should be initiated as soon as possible, as patients who have had splenectomies are immunosuppressed, and at increased risk for infection with encapsulated organisms.

This patient was admitted to the general medicine floor and provided with 2 liters of oxygen by nasal cannula to maintain an oxygen saturation greater than 95%. Within 48 hours the patient's respiratory status, pulse rate, and oxygen saturation had returned to normal. The nausea, vomiting, and diarrhea had resolved. Her vaccination status was confirmed with the primary medical doctor who indicated the patient had received the pneumococcal vaccine. The patient was discharged without any further complications after 5 days of therapy.

Further reading

Vardakas KZ, et al. Respiratory fluoroquinolones for the treatment of community-acquired pneumonia: a metanalysis of randomized controlled trials. *CMAJ* 2008;**179**(12):1269–77.

Sartin JS, et al. Implementing CAP guidelines: impediments and opportunities. *WMJ* 2007;**106**(4):205–10.

File TM. Community-acquired pneumonia. *Lancet* 2003;**362**:199

Halm EA, Teirstein AS. Management of community-acquired pneumonia. *N Engl J Med* 2002;**347**:2039–45.

Mandell LA, Wunderink RG, Anzueto A, et al. Infectious Diseases Society of America/American Thoracic Society Consensus Guideline on the Management of Community-Acquired Pneumonia in Adults. *Clin Infect Dis* 2007;**44**:S27–72.

Fein MJ, Auble TE, Yealy DM, et al. A prediction rule to identify low-risk patients with community-acquired pneumonia. *N Engl J Med* 1997;**336**:243–50.

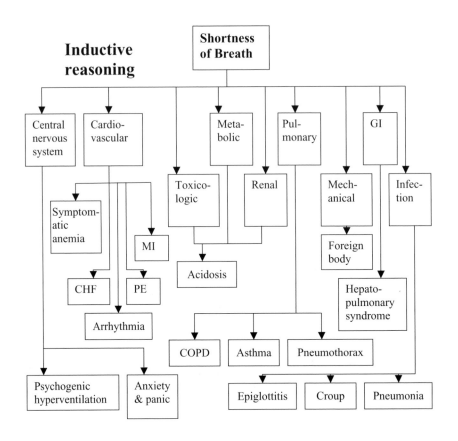

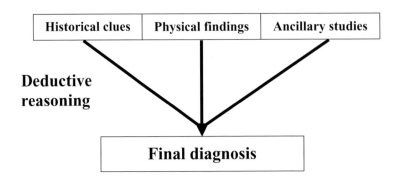

Chief complaint: traumatic injuries

Wendy DeMartino, Chad Lewis, Shellie Asher, Rebecca Jeanmonod, Mara McErlean, Donald Jeanmonod, Chame Blackburn, Edward Amores, Tyler Kenning, Ravi Ghandi

Case #1

History

> A 26-year-old helmeted male rider of a motorcycle arrives to the trauma bay by helicopter ambulance. The patient was reported to be traveling at a high rate of speed on a major highway when he lost control of his motorcycle, striking the guardrail before veering back into traffic and being hit by a car. The patient reportedly lost consciousness. He was intubated on scene for a Glasgow coma scale of 4. The patient was noted to be hypotensive by prehospital personnel with the highest heart rate of 132 and lowest blood pressure of 76/42. He has two large bore intravenous lines established and saline running in as fast as possible. Identified injuries include abrasions and contusions over the bilateral upper extremities, chest and abdomen. The patient has an open lower extremity fracture which has been splinted.

Past medical history

It is unknown whether the patient has any medical problems.

Medications

His medication use is unknown.

Allergies

It is unknown whether the patient has any allergies.

Physical exam and ancillary studies

- *Vital signs:* the patient's temperature is 36.3°C, his heart rate is 122 bpm, his blood pressure is 84/58. He is being bagged at a respiratory rate of 16, and his oxygen saturation is 98% on 100% oxygen.

Case Studies in Emergency Medicine, ed. R. Jeanmonod, M. Tomassi and D. Mayer.
Published by Cambridge University Press © Cambridge University Press 2010.

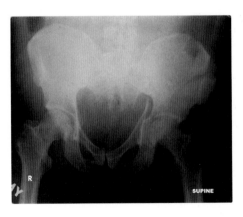

Figure 5.1. This pelvic X-ray shows multiple pelvic fractures, including the left iliac wing and left acetabulum. The pubic symphysis reveals superoinferior shift, consistent with a shearing injury and an unstable pelvis.

- *General:* the patient is on a backboard and in a cervical collar. He is intubated. He has no spontaneous movements.
- *Primary survey:* the patient is intubated with an 8–0 endotracheal tube, which is 23 cm at the lip. His breath sounds are slightly decreased on the left. He has no appreciable chest wall crepitus. The patient has weak radial and femoral pulses. There is oozing from a gauze dressing above the left ankle. There are weak dorsalis pedis pulses.
- *Head and neck:* the patient's pupils are 3 mm and reactive. His tympanic membranes are clear. There is no intraoral trauma. His neck is in a cervical collar.
- *Cardiovascular:* the patient is tachycardic, and his peripheral pulses are thready.
- *Lungs:* his breath sounds are diminished on the left. There are rhonchi noted on the left, as well.
- *Abdomen:* the patient has decreased bowel sounds. His abdomen is firm. His rectal exam reveals a normal prostate with no blood.
- *Pelvis:* the patient's pelvis is unstable to anterior–posterior compression. He has no blood at his urethral meatus.
- *Extremities and skin:* the patient has dorsal swelling at the right wrist. He has multiple abrasions and contusions of the bilateral upper extremities. There is an open fracture of the left distal tibia and fibula. His right lower extremity is unremarkable.
- *Back:* there are no step-offs or bony abnormalities on back exam.
- *Pertinent labs:* the patient's complete blood count is remarkable for a white blood cell count of 16.2 and a hematocrit of 27.4%. His electrolytes, glucose, and renal function are normal. His alkaline phosphatase is 120, his ALT is 206, and his AST is 256.
- *Imaging:* the patient's chest X-ray reveals no abnormalities. His pelvic X-ray is shown in Figure 5.1. Bedside ultrasound was performed to assist in the diagnosis of this patient. The images are shown in Figures 5.2 and 5.3.

Questions for thought

- What are the appropriate initial actions to take to stabilize this patient?
- After performing the primary and secondary surveys, what could be the immediately life-threatening diagnoses? What could be causing the hypotension?

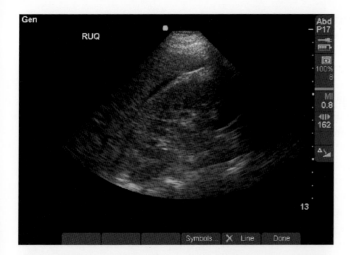

Figure 5.2. This ultrasound shows fluid (which is black, or anechoic) around the right kidney, in Morison's pouch. With this history, this probably represents blood.

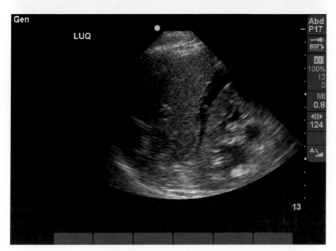

Figure 5.3. This ultrasound view shows fluid between the left kidney and the spleen, consistent with intraabdominal bleeding.

- What exam clues might suggest that hemorrhagic shock is a more likely etiology than neurogenic shock as a cause for the hypotension?
- What bedside tests can be used to assist with the diagnosis?
- How would management differ between the stable and unstable patient?

Diagnosis

Hemoperitoneum and pelvic fracture.

Discussion

- *Background:* the FAST examination stands for the Focused Assessment with Sonography for Trauma. Ultrasound has been used in the assessment of trauma patients in Europe since the late 1970s and has been used in the United States since the early 1990s. The

FAST examination consists of ultrasound views of dependent portions of the thoracic and abdominal cavities assessing for free fluid, which in the setting of trauma could represent hemoperitoneum, hemopericardium, or hemothorax. The FAST examination can be incorporated into the secondary survey to help with management decisions in the unstable trauma patient.

- *The examination:* multiple studies using CT scans or operative findings as the gold standard have demonstrated that FAST has a sensitivity in the high 80s to low 90s and specificity in the mid 90s regardless of whether the study is performed and interpreted by a radiologist, a surgeon, or an emergency physician. The standard examination consists of four views, including a right upper quadrant view of Morison's pouch, the left upper quadrant view of the splenorenal space and subphrenic space, the pelvic view of the rectovesicular pouch in men or the pouch of Douglas in women, and either the parasternal or subxiphoid cardiac view. The ultrasonographer is looking for anechoic free fluid within these quadrants, which is presumed to represent free blood in the setting of the trauma patient. The ultrasound is not sensitive for detecting encapsulated solid organ injury or injury to retroperitoneal organs. However, it is a rapidly performed, non-invasive, easily repeatable, bedside test. It offers the advantage of having no known risks to the patient, as it does not use radiation. The examination can be extended to include anterior thoracic views to detect pneumothorax with a sensitivity that is greater than the supine chest X-ray.

Clinical course

The diagnosis of intraabdominal bleeding was made by careful adherence to trauma resuscitation and evaluation guidelines, including appropriate ancillary studies.

Historical clues	Physical findings	Ancillary studies
• High-speed, unprotected motorcycle accident (MCA)	• Tachycardia	• Low hematocrit
• Prehospital tachycardia	• Hypotension	• Elevated LFTs
• Prehospital hypotension	• Left lung rhonchi	• Left pleural effusion
	• Firm abdomen	• Positive FAST exam
	• Unstable pelvis	
	• Open left ankle fracture	

Based on the findings of the FAST exam demonstrating free fluid on the right upper quadrant and left upper quadrant views and the patient's continued hypotension despite resuscitation, a decision was made to transport the patient directly to the operating room. On exploratory laparotomy, the patient was found to have active bleeding from the liver as well as the spleen. A large pelvic blood collection was noted as well. The patient underwent splenectomy and control of bleeding from the liver and pelvis and was taken to the surgical intensive care unit. Follow-up CT scans of the abdomen, pelvis and head demonstrated a renal laceration and small subdural hemorrhage.

Traumatic mechanisms can be accompanied by multiple internal and external injuries. It is very easy to become distracted by the open extremity injuries, which is part of the reason that trauma care proceeds in an algorithmic manner. In this patient, the airway had been secured in the prehospital setting. One notes the abnormal breath sounds on the left, but the patient appears to be oxygenating sufficiently. In this case, one does not pass beyond the circulation exam. Based on the physical examination, one can identify a number of potential sources of bleeding including the abdomen, the pelvis, and the open distal tibia and fibula fracture.

Further reading

Rose JS. Ultrasound in abdominal trauma. *Emerg Med Clin North Am* 2004;**22**:581–99.

Jehle D, Heller M, eds. *Ultrasonography in Trauma: The FAST*. Dallas, TX: American College of Emergency Physicians, 2003.

Case #2

History

A 3-year-old child is brought to the ED by emergency medical services. He is accompanied by his father. The father states that the child was well when he put him to bed earlier in the evening. He went to check on the child and noted the child was breathing irregularly, so he called an ambulance. The child received bag-valve-mask ventilation during the short transport to your hospital. No additional details are available other than that the child has had a recent upper respiratory infection. The child and his parents have recently re-located to this area and have not yet established primary care.

Past medical history

The child was born prematurely and had a birth weight of 3 lb 10 oz. He was in the neonatal intensive care unit, and his course was uncomplicated. He is missing his most recent set of immunizations.

Medications

The patient takes no medications.

Allergies

He has no known allergies.

Physical exam and ancillary studies

- *Vital signs:* on exam, the patient is afebrile. His heart rate is 105 bpm, he is being ventilated at a rate of 20, his blood pressure is 110/60, and his oxygen saturation is 96% with 100% oxygen.
- *General:* he is a thin, unresponsive toddler with poor muscle tone.
- *Head and neck:* the patient has no signs of trauma on initial exam.
- *Cardiovascular:* he has a regular heart rate, with faint peripheral pulses.
- *Lungs:* the patient's exam shows equal chest rise and clear lungs on bagging.
- *Extremities and skin:* his skin is cool and dry, with poor tone in all four extremities.
- *Pertinent labs:* the patient's complete blood count shows a white blood cell count of 12 000 and a hematocrit of 36.5%. His electrolyte panel is normal except for a bicarbonate of 16.
- *EKG:* his EKG shows a normal sinus rhythm with no acute changes.
- *Radiographs:* the patient's chest and arm X-rays are shown in Figures 5.4 and 5.5.

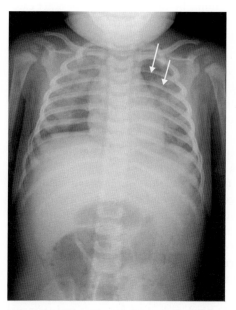

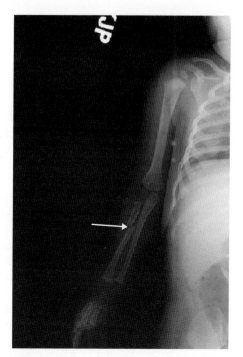

Figure 5.4. This radiograph demonstrates healing right posterior rib fractures, as evidenced by bony callus.

Figure 5.5. This radiograph demonstrates a fracture of the right radius.

Questions for thought

- What are the appropriate initial actions to take to stabilize this patient?
- Once stable, what are other diagnostic tools you can use to make a diagnosis?
- What medications should be avoided in this patient?
- How does one urgently treat this condition in the emergency department?
- What is definitive treatment of this condition?

Diagnosis

Child abuse.

Discussion

- *Epidemiology:* children 3 years of age and younger are most vulnerable to child abuse, and this age group accounts for more than 80% of fatalities. Although many more children are the victims of neglect and non-fatal abuse, a conservative estimate of the death rate due to child abuse is 2 children per 100 000. Death is most often due to head injury and frequently follows a pattern of abuse. Male caretakers are most often responsible for deaths from child abuse.

- *Pathophysiology*: most abuse occurs within the home by custodial parents or other caretakers. Abuse can be physical, emotional, sexual, any form of neglect, or any combination of these. Adult survivors of child abuse are more likely to abuse children themselves.
- *Presentation*: presentation can be dramatic, such as this case. Subsequent full examination after the child is stabilized would reveal retinal findings of hemorrhage and edema consistent with violent shaking. A more thorough physical exam after intubation would also reveal instability of the bones of the forearm. Skeletal films might demonstrate occult and healing fractures.
- *Diagnosis*: the diagnosis of child abuse is based on clinical suspicion in children who are not able to voice complaints or provide a history. Interview of parents separately, or of other family members or social contacts, might reveal inconsistencies in history that would make child advocacy workers more concerned about child abuse. The eye findings of Shaken Baby Syndrome are pathognomonic for child abuse. Multiple fractures at different stages of healing are rare except in the setting of child abuse. Fractures that occur at the metaphyses may be difficult to recognize on plain films but are diagnostic of child abuse. Transverse fractures of the forearm may correlate with defensive injuries and spiral fractures of the long bones are suggestive of twisting injuries and are rarely associated with accidental trauma.
- *Treatment*: all potential victims of child abuse need evaluation for acute and subacute injuries and general nutritional status. Evaluation for sexual abuse is performed on the basis of history and clinical suspicion. Treatment is directed at the specific injury. Subsequent determination is made as to whether the child is safe to be discharged from the ED. Referral to local or state child protective agencies is mandatory. The primary care physician should be included in all follow up plans.
- *Definitive therapy*: definitive therapy is tailored to the presenting complaint and injury.

Clinical course

This child was believed to be abused based on the inconsistency of his history, his physical exam, and the results of ancillary studies.

Historical clues	Physical findings	Ancillary studies
• History not consistent with exam findings	• Retinal findings consistent with Shaken Baby Syndrome • Exam suggestive of extremity fracture	• Fractures at various stages of healing • New transverse fracture of the forearm

This patient was recognized to require urgent airway management. He stabilized after intubation. The parents were interviewed separately and confessed to shaking the child when he would not go to sleep. He was admitted to the pediatric intensive care unit. He survived his acute injury, but required a tracheostomy for protracted ventilatory support and eventual feeding tube placement. He was placed in a chronic care facility at the time of discharge. He slowly improved in the chronic care facility. His younger siblings were placed in foster care.

Further reading

Wu SS, Ma C-X, Carter RL, et al. Risk factors for infant maltreatment: a population-based study. *Child Abuse Negl* 2004;**28**(12):1253–64.

Finkelhor D, Wolak J, Berliner L. Police reporting and professional help seeking for child crime victims: a review. *Child Maltreat* 2001;**6**(1):17–30.

Widom CS, Weiler BL, Cottler LB. Childhood victimization and drug abuse: a comparison of prospective and retrospective findings. *J Consult Clin Psychol* 1999;**67**:867–80.

Case #3

History

A 25-year-old presents to the ED complaining of left shoulder pain. The patient states that he was snowboarding earlier today when he caught an edge and fell forward on his left arm. Since that time, he has had left shoulder pain, and has been unable to move his left shoulder. The patient did not injure any other part of his body. He is right-hand dominant. He has never had a shoulder injury before. His review of systems is otherwise negative.

Past medical history

The patient has no significant past medical history.

Medications

The patient takes no medications daily.

Allergies

The patient has no known drug allergies.

Social

The patient smokes half a pack of cigarettes daily. He drinks socially. He denies recreational drug use.

Physical exam and ancillary studies

- *Vital signs:* the patient's temperature is 36.8°C, his heart rate is 88 bpm, his blood pressure is 145/81, his respiratory rate is 13, and his room air oxygen saturation is 100%.
- *General:* the patient appears to be in general good health, but also seems very uncomfortable. He is holding his left arm internally rotated, slightly abducted, and flexed at the elbow.
- *Head and neck:* the patient has no evidence of head trauma. His neck is supple and non-tender, with no jugular venous distension.
- *Cardiovascular:* his heart has a regular rate and rhythm without murmur, rub, or gallop. His injured arm has +2 radial pulse.
- *Lungs:* the patient's chest wall is non-tender with equal expansion. His lungs are clear bilaterally.
- *Abdomen:* his abdomen is soft and non-tender. There are no peritoneal signs. He has no organomegaly.
- *Extremities and skin:* the patient's extremities are warm and well perfused. He has no edema, with normal capillary refill. His left arm is non-tender to palpation. He has flattening beneath his acromion, and his humeral head is palpable anterior to the glenoid.

He is unable to range the shoulder. His elbow and wrist have intact range of motion. He has no clavicular tenderness.

- *Neurologic:* the patient's cranial nerves are intact. He has intact strength and sensation in his lower extremities, with normal deep tendon reflexes. His sensation and reflexes are intact in his upper extremities. He cannot participate in strength testing of his left upper extremity secondary to pain.
- *Pertinent labs:* no labs are performed.

Questions for thought

- What is the patient's diagnosis?
- What are other diagnostic tools you can use to make a diagnosis?
- Does the patient require additional diagnostic testing in the emergency department?
- What is the appropriate treatment of this patient in the ED?
- What is the appropriate disposition for this patient?
- What is the definitive treatment of this condition?

Diagnosis

Left anterior shoulder dislocation.

Discussion

- *Epidemiology:* shoulder dislocations account for 50% of all joint dislocations. This is probably secondary to the high mobility of the joint, and therefore its predisposition to become unstable. Shoulder dislocations are more common in people under the age of 40, and they are anterior in position 90% of the time.
- *Pathophysiology:* shoulder dislocations can be either traumatic or atraumatic. Atraumatic shoulder dislocations usually occur in people with a history of previous dislocation and those with underlying joint abnormalities. They can also occur from forceful muscle contraction, as may occur with seizure activity. Traumatic shoulder dislocations are commonly secondary to sporting injuries or major trauma. The usual mechanism is a fall directly on the shoulder or on an outstretched hand. The shoulder typically dislocates anteriorly, where the joint capsule is the thinnest. In greater than 90% of shoulder dislocations, the patient avulses the labrum from the glenoid rim (Bankart lesion), and this injury is important to identify, as it affects the treatment and prognosis of the injury.
- *Presentation:* the majority of patients present shortly after the dislocation occurs. Rarely in patients who have seized or in those who are intoxicated, presentation may be delayed hours or days. Most patients complain of pain in the shoulder, and some will have tingling in the lateral aspect of their shoulder or lower in their arm from stretch on the brachial plexus. Patients with anterior dislocations will have flattening of their shoulder just beneath the acromion, and will have the humeral head palpable anteriorly. Patients with inferior dislocations will present with their arms fully flexed and will be unable to extend their arms down to their sides. Posterior dislocations can be difficult to diagnose,

as it is more difficult to palpate the humeral head posteriorly and X-rays may be misleading. Patients with shoulder dislocation will have limited motion at the joint.

Beyond physical exam, patients will have X-ray findings consistent with a dislocated shoulder. However, when the clinical diagnosis is certain, X-rays are not always necessary. About 20% of patients with shoulder dislocations have shoulder fractures, and these are important for long-term prognosis, rehabilitation, and treatment, but have not been shown to alter ED treatment and course. Therefore, some ED practitioners do not radiograph shoulder dislocations when they are certain of the diagnosis.

- *Treatment:* treatment of shoulder dislocation is reduction of the injury. In the ED, this entails providing adequate analgesia and performing one of the many maneuvers acceptable for reduction. Analgesia can be provided by intraarticular local anesthesia, which has been shown to have reduced complications and similar success to conscious sedation. Conscious sedation is another alternative, which is usually successful, but increases the cost of the visit and the length of ED stay. Finally, there are some methods (scapular manipulation, external rotation, and the Milch technique) which are considered less painful and may be attempted without full sedation. After reduction, if the provider is certain the shoulder has been reduced, there is no indication for X-rays. Whenever possible, the patient should be placed in a splint that maintains $10°$ of external rotation at the shoulder to promote healing of the Bankart lesion. This method of immobilization has been shown to be superior to simple sling placement.
- *Definitive therapy:* all patients should be referred to orthopedic surgery. The recurrence rate of shoulder dislocation is very high. Patients under the age of 20 have a recurrence of about 90%, those under 30 have a recurrence rate of about 70%, and those under 40 have a recurrence rate of about 60%. Surgical treatment has been shown to have a better overall long-term outcome than conservative management with sling immobilization, and therefore orthopedic referral is the appropriate next step.

Clinical course

The keys to this patient's diagnosis are careful attention to history and physical exam.

Historical clues	Physical findings
• Fall on outstretched arm	• No bony tenderness
• Shoulder pain	• Flattening of shoulder contour
• Decreased range of motion	• Humeral head palpable anterior to glenoid
	• Neurovascularly intact

This patient was suspected of having an acute anterior shoulder dislocation based on his history and exam. The provider decided to forgo radiographs, as he did not want to delay the time to treating the patient. The patient received 15 mL of lidocaine injected into his shoulder joint capsule. After waiting for 10 minutes, the medical provider reduced the shoulder using external rotation. The patient was splinted in external rotation and given a prescription for pain medication.

He followed up at 5 days with orthopedics, who ordered an MRI of his shoulder. This demonstrated evidence of a Bankart lesion as well as a greater tuberosity fracture. The patient went on to have early surgical repair of his shoulder. At 6 months follow-up, he reported no disability and no recurrence.

Further reading

Chalidis B, Sachinis N, Dimitriou C, Papadopoulos P, et al. Has the management of shoulder dislocations changed over time? *Int Orthop* 2007;**31**(3):385–9.

Law BK, Yung PS, Ho EP, Chang JJ, et al. The surgical outcome of immediate arthroscopic Bankart repair for first time anterior shoulder dislocation in young active patients. *Knee Surg Sports Traumatol Arthrosc* 2008;**16**(2):188–93.

Itoi E, Hatakeyama Y, Sato T, Kido T, et al. Immobilization in external rotation after shoulder dislocation reduces risk of recurrence. A randomized controlled trial. *J Bone Joint Surg Am* 2007;**89**(10):2124–31.

Kuhn JE. Treating the initial anterior shoulder dislocation – an evidence-based medicine approach. *Sports Med Arthrosc* 2006;**14**(4):192—8.

Shuster M, Abu-Laban RB, Boyd J. Prereduction radiographs in clinically evident anterior shoulder dislocation. *Am J Emerg Med* 1999;**17**(7):653–8.

Hendey GW. Necessity of radiographs in the emergency department management of shoulder dislocations. *Ann Emerg Med* 2000;**36**(2): 108–13.

Case #4

History

A 20-year-old woman presents to the ED in the late morning stating that she suspects she has been sexually assaulted. Her memory is "fuzzy" regarding the events but says she remembers attending a party at a fraternity house near campus where she had a beer and two shots. She was much more intoxicated than she expected, having consumed similar amounts in the past with "no problem." She remembers being helped into a bedroom upstairs by "Tom," whom she had met a few times around campus. She woke this morning at the house wearing nothing but a man's T-shirt. No one was in the room with her and she immediately called a friend who came to get her and brought her here. Her physical complaints are a pounding headache, some nausea, and some discomfort in both the vaginal and anal areas. While she is waiting in the ED, she receives a text message from Tom stating "U were real good 2 me last nite."

Past medical history

The patient has no medical problems but does have a history of depression and anxiety. Her last menstrual period was 2 weeks ago. Her last consensual intercourse was 1 month ago and her usual method of contraception is condoms. She smokes cigarettes occasionally, going through a pack every week. She admits to heavy alcohol use on the weekends. She does not use illicit drugs. She is a college student living on campus.

Medications

The patient takes sertraline and zolpidem.

Allergies

She has no known drug allergies.

Physical exam and ancillary studies

- *Vital signs:* the patient's temperature is 37.0°C, her pulse is 91 bpm, her blood pressure is 111/68, her respiratory rate is 20, and her room air oxygen saturation is 99%.
- *General:* she is awake and alert but quiet. She is occasionally tearful.
- *Head and neck:* her head and neck show no signs of trauma. Her neck is supple with no midline tenderness. Her mucous membranes are slightly dry, with no lesions noted in her mouth.
- *Cardiovascular:* her heart has a regular rate and rhythm. Her pulses are normal.
- *Lungs:* the patient's lungs are clear bilaterally.
- *Extremities and skin:* her extremities are warm and dry with normal capillary refill. There are no external signs of trauma.

- *Genital:* she has normal external genitalia. She has some tenderness upon palpation of the labia minora at the posterior forchette, but there are no visible signs of injury. There is a small amount of white discharge noted in the vaginal vault. There is no cervical motion tenderness. There is some redness and tenderness around her anal area. The patient refuses a rectal exam.

Questions for thought

- What are the medical, emotional, and legal needs of this patient?
- What physical exam findings are suggestive of the diagnosis?
- What risk factors are associated with this condition?
- What are appropriate actions to treat this patient and minimize risks?
- What responsibility do you have as a medical provider to also collect evidence at the time of the exam?

Diagnosis

Drug-facilitated sexual assault.

Discussion

- *Epidemiology:* sexual assault is defined as any sexual act performed by one person (or more than one person) on another without consent. It is impossible to determine the precise epidemiology of sexual assault since actual reporting definitions vary and it is thought to be a vastly underreported crime. However, approximately 1 in 4 women and 1 in 6 men will be the victims of sexual assault in their lifetimes. The majority (50–90%) of victims know their assailant. Some risk factors include: teenage and college-aged women (3.5 times more likely to be victims of sexual assault), previous history of sexual assault, and alcohol or drug use.
- *Presentation:* some patients will present with a clear recollection of events and are able to give an adequate history of the sexual assault. However, it is very common for patients to be vague because of either embarrassment, shame, poor recollection of events secondary to emotional trauma, or memory impairment due to alcohol or drug use, including "date-rape" drugs. Other patients may present for totally unrelated or "pretense" complaints, in hopes that the medical provider may be the one to address the subject.
- *Diagnosis:* diagnosis is generally made by the patient's history. While a thorough physical exam is performed, the presence or absence of injuries (body or genital) does not confirm or exclude sexual assault. Drug-facilitated sexual assault should be suspected in patients who have amnesia, memory impairment, reports of feeling more intoxicated than expected, or had clothing or location altered without their recall.
- *Treatment:* the treatment of sexual assault patients is optimally provided by trained examiners since evaluation and forensic evidence collection can be specialized and time-intensive. Many hospitals have SAFE or SANE providers for this purpose (Sexual Assault Forensic/Nurse Examiner). However, the majority of sexual assault patients present to centers without special programs, thus it is important for all emergency providers to

be familiar with the special needs of this population. Four treatment areas need to be addressed with sexual assault patients:

1. Acute medical care – any acute conditions should be addressed (fractures, soft-tissue injuries, vomiting, etc.).
2. Psychological support – patients should be treated in an emotionally supportive manner without any personal blame implied by the provider. Optimally a rape crisis advocate or other support person should be present from the beginning.
3. Post-exposure prophylaxis – sexual assault patients are at risk for pregnancy, HIV, hepatitis, and sexually transmitted infections. All patients should be offered post-coital contraception up to 120 hours after the assault (levonorgestrel, Ovral or Plan B). HIV prophylaxis should be given as soon as possible and is generally not effective when given more than 36–72 hours after sexual assault. Patients need to complete 28 days of treatment (lamivudine/zidovudine and tenofovir). For those previously unimmunized, the hepatitis B vaccine series should be started. Medications to prevent sexually transmitted infections such as chlamydia and gonorrhea can also be offered (cefixime and doxycycline or equivalent).
4. Forensic evidence collection – patients who present to the emergency department after sexual assault within 3–7 days (depending on local protocol) should also be offered forensic evidence collection. Most states have a specialized protocol and "kit" for this purpose. Clothing, trace evidence, and swabs from the patient's mouth, vagina, anus, and other areas guided by history and exam are taken for analysis by the forensic lab. In addition, when drug-facilitated sexual assault is suspected, blood and urine samples should be collected for forensic toxicological screening.

- *Definitive therapy:* in addition to emergency care and the initiation of post-exposure prophylaxis, patients should be referred for outpatient follow-up to assess compliance and problems with medications and for testing of HIV, pregnancy, and STDs. All patients should be referred to rape crisis centers for counseling and advocacy. Providers need to cooperate with the legal system, including providing complete and clear documentation and court testimony if needed.

Clinical course

The patient's diagnosis was supported by her history and physical exam findings.

Historical clues	Physical findings
• No recollection of event	• Discharge in vagina consistent with ejaculate
• Pain in genitals	• Local genital pain and erythema

She was seen and examined in the ED and offered post-exposure prophylaxis for pregnancy, HIV, and sexually transmitted diseases. She had a rape crisis advocate present during the interview and exam and was scheduled for follow-up counseling. The patient received aid at her request in making a police report. Forensic evidence was collected and turned over to law enforcement. A DNA profile was obtained from the vaginal and perianal swabs and matched the suspect who had texted the patient. The patient also had evidence of gamma-hydroxybutyrate ingestion, a known date-rape drug. The perpetrator had bragged about the exploit to his friends, who later gave testimony against him. Initially he had insisted that the encounter was consensual but when confronted with the evidence, he agreed to a plea bargain. He served jail time and is required to register on the sex-offender registry.

Further reading

American College of Emergency Physicians. Evaluation and Management of the Sexually Assaulted or Sexually Abused Patient. October 2002. Retrieved December 20, 2008, from www.acep.org/practres.aspx?id=29562.

Centers for Disease Control and Prevention, US Department of Health and Human Services. Sexual assault and STDs. *Sexually Transmitted Diseases Treatment Guidelines*. 2006. Retrieved December 20, 2008, from www.cdc.gov/std/treatment/2006/sexual-assault.htm.

Interactive Media Laboratory, Dartmouth Medical School. Sexual assault – forensic and clinical management. A virtual clinical program based on the national protocol for sexual assault medical forensic examinations. DVD. 2008. Available at www.iafn.org.

Seneski PC, et al. *Color Atlas of Sexual Assault*. Philadelphia, PA: Mosby 1997.

US Department of Justice, Office of Violence Against Women. A national protocol for sexual assault medical forensic evaluations adults/adolescents. September 2004, NCJ 206554. Retrieved December 20, 2008, from www.ncjrs.org/pdffiles1/ovw/206554.pdf.

Case #5

History

A 23-year-old woman presents to the ED with her husband. She is bleeding from the volar aspect of her right forearm. She reportedly came home earlier that evening to find a strange woman visiting with her husband. She became enraged and punched the bathroom mirror, shattering it. Since then she has felt something "sharp" in her arm. She denies head injury or other trauma. Her last meal, consisting of two slices of pizza with soda, was approximately 3 hours before arrival.

Past medical history

She has a history of childhood asthma and has had an appendectomy. Her last tetanus vaccination was 3 years ago, given after she stepped on a nail.

Medications

The patient takes no medications. She has not used an inhaler for her asthma for over 10 years.

Allergies

She has no known allergies.

Social History

The patient drinks socially two to three times weekly. She denies tobacco or illicit drug use.

Physical exam and ancillary studies

- *Vital signs:* the patient's temperature is 36.7°C, her heart rate is 92 bpm, her blood pressure is 112/75 mmHg, her respiratory rate is 12, and she has a room air oxygen saturation of 98%.
- *General:* the patient is well-appearing, in no acute distress.
- *Head and neck:* the patient is normocephalic, atraumatic. Her cervical spine is non-tender with full range of motion. Her extraocular movements are intact, and her oropharynx is clear.
- *Chest:* there are no lesions noted upon inspection of her upper chest, back, and axillae.
- *Cardiovascular:* her heart has a regular rate and rhythm with normal heart sounds. There are no murmurs, rubs, or gallops. Her distal pulses are palpable, including bilateral radial pulses.
- *Lungs:* the chest wall has equal expansion without retractions. The patient's breath sounds are equal and clear without expiratory wheezes.
- *Abdomen:* the patient's abdomen is soft and non-tender. There are no masses or organomegaly.

- *Extremities and skin:* her skin is warm and dry. There is a slowly bleeding laceration on the volar aspect of her right arm, approximately 8 cm long. There is no pulsatile bleeding.
- *Neurologic:* the patient is moving all extremities. On detailed exam of her right upper extremity, she has full range of motion at the shoulder, elbow, and wrist. There is no palpable deformity of the radius or ulna, and no foreign body is noted with gentle palpation over the laceration. She is able to flex and extend her wrist against resistance. She can oppose her thumb to each finger, cross her second and third fingers, and abduct her thumb in the plane of her palm. She can pronate and supinate her forearm. She is able to flex and extend all metacarpophalangeal and interphalangeal joints against resistance.
- *Psychiatric:* the patient appears to be somewhat angry but is cooperative with examination. She is oriented to self, place, and time.
- *Radiographs:* an AP view of the forearm shows a triangular-shaped radio-opaque fragment of glass approximately 4 cm long and 2 cm wide at its base wedged in between the radius and ulna.
- *Bedside ultrasound:* the edge of the glass is noted to lie approximately 1.5 cm below the skin surface.

Questions for thought

- What are the appropriate techniques for removal of the foreign body?
- Why must one examine the patient's neurovascular function before and after removal?
- What is the danger of missing a retained foreign body?
- Are antibiotics indicated?
- When should this patient be seen in follow-up?
- What are the considerations involved in wound closure?

Diagnosis
Retained foreign body.

Discussion

- *Epidemiology:* it is difficult to say how often a retained foreign body in the setting of trauma is missed. In one study reviewing insurance claims over a 7 year period for retained foreign bodies, 53% of suits were for retained glass; only 35% of these patients had X-rays done to search for foreign bodies.
- *Pathophysiology:* retained foreign bodies occupy space within a natural or created cavity, exerting pressure on adjacent structures. Sharp objects such as retained glass can lacerate muscle fibers, blood vessels, or nerves. Further, foreign bodies may serve as a nidus for infection or inflammation.
- *Presentation:* most patients with a traumatic retained foreign body will have a visible wound; very thin sharp objects such as needles may be missed on physical exam. Radio-opaque objects are easily detected on X-rays, and many non-radio-opaque objects can be visualized using bedside ultrasound. Patients with a history of recent injury may not

181

be aware of a retained foreign body, possibly presenting with persistent pain, infection within a recently closed wound, or a sensation of a retained foreign body.

- *Treatment:* advanced trauma life-support protocols should be followed in patients presenting with traumatic injuries. Once stability is ensured, wounds with potential foreign bodies should be evaluated thoroughly. After neurovascular status is evaluated, the wound can be anesthetized locally to allow for careful probing. A tool such as a hemostat or forceps may make it easier to grab and remove a foreign body embedded within a wound. Caution must be taken to avoid causing further injury such as vessel or nerve laceration with object removal. If there is any doubt of complete foreign body removal after probing, X-ray imaging or bedside ultrasound should be considered. All glass and metal is radio-opaque; objects such as wood or plastic are usually detected with ultrasound. After removal, wounds can be irrigated and closed, with attention paid to bleeding vessels. Repeat neurovascular assessment is indicated, and tetanus status should be updated if necessary.
- *Definitive therapy:* follow-up care should include having the patient return for a wound check within a couple of days, especially in patients at high risk for infection, such as diabetic patients, or in high-risk wounds, such as those contaminated with dirt. Splinting may be necessary to immobilize the injury during healing. Patients should be given very specific instructions regarding the need to return to the ED for signs of infection, hematoma formation, or the development of neurologic deficits.

Clinical course

This patient was suspected of having a retained foreign body based on her mechanism of injury, and radiographs confirmed this.

Historical clues	Ancillary studies
• History of striking glass	• Foreign body visualized on plain film
• Laceration present	• Foreign body localized with bedside ultrasound

This patient was noted to have a retained foreign body with wound probing after a thorough neurovascular exam. An X-ray of her forearm demonstrated the shape, size, and orientation of the fragment of glass, which proved useful in planning removal as well as ensuring that there was only one retained foreign body. Once removed, the glass fragment was inspected and compared to the film to ensure that it was removed in its entirety. This was further confirmed with repeat bedside ultrasound evaluation, showing no other glass fragments.

The patient's wound was then irrigated and probed to look for any possible missed tendon, vessel, or muscle belly lacerations. The fascia was re-approximated with absorbable suture and the skin closed with nylon suture. Repeat neurovascular exam after closure was unchanged. Her wrist was splinted in neutral position and she was told to remove the splint in 3 days. She was asked to return in 10–14 days for suture removal, sooner if she noted any signs of infection.

Further reading

Eckerline CA, Blake J, Koury RF. Chapter 43. Puncture wounds and bites. In Tintinalli JE, Kelen GD, Stapcyznski JS, eds., *Emergency Medicine: A Comprehensive Study Guide*, 5th edition. New York: McGraw-Hill, 2000.

Case #6

History

A 26-year-old female presents to the ED via emergency medical services. She was an unbelted passenger in the rear seat of a vehicle that was rear-ended with significant intrusion into the cabin of the vehicle. The patient had to be extricated from the vehicle and was brought into the ED boarded and collared. At the time of exam, the patient complains of severe lower back pain and neck pain. She denies any loss of consciousness. She has no nausea or vomiting, visual changes, lightheadedness or dizziness, abdominal pain, or prior injuries to her back or neck. She denies any numbness or tingling in her extremities or any urinary or bowel incontinence. She states that the pain is constant and sharp and increases with any movement. She has not attempted to ambulate as she was extricated at the scene.

Past medical history

She is otherwise well.

Medications

The patient only takes birth control pills.

Allergies

She is allergic to latex.

Physical exam and ancillary studies

- *Vital signs:* the patient's temperature is 36.9°C, her blood pressure is 115/79, her pulse is 86 bpm, her respiratory rate is 16, and her oxygen saturation is 99% on room air. Her pain is rated 8/10.
- *General:* she is alert and oriented, and seems uncomfortable.
- *Head and neck:* the patient's pupils are equally round and reactive. Her head is atraumatic. She has no malocclusion or trismus. Her neck is exquisitely tender to palpation over C2 and C3 as well as the paravertebral muscles bilaterally.
- *Cardiovascular:* her heart has a regular rhythm, without murmurs, rubs, or gallops. Her radial and posterior tibial pulses are 2+ bilaterally.
- *Respiratory:* the patient's lungs are clear to auscultation with bilaterally equal breath sounds.
- *Abdomen:* her abdomen is non-tender, with normal bowel sounds. There is no seatbelt sign.
- *Musculoskeletal:* her arms and legs are non-tender with full range of motion. There is no instability or increase in pain with pelvic rocking. Her back is exquisitely tender to palpation at the T10–T11 level. There are no step-offs or deformity.

- *Neurologic:* her light touch sensation is intact. Her strength is 5/5 in her bilateral lower extremities.
- *Initial evaluation:* the patient is carefully rolled onto a slider, maintaining alignment of her spine. The decision is made to place an IV for pain management so that the patient will not have to sit up in order to drink. Plain X-rays are ordered of the patient's cervical, thoracic, and lumbar spine. She is given IV lorazepam and ketorolac for her pain. The patient receives minimal relief with those medications and is given oxycodone and cyclobenzaprine. This resolves her neck pain completely, but she continues to have severe mid-thoracic back pain.
- *Radiologic studies:* the patient's cervical and lumbar spine films show no evidence of fracture or dislocation. Her thoracic spine films shows a possible fracture to the anterosuperior aspect of the T12 vertebral body.

Questions for thought

- How can the provider clear the cervical spine clinically?
- What is the most likely fracture to occur with this mechanism of injury?
- What is the best radiologic study for confirmation of suspected spinal fracture?

Diagnosis

T12 compression fraction.

Discussion

- *Epidemiology:* motor vehicle collision is one of the most common causes of thoracic and lumbar spinal injury. The incidence of thoracolumbar fractures after blunt trauma has been cited to be as low as 2–7.5%, with 40% of these injuries related to crashes. Overall, the most common type of motor-vehicle-related spine and spinal cord injury involves the cervical spine with a 3-fold reduction of cervical spine fractures in restrained drivers. When restrained automobile occupants sustain a major spine injury, it is most commonly located in the lumbar spine. Four-fifths of front seat occupants with a motor vehicle crash-related lumbar fracture were restrained at the time of impact.
- *Pathology:* there are several different types of thoracic spine fractures. The management of thoracic fracture depends on the type. Compression fractures are usually stable, involving only the anterior column. These have a low incidence of neurologic sequelae. Management of this type of fracture is usually conservative and may involve bracing and physical or occupational therapy. A compression fracture may have a burst component leading to spinal cord damage from intrusion of the bone into the neural canal. There can also be displacement of the pedicles or fracture of the laminae with associated neurologic deficits. Management of these types of fractures will be more aggressive and may include surgical management. Chance, or flexion-distraction fractures can lead to nerve root injuries and have a higher incidence of neurologic deficit than compression or burst fractures. Fracture dislocations are usually caused by forces that cause a translation of the vertebrae leading to severe neurologic deficits.

- *Clinical presentation:* evaluation of a patient involved in a motor vehicle collision includes eliciting a careful history and systematic assessment. After airway, breathing, and circulation assessments, disability assessment requires a careful spine and neurologic examination. A patient who complains of back pain should be boarded and collared if that was not performed at the scene. The most common clinical sign of spinal injury is the presence of back pain and midline tenderness. Radiologic evaluation is indicated in those patients. CT has been found to be more sensitive than plain radiographs for evaluation of thoracolumbar spine injuries after blunt trauma. Once the fracture is identified, it is important to look for other injuries, particularly in the abdomen and chest. A patient without spine pain, no point tenderness on the spine, and no competing pain, who is neurologically stable and not intoxicated, can have their spine cleared clinically.
- *Treatment:* treatment of thoracic spine fractures depends on severity and extent of the injury. Fractures without neurologic deficit that are inherently stable can be managed conservatively. It has been said that for fractures with deviation greater than 30°, MRI should be performed to assess associated damage to the posterior ligamentous complex. In that case, surgical treatment may be indicated to stabilize the spine. Unstable fractures not requiring reduction may be treated with a rigid brace as well as bed rest. The stable type of fractures, such as compression type, can be treated with a simple extension orthosis or brace to limit flexion. Early mobilization is often combined with the bracing and therapy for earlier resolution of symptoms. More severe injuries require more rigid immobilization such as the Boston brace, which protects the spine below T7. Upper thoracic spine injuries are more difficult to treat with bracing as patients do not tolerate immobilization well. A halo may be needed for proper immobilization in non-operative treatment of the upper thoracic spine. Burst fractures and flexion-distraction injuries of the thoracic spine should be managed with the assistance of experienced spine surgeons.

Clinical course

The keys to this patient's diagnosis are careful attention to her history, physical exam, and ancillary studies.

Historical clues	Physical findings	Ancillary studies
• Recent motor vehicle trauma • Severe mid-back pain	• Tenderness over the thoracic spinous processes	• Lateral X-rays of the thoracic spine demonstrating fracture

The patient's fracture was poorly visualized on thoracic plain films, so she underwent CT. She was kept in proper alignment and put on a slider board. Since her neck pain had resolved completely and she had no pain to palpation of her neck, the c-spine collar was removed. She was given morphine 4 mg intravenously for pain. Her CT confirmed a compression fracture of the anterosuperior aspect of T12 without any fragments or intrusion into the spinal canal. A consultant from neurosurgery saw the patient and admitted her to the hospital, where she was placed in a brace. X-rays in the brace showed a stable T12 compression fracture. The patient was seen by physical therapy prior to discharge in a brace.

Further reading

Bradley LH, Paullus WC, Howe J, et al. Isolated transverse process fractures: spine service management not needed. *J Trauma* 2008;**65**(4):832–6; discussion 836.

Vives MJ, Kishan S, Asghar J, et al. Spinal injuries in pedestrians struck by motor vehicles. *J Spinal Disord Tech* 2008;**21**(4):281–7.

Markogiannakis H, Sanidas E, Messaris E, et al. Motor vehicle trauma: analysis of injury profiles by road-user category. *Emerg Med J* 2006;**23**(1):27–31.

Robertson A, Branfoot T, Barlow IF, et al. Spinal injury patterns resulting from car and motorcycle accidents. *Spine* 2002;**27**(24):2825–30.

Case #7

History

A 20-year-old male was skateboarding and fell on his outstretched hand. He complains of left wrist pain which has not improved with ibuprofen. He denies any other injuries or complaints. He has no elbow, shoulder, neck, or back pain. There is no numbness, weakness, or tingling. His pain is rated 8/10.

Past medical history

He has no significant past medical history.

Medications

He takes no daily medications. He took ibuprofen 1 hour ago.

Allergies

The patient has no known drug allergies.

Social

The patient does not use tobacco. He drinks alcohol occasionally, but has had none today. He is a full-time student.

Physical exam and ancillary studies

- *Vital signs:* the patient's temperature is 37.0°C, his heart rate is 72 bpm, his blood pressure is 136/63, his respiratory rate is 17, and his room air oxygen saturation is 100%.
- *General:* he appears uncomfortable, but is not toxic.
- *Head and neck:* the patient has no signs of trauma. His cervical spine is non-tender, with normal range of motion.
- *Cardiovascular:* his heart has a regular rate and rhythm. There is no murmur. He has equal distal pulses.
- *Lungs:* his lungs are clear without rales, wheezes, or rhonchi.
- *Abdomen:* the patient's abdomen is soft and non-tender. His bowel sounds are normal.
- *Extremities and skin:* the patient complains of pain in the left wrist. There is no obvious deformity. His distal strength, sensation, and capillary refill are normal. The radial pulse is 2+. There is tenderness at the anatomic snuffbox with minimal swelling. There is pain with axial load of the thumb. He has decreased range of motion of the wrist secondary to pain. There is an abrasion across the base of the palm, without active bleeding.

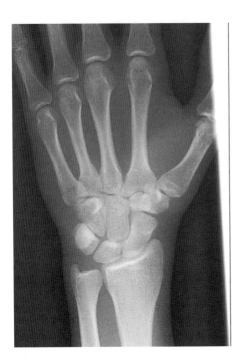

Figure 5.6. This radiograph of the left wrist was interpreted as normal.

- *Neurologic:* the patient has normal strength and sensation.
- *Radiographs:* an X-ray of the left wrist is shown in Figure 5.6.

Questions for thought

- What is your interpretation of the wrist X-ray?
- What should be your next step in management?
- What is the appropriate disposition for this patient?
- What complications should you discuss with the patient?

Diagnosis

Scaphoid fracture.

Discussion

- *Epidemiology:* the scaphoid is the most frequently fractured carpal bone. Scaphoid fractures typically occur in young and middle-aged adults.
- *Anatomy and pathophysiology:* the most common mechanism for scaphoid fracture is fall on an outstretched hand (FOOSH). The majority of fractures involve the waist of the scaphoid. The relatively poor blood supply to the scaphoid, particularly the proximal portion, increases the risk of complications after fracture.

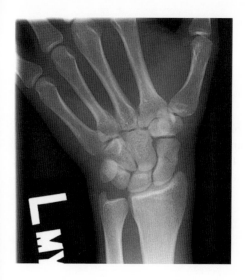

Figure 5.7. Scaphoid view of the wrist demonstrating fracture through the waist of the scaphoid.

- *Presentation:* patients typically present with wrist pain after a fall on an outstretched hand. Patients who have delayed seeking medical evaluation or who have had a missed diagnosis may present with a remote history of trauma and persistent wrist pain. Physical exam typically reveals maximal tenderness in the anatomic snuffbox, between the extensor pollicis brevis and abductor pollicis longus tendons. Pain may also be exacerbated by radial deviation of the wrist or axial loading of the first metacarpal.

- *Diagnosis:* plain-film radiography is the first line for diagnosis. Wrist X-rays should be obtained with a minimum of three views. Scaphoid views are often performed with the wrist held in ulnar deviation to elongate the scaphoid and improve accuracy (see Figure 5.7). CT scans of the wrist are sensitive for scaphoid fracture and may be done if indicated.

- *Treatment:* emergency treatment consists of pain management and immobilization of the scaphoid with a thumb spica splint or cast. Immobilization is mandatory for any patient suspected of having a scaphoid fracture, even with normal radiographs, as up to 15% of scaphoid fractures may be missed on plain film. Patients should be referred to an orthopedist or other hand surgeon for definitive immobilization and follow-up studies. Repeat plain radiography 2 weeks after injury will often show signs of healing and reveal a fracture not previously detectable by plain film.

- *Definitive therapy:* most scaphoid fractures heal with prolonged immobilization (casting). Treatment failures (non-healing) may be treated operatively.

- *Complications:* complications include malunion, delayed union, nonunion, and avascular necrosis. These may result in prolonged pain, limited wrist mobility, osteoarthritis, and decreased grip strength. The overall complication rate is increased if the patient delays seeking medical evaluation, if the fracture is missed, and if the fracture is not properly immobilized. The risk of avascular necrosis increases with more proximal fractures.

Clinical course

The keys to this patient's diagnosis are careful attention to history, physical exam, and ancillary studies.

Historical clues	Physical findings	Ancillary studies
• Fall on outstretched hand	• Anatomic snuffbox tenderness and swelling	• Wrist X-ray interpreted as normal
	• Pain with axial load of the thumb	• Additional scaphoid views reveal fracture

The patient was recognized to have a scaphoid fracture by X-ray in addition to clinical criteria of anatomic snuffbox tenderness and pain with axial load of the first metacarpal. He was placed in a thumb spica splint and referred for orthopedic follow up within 2 days. He was then casted by orthopedics and healed without complications.

Further reading

Hoynak B. Fractures, wrist. Retrieved March 5, 2008, from eMedicine.com.

Case #8

History

A 23-year-old male is brought to the ED via ambulance after being involved in a high-speed motorcycle accident. According to the emergency medical service team, the accident occurred approximately 2 hours before he was brought to the ED. The patient had full recollection of the event. He reported trying to make a right turn when the bike slid out from under him and dragged his right leg under the rear tire. The patient's major complaint is pain and deformity of the right leg. He reports that he is unable to move his knee, ankle, or foot. He is very concerned that he has been bleeding "uncontrollably" from his leg.

Past medical history

The patient has no other medical problems, but does report smoking one pack per day and socially drinks alcohol.

Medications

He takes a daily multivitamin.

Allergies

The patient has no known drug allergies.

Physical exam and ancillary studies

- *Vital signs:* the patient's temperature is 99.2°F, his heart rate is 124 bpm, his blood pressure is 108/51, his respiratory rate is 31, and his room air oxygen saturation is 99%.
- *General:* he is awake and alert.
- *Head and neck:* the patient's pupils are equally round and reactive to light, and his cranial nerves are intact. The patient's mucous membranes are moist. His neck is supple.
- *Cardiovascular:* the patient's heart has a regular tachycardia, without murmurs, rubs, or gallops.
- *Lungs:* his lungs are equal and clear bilaterally on auscultation.
- *Extremities and skin:* the patient's right lower extremity has a significant deformity 2–3 cm above the knee. The skin injury at this level is significant, with a near complete circumferential exposure. The femur is exposed and fractured through the opening and the remainder of the extremity is attached by a 4 cm skin bridge on the medial side. The ankle and toes are pale and dusky. The patient is unable to dorsiflex or plantar flex his ankle or his toes. There is no capillary refill in the nail beds of the toes. There is no palpable popliteal pulse nor Doppler pulses of the dorsalis pedis or posterior tibial arteries. The patient has no sensation below the level of the injury.

- *Pertinent labs:* the patient's complete blood count is remarkable for a white cell count of 17.6 and a hematocrit of 38.4%. The remainder of the metabolic profile and cell counts are normal.
- *Radiographs:* a radiograph of the patient's right femur shows a comminuted fracture of the distal femur at the supracondylar ridge. There is air at the fracture site. His other films are unremarkable.

Questions for thought

- What are the appropriate initial actions to take to stabilize this patient?
- Once stable, what are other diagnostic tools you can use to make a diagnosis?
- How does one urgently treat this condition in the emergency department?
- What is definitive treatment of this condition?

Diagnosis

Near complete traumatic amputation with vascular injury.

Discussion

- *Presentation:* the presentation for traumatic amputation should be immediately obvious. The patients are usually involved in high-speed motor vehicle or motorcycle accidents, industrial or farm injuries, or rifle injuries when hunting or in the military. The initial clinical efforts should be focused on the principles of stabilization: airway, breathing, circulation. Life-threatening injuries should be examined and ruled out. The fractured limb, distracting though it may be, is often not the most significant injury the patient has.
- *Additional studies:* patients with traumatic amputations should be treated as major trauma patients until proven otherwise. In addition to all clinically necessary studies, it is important to get radiographs of the amputation stump as well as the amputated part, even if it is no longer attached to the patient. Other studies such as peripheral vascular resistance (PVR) can be useful to assess the distal extent of the vascular injury. If PVR is inconclusive, angiogram can help determine vascular transection or patency. This is often an important pre-operative step, as a surgeon will need to know the vascular anatomy in order to attempt reanastomosis.
- *Consultations:* an orthopaedic surgeon should be consulted for the open fracture and to help determine management. Trauma surgery should evaluate the patient on the mechanism of injury and can also help coordinate planning for surgery and definitive care. A vascular surgeon needs to be consulted to discuss viability options for the extremity.
- *Treatment:* once all life-threatening injuries are ruled out, treatment may focus on the amputated or near-amputated extremity. Bleeding should be controlled as much as possible with compressive dressings, pressure, and elevation. If bleeding vessels of the extremity are directly visualized clamping with a hemostat is an option. The patient should be given narcotic analgesia. Antibiotics are indicated for open fractures. If the patient has not had a tetanus booster within 5 years, update is warranted.

- *Definitive therapy:* primary amputation is the treatment of choice for a nonviable limb. The risk of muscle necrosis, sepsis, renal failure, and death is very high if a nonviable limb is not removed. Replantation is an option for good surgical candidates with clean wounds who are hemodyanically stable. The Mangled Extremity Severity Score (MESS) is a scoring system that helps guide the replantation decision in the lower extremity. Points are given for advancing age, presence of shock, degree of energy and contamination of the mechanism, and degree of limb ischemia. The higher the score, the less likely replantation will be successful. Whether a limb is replanted or not, it is also important to have a rehabilitation physician and a prosthetist involved early for patient support and planning.

Clinical course

This patient's partial amputation was obvious on arrival based on his physical exam. A comprehensive diagnostic plan was initiated to rule out other injuries, which was essentially unremarkable. Vascular surgery determined that there was no blood flow to the lower extremity below the level of the injury. All attendings were present for a discussion with the patient and his family. The risk of infection, multiple reoperations, and potential for later amputation were all discussed. The patient elected to undergo a primary amputation which was performed by the orthopedic surgeon. Post-operatively, he was fitted with a prosthesis after his stump had healed. He has since been doing well, with no further complications.

Further reading

Helfet DL, et al. Limb salvage versus amputation. Preliminary results of the Mangled Extremity Severity Score. *Clin Orthop Relat Res* 1990;**256**:80–6.

Bucholz RW, Heckman JD, Court-Brown CM, eds. *Rockwood and Green's Fractures in Adults*, 6th edition. Philadelphia, PA: Lippincott Williams & Wilkins, 2006.

Case #9

History

The charge nurse receives a radio call that the air ambulance is 5 minutes out with an 18-year-old female. She is being airlifted from 100 miles up the interstate, where she had been involved in a serious motorcycle accident. According to the flight medics, she had been a passenger on a motorcycle driven by a male driver. Witnesses stated they had spun out traveling approximately 85 miles per hour and impacted a guard rail. The driver had been pronounced dead at the scene. Although she had been wearing a helmet with a face shield, the patient was not wearing any protective gear. The medics stabilized her on scene with oxygen by facemask but did not intubate her, as she was breathing spontaneously. She arrives in the ED on a backboard with a cervical collar, with two large-bore peripheral IVs in place with normal saline running wide open into each.

Past medical history

The patient's past medical history is unknown.

Medications

It is not known whether she takes any medications.

Allergies

It is unknown whether the patient has any allergies.

Physical exam and ancillary studies

- *Vital signs:* the patient's temperature is 35.9°C, her pulse is 90 bpm, her respiratory rate is 14 and labored, her blood pressure is 100/62, and her oxygen saturation is 96% on 100% oxygen via facemask.
- *General:* the patient is essentially unconscious. Her clothes are cut off. Her eyes open to sternal rub. She makes gurgling moans but does not speak, and withdraws from pain but does not localize.
- *Head and neck:* the patient's head shows no trauma. Her pupils are 6 mm and sluggishly reactive bilaterally. Her ears have a normal conus, with no blood or otorrhea. She has a nasal trumpet in her left nostril. There is ongoing epistaxis. Her oropharynx is clear. Her trachea is midline, with no jugular venous distension.
- *Cardiovascular:* the patient's heart is tachycardic and regular.
- *Lungs:* her lungs are clear to auscultation bilaterally.
- *Abdomen:* the patient has a 3×3 cm hematoma over her right abdomen. She has minimal bowel sounds. Her abdomen is otherwise non-tender and non-distended on palpation.

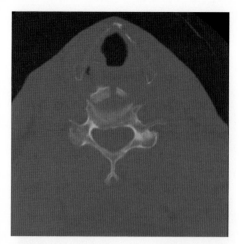

Figure 5.8. This CT of the patient's cervical spine shows disruption of the vertebral body of C5.

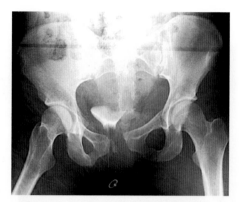

Figure 5.9. The pelvic radiograph reveals left superior and inferior rami fractures as well as disruption of the symphysis and a likely open-book pelvic fracture.

- *Extremities and skin:* all of the patient's extremities are cold and mottled. She has 1+ pulses in her right upper and lower extremities. Her left leg has a severe crush injury, but is not amputated. It is pulseless beyond the knee. Her left arm has trauma at her wrist and hand. Digits 3–5 are mutilated, and there is no radial pulse. There are no step-offs or abnormalities on spine exam. Her pelvis has slight "rock" to pressure, right greater than left.
- *Genitourinary:* the patient has good rectal tone. There is no blood at the urethra.
- *Neurology:* the patient's Glasgow coma scale (GCS) is 7. Her reflexes are normal and equal bilaterally at the patella and Achilles. Her Babinski reflex is negative.
- *Radiographs:* radiographs of the patient's pelvis, hand, and femur, as well as a representative cut from her cervical spine CT, are shown in Figures 5.8–5.11.

Questions for thought

- What is the initial approach to the patient with multi-system trauma?
- How does the emergency physician prioritize treatment of serious injuries? Which of these injuries warrant immediate treatment, and which can be triaged to later?
- What is the role of consultants in the ED, and what is their part in a trauma activation?

Diagnosis

Multi-system trauma secondary to high-speed motorcycle accident.

Discussion

- *Epidemiology:* 30% of ED visits are due to unintentional injuries (poisonings, falls, MVAs/MCAs, assaults, industrial/agricultural accidents, etc.). The prevalence of unintentional injuries has remained stable over the past 40 years, and is now increasing at a rate

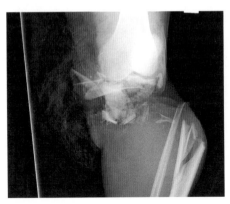

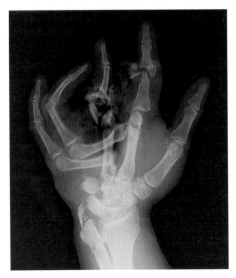

Figure 5.10. The plain film of the patient's knee demonstrates a severely comminuted open proximal tibia and fibula fracture, with greater than 100% displacement.

Figure 5.11. The patient's hand radiograph reveals multiple fractures and dislocations involving all her fingers except for her thumb as well as her ulna and several carpal bones.

of about 1% per year. As of 2005 accidents and injuries accounted for 112 000 deaths per year in the United States. Nearly 40% of these deaths were due to motor vehicle fatalities. Accidents and injuries remain the primary cause of death among persons under 45 years of age. Traumatic injuries tend to peak in the summer months, when people are outside and traveling.

- *Pathophysiology:* multi-system trauma occurs when any system in the body is exposed to high force, whether blunt or penetrating trauma. There are serious and immediately deadly conditions (airway compromise, cardiac tamponade, aortic dissection, tension pneumothorax, massive internal or external bleeding), which need to be immediately identified and treated before the less serious injuries (intracranial bleeding, spinal cord injury, extremity trauma including amputations, burns, lacerations, facial trauma) are addressed. Shock is the inability of the body to maintain adequate tissue perfusion due to hypovolemia.

- *Presentation:* the presentation of multi-trauma is broad and the best approach to the patient is to begin with a history from a family member, bystander, or prehospital personnel. Identify the cause of the trauma, pertinent facts of the trauma (passenger restraint, ejection, intrusion into passenger compartment, fatality at the scene), or any known medical condition or allergies that were pre-existing. The history from paramedics is invaluable and can give clues on the nature of the injuries sustained.

- *Diagnosis:* in the patient with multi-system trauma, the initial examination, called the primary survey, always comes first and is structured so that problems encountered are treated as they are diagnosed. The primary survey consists of:

  · Airway – does the patient have a patent, self-maintained airway, or do we need to intubate?

- Breathing – is the patient breathing spontaneously or do we need to breathe for them? Are breath sounds equal bilaterally? Is there equal chest wall motion or crepitus (a sign of flail chest)? Is the trachea midline?
- Circulation – is the patient's cardiovascular system functioning properly? Is there massive hemorrhage that must immediately be controlled? Are two large-bore IVs in place and rapidly infusing crystalloid fluids?
- Disability – is there neurologic compromise (from a fractured cervical spine or intracranial hemorrhage) which needs to be addressed? What's the patient's GCS? Are the pupils equally reactive?
- Exposure/environmental factors – is the patient fully undressed and are we addressing environmental factors (body temperature extremes) which could be imminently lethal?

This is followed by the secondary survey, in which the undressed patient is examined head to toe, including logrolling onto her side to check for back trauma and performing a quick rectal and genitourinary exam. A focused abdominal sonogram for trauma (FAST) is performed at the bedside, checking for evidence of hemorrhage.

Additional diagnostic testing includes radiographs, which are ordered based on patient complaints, physical exam findings, and nature of the mechanism. CT scan is commonly used to assess the extent of traumatic injuries to the head, neck, chest, abdomen, and pelvis.

- *Treatment:* treatment begins by securing an airway, either physically using a chin-lift or jaw-thrust maneuver, temporary oral or nasal airway or laryngeal-mask airway, or definitive with orotracheal or nasotracheal intubation or surgical crichothyrotomy. Adequate breathing may be spontaneous, but some patients require mechanical assistance. Circulation should be supported with two large-bore (16–18 gauge) peripheral IVs and warmed normal saline should be rapidly infused, with blood products given in cases of heavy bleeding. Tension pnuemothorax and hemothorax should be treated either initially by needle decompression or with a large-bore chest tube. Cardiac tamponade should be treated by needle drainage. Rarely an urgent ED thoracotomy will be required in the patient with vital signs present in the field and absent in the ED. Fractured pelvis and extremity fractures or dislocations should be splinted or placed in traction. Significant internal bleeding leading to hypotension may require immediate surgical laparotomy.

Clinical course

The approach to this patient's care included a brisk history and physical examination, intubation, fluid resuscitation, radiographic studies, and definitive trauma and orthopedic surgical care.

Historical clues	Physical findings	Ancillary studies
• History of high-speed motorcycle accident	• Depressed Glasgow coma scale	• Pelvic fracture on X-ray
• Death at the scene	• Unstable pelvis	• Cervical spine fracture on CT
• Decreased level of consciousness	• Obvious bony injuries	• Extremity fractures

Even though this patient was protecting her own airway upon arrival in the ED, her Glasgow coma scale of 7 necessitated intubation. Her secondary survey was significant for positive pelvic rock and severe left upper and lower extremity trauma, with decreased pulses in both extremities. The FAST scan was negative in all four quadrants and a Foley catheter was placed which showed normal urine without gross blood. Her pelvis was stabilized by crosstable sheeting, and her extremities were loosely splinted by the orthopedist.

This patient received aggressive fluid resuscitation. She was taken to the OR for orthopedic repair and stabilization of her cervical, pelvic, and extremity fractures. She had a head CT, which showed no injury. Post-operatively, the patient remained in the SICU until she was more awake. She had some memory deficits and cognitive problems still remaining, but was ultimately discharged to a rehabilitation facility.

Further reading

Cornwell E. Initial approach to trauma. In *Tintanelli's Emergency Medicine*, 6th edition. New York: McGraw-Hill, 2004.

Nawar EW, Niska RW, Xu J. National Hospital Ambulatory Medical Care Survey: 2005 emergency department summary. *Adv Data* 2007;**386**:1–32.

CDC Injury Data and Resources. Retrieved January 8, 2008, from www.cdc.gov/nchs/injury.htm.

Case #10

History

A 21-year-old man presents to the ED after having his right foreleg pinned between two car fenders. He was sitting on the hood of a parked car with his left foot resting on its front fender and his right leg dangling below the fender. The car parked in front of the car he was sitting on backed up to pull out of its parking spot, pinning his right foreleg between its rear fender and the front fender of the car he was sitting on. He states he "felt his bones crack," noted immediate intense pain and was unable to stand on his right leg. When he tried to put weight on his right leg, he noted the lower third of his foreleg "gave out" and formed a 90° angle. He then lifted his leg and the angle decreased to less than 20°. He called his girlfriend, who brought him in to the ED by car. He denies head injury or other trauma. His last meal, consisting of a chicken sandwich and a beer, was approximately 2 hours before arrival.

Past medical history

He has no significant past medical or surgical history.

Medications

The patient takes no medications.

Allergies

He has no known drug allergies.

Social history

The patient drinks socially 2–3 beers or drinks two nights a week. He admits occasional cigarette use when he drinks and sometimes smokes marijuana but denies other illicit drug use.

Physical exam and ancillary studies

- *Vital signs:* the patient's temperature is 37.2°C, his heart rate is 92 bpm, his blood pressure is 130/88 mmHg, his respiratory rate is 16, and his room air oxygen saturation is 99%.
- *General:* the patient appears uncomfortable and is wincing in pain. His airway, breathing, and circulation are intact.
- *Head and neck:* the patient is normocephalic with no signs of trauma. His cervical spine is non-tender with full range of motion. His extraocular movements are intact, and his oropharynx is clear.
- *Chest:* there is no injury noted upon inspection of the patient's upper chest, back, and axillae.

199

- *Cardiovascular:* his heart has a regular rate and rhythm with normal heart sounds. He has no murmurs, rubs, or gallops. His distal pulses are palpable including bilateral posterior tibial pulses.
- *Lungs:* the chest wall has equal expansion without retractions. His breath sounds are equal and clear.
- *Abdomen:* the patient's abdomen is soft and non-tender. There are no masses or organomegaly.
- *Extremities and skin:* his skin is warm and dry. There is no bruising or signs of trauma to his arms or left leg. There is bruising around the lower half of his right foreleg. There is obvious bony deformity with approximately 10° of valgus angulation of the distal third of the lower leg relative to the proximal. His right lower leg is slightly more tense to palpation than his left leg. No temperature difference or breaks in the skin are appreciated. His femoral and popliteal pulses are easily palpated bilaterally. Dorsalis pedis and posterior pulses remain palpable bilaterally although are less pronounced on the right.
- *Neurologic:* the patient is moving his upper extremities and left leg easily. He notes leg pain with passive plantar and dorsiflexion at the metatarsophalangeal joints of his right foot. He is able to wiggle the toes of his right foot but notes a slight tingling when he does so.
- *Radiographs:* an AP view of the right tibia and fibula shows a comminuted fracture of the tibia and a transverse fracture of the fibula, at approximately the junction of the middle and distal thirds of both bones.
- *Compartment pressure measurements:* compartment pressures were measured using the Stryker© Stic pressure monitor. The pressure immediately adjacent to the fracture is 22 mmHg for the anterior compartment, 25 mmHg for the deep posterior compartment, 18 mmHg for the superficial posterior compartment, and 12 mmHg for the lateral compartment.

Questions for thought

- What are the earliest signs of elevated compartment pressure?
- Why should each compartment in the area of the fracture be measured individually?
- What steps can be taken in the emergency department to decrease compartment pressures in patients at risk for compartment syndrome?
- At what compartment pressure is fasciotomy indicated, regardless of presence or absence of symptoms?
- What is the ischemic time for irreversible nerve or muscle damage?

Diagnosis

Acute compartment syndrome.

Discussion

- *Epidemiology:* it is difficult to estimate the incidence of acute compartment syndrome in traumatic injuries, as many go undetected or are underreported. Approximately 69%

of reported cases of acute compartment syndrome are due to trauma, with 36% of these occurring in the setting of tibial fractures, almost 10% occurring in the setting of distal radius fractures, and 23% being due to soft tissue injuries without fracture. Comminuted fractures pose a higher risk than non-comminuted fractures; anticoagulation also increases the risk of acute compartment syndrome in trauma.

- *Pathophysiology:* in acute compartment syndrome, increased tissue pressure within a confined osseofascial compartment impedes capillary vascular flow to below that which is necessary for tissue viability. Causes of elevated pressure include increased volume or decreased space within a compartment. As compartment pressure is increased, venous pressure is also increased, which in turn decreases the arteriovenous (A-V) gradient. Subsequently, capillaries collapse; cells become hypoxic and release proteins, causing tissue edema. With edema there is further elevation of intracompartmental pressure, greater vascular compromise and hypoxia, and further cell damage leading to eventual muscle ischemia and necrosis.
- *Presentation:* most patients with acute compartment syndrome in the setting of trauma will have a fracture noted on X-ray, although elevated compartment pressures may be seen with isolated vascular injuries not involving fractures. Clues to the development of acute compartment syndrome include pain out of proportion to injury, pain with passive stretch of involved muscles, muscle weakness, anesthesia, paresthesia, decreased two-point discrimination, swelling, and tense skin. Decreased capillary refill and decreased pulses are late findings.
- *Treatment:* advanced trauma life-support protocols should be followed in patients presenting with traumatic injuries. Once stability is ensured, injuries associated with potentially elevated compartment pressures should be thoroughly evaluated. Ask about symptoms and assess for pain with gentle passive stretching of the involved muscles. Palpate pulses, check capillary refill, assess skin temperature and tension, and complete a motor and sensory exam. Lower the leg to heart level, as elevation can reduce arterial inflow and decrease the arteriovenous gradient. Correct hypotension to improve perfusion pressure. Remove any circumferential bandages; split and spread any casts.
- *Definitive therapy:* measure compartment pressures with a catheter device such as the Stryker© Stic pressure monitor to confirm your clinical exam, trend pressures, or evaluate suspected elevated compartment pressure in the obtunded patient. Pressure measurements are most accurate when very close to the fracture site. Refer for immediate fasciotomy if intracompartmental pressure is greater than 30 mmHg without signs, lower if there are any signs of elevated pressure. Diastolic pressure minus intracompartmental pressure (Δp) of less than 30 mmHg is also an indication for fasciotomy. Permanent damage to muscle tissue may occur within 6 hours of ischemia, while peripheral nerves may be irreversibly damaged within 75 minutes.

Clinical course

The key to not missing acute compartment syndrome is maintenance of a high index of suspicion. In this case, detection of the early clues of elevated compartment pressure permitted rapid confirmation of our suspicions.

Historical clues	Physical findings	Ancillary studies
• Recent trauma with tibia and fibula fracture	• Tense skin • Pain with passive muscle stretch • Tingling with toe movement • Slightly decreased pulses	• Film showing a comminuted tibial fracture and a transverse fibular fracture • Elevated compartment pressure

This patient was found to have elevated compartment pressures in all four foreleg compartments using a Stryker© Stic pressure monitor. His leg was kept at heart level while in the emergency department and two large-bore IV lines were placed with a 1 liter bolus of lactated Ringer's solution given. Opiate analgesia was provided and the patient was placed on nothing by mouth (NPO) dietary status. Labs were drawn and sent, including CPK and myoglobin.

The patient was admitted to the orthopedic trauma service, where an external fixator was placed to align his tibial and fibular fractures. Fasciotomy of all four foreleg compartments was accomplished with a single lateral incision overlying the middle and distal fibula, deepened anteriorly and posteriorly to decompress all four compartments. The patient eventually needed skin grafting to close the fasciotomy site but showed no permanent motor or sensory deficits.

Further reading

Ruiz E. Chapter 270. Compartment syndromes. In Tintinalli JE, Kelen GD Stapcyznski JS, eds., *Emergency Medicine: A Comprehensive Study Guide*, 5th edition. New York: McGraw-Hill, 2000.

Case #11

History

A 22-year-old male presents to the ED after falling approximately 15 feet to the ground. The patient was drinking alcohol at a fraternity party when one of his friends accidentally shoved him over the railing of a second-storey deck. Emergency medical service responders found him lying on his back. He was complaining of severe neck pain and could not move his extremities. He complained of numbness in his arms and legs. He had an abrasion on his right shoulder but no other external signs of trauma. He appears intoxicated but denies loss of consciousness and remembers the details of the fall. The paramedics applied a cervical collar, placed the patient on a rigid backboard, and transported him to the ED.

Past medical history

The patient has moderate persistent asthma that has been treated since childhood. He has seasonal allergies to pollen and some grasses.

Medications

The patient's medications include ranitidine, advair, and albuterol.

Allergies

He has no known drug allergies.

Physical exam and ancillary studies

- *Vital signs:* the patient's current temperature is 38.4°C. His blood pressure is 92/56 mmHg, his pulse is 58 bpm, his respiratory rate is 26, and his oxygen saturation is 96% on 2 liters of nasal cannula oxygen.
- *General:* the patient is anxious and appears intoxicated. He is in moderate distress. He has shallow respirations and is breathing rapidly.
- *Head and neck:* the patient's pupils are equal, round, and reactive to light. He has no hemotympanum or periorbital ecchymosis. The patient's neck has tenderness to palpation from C4 to C6. There is palpable deformity at C5. The trachea is midline and there is no crepitus.
- *Cardiovascular:* the patient's heart is bradycardic with a normal S1 and S2. He has no murmur, rub, or gallop.
- *Respiratory:* the patient's breath sounds are equal bilaterally. He has mild expiratory wheezing throughout both lung fields. There are no rales or rhonchi.
- *Abdomen:* the patient's abdomen is soft, non-tender to palpation, and non-distended. His bowel sounds are normal.
- *GU/rectal:* the patient has no rectal tone. There is no gross blood on digital rectal exam.

- *Extremities:* his hips are stable to compression and extraction. The patient is able to raise his shoulders but cannot lift his arms against gravity. His lower extremities are flaccid.
- *Skin:* the patient's skin is pink, warm, and dry to the touch. There is a 2 cm superficial abrasion on his right shoulder.
- *Neurologic:* the patient's cranial nerves are intact. The patient loses sensation approximately 2 inches above the nipple line bilaterally. He has some sensation in the arms. The patient has minimal biceps brachii reflexes. The rest of the patient's deep tendon reflexes are absent.
- *Pertinent labs:* the patient's blood work is unremarkable except for a pCO_2 of 55 and pH of 7.28. The patient's bicarbonate is 25.
- *EKG:* the patient's EKG shows sinus bradycardia with a normal axis and no ectopy.
- *Ultrasound:* the patient's bedside FAST exam is negative for free fluid.
- *Radiographs:* the patient's chest X-ray shows decreased lung expansion. The CT scan of his cervical spine demonstrates a C5–C6 fracture-dislocation with marked anterior and lateral compression of the spinal cord at that level.

Questions for thought

- What type of injury does this history suggest?
- What are the most common causes of this type of injury and who is at risk?
- Why is this patient's heart rate and blood pressure low in this time of emergency?
- Why are the patient's respirations rapid and shallow?

Diagnosis

Traumatic spinal cord injury (TSCI).

Discussion

- *Epidemiology:* traumatic spinal cord injury in the United States has an incidence of 40 per million persons per year. The most common causes of TSCI are high-speed motor vehicle crashes, falls from height, violence, and sports-related. Males continue to constitute 80% of cases. The most frequent victim of TSCI is a young male with a median age of 38. Alcohol is involved in approximately 25% of cases. Patients with underlying disease of the spine such as spinal arthropathy, cervical spondylosis, and osteoporosis are more susceptible to traumatic spinal cord injury.
- *Pathophysiology:* most spinal cord injuries occur in conjunction with vertebral column injury. The spinal cord can be damaged when vertebral bones are fractured or joints are dislocated. Most vertebral injuries involve both fractures and dislocations. The type of fracture and spinal cord injury sustained is dependent on the amount and direction of force applied to the vertebra at the time of injury. Certain types of fractures are considered unstable and are more likely to cause spinal cord injury if they are not stabilized. The spinal cord can also be injured when spinal ligaments are torn. Disrupted or herniated intervertebral disks can compress the spinal cord and cause injury and ischemia.

The pathophysiology of TSCI is often divided into primary and secondary injury. The primary SCI occurs at the time of the trauma and is caused by the forces applied to the spinal canal. These forces cause pathologic compression, flexion, extension, and/or rotation of the spine. The traumatic forces to the spine can result in compression, contusion, and/or shear injury to the spinal cord. The spinal cord may appear radiographically and pathologically normal immediately following the primary SCI. Secondary SCI is thought to be caused by the body's natural inflammatory response to injury. Secondary injury begins within minutes of the SCI and evolves over several hours. The mechanism of this type of injury is not completely understood. It is thought to be related to ischemia, edema, hypoxia, excitotoxicity, apoptosis, and abnormal ion exchange. Secondary injury may present as progressive neurologic deterioration in a patient with an incomplete SCI. Maximal cord edema develops from day 3 to 6 and begins to recede around day 9. Central hemorrhagic necrosis often replaces cord edema.

- *Presentation:* alert patients with spinal cord injury often have pain at the site of bony fracture. Many patients will have brain and systemic injuries in addition to TSCI. These patients may have a limited ability to report their symptoms. A high level of suspicion based on mechanism (fall from height, high-speed motor vehicle crash, electrical injury) is necessary. Approximately 50% of TSCI involve the cervical spine and result in quadriplegia or quadriparesis.

Patients with complete spinal cord injuries tend to have sensation spared above the level of the injury. They have decreased sensation in the level immediately below the injury. Below this level, their sensation is absent. There is no sensation from S2–S4 (no sacral sparing). A patient with a complete cord injury will have decreased motor function of the muscles supplied by the cord immediately below the site of injury and complete paralysis of the more caudally supplied muscles. Their muscles are flaccid and deep tendon reflexes are absent in the acute setting. Males with complete cord injury may develop priapism and lack a bulbocavernosus reflex. Complete cord injured patients usually develop urinary retention.

A patient with an incomplete spinal cord injury may have various degrees of sensation and motor function preserved caudal to the level of injury. Frequently sensation is preserved to a greater extent than motor function due to the more protected, peripheral location of the sensory tracts in the spinal cord. The patient's anal sensation is intact and the bulbocavernosus reflex is present.

Patients with a central cord syndrome will present with greater impairment of motor strength in the upper extremities than the lower extremities. This is a forced hyperextension injury that usually occurs in the elderly patient with spondylosis or spinal stenosis. These patients have a variable loss of bladder function and sensation caudal to the injury. Anterior cord syndrome is caused by a hyperflexion injury that disrupts blood flow in the anterior spinal artery. Patients with this type of spinal cord injury will present with loss of pain and temperature sensation and complete paralysis of their muscles distal to the lesion. These patients will have preserved dorsal column function and will be able to sense vibration, light touch, and position. A patient with a penetrating injury to the spinal cord may present with hemisection of the cord, a syndrome known as Brown-Séquard. The patient with this injury will have motor paralysis and loss of dorsal column function ipsilateral and distal to the injury. This patient will experience loss of pain and temperature sensation contralateral and distal to the injury.

The patient with a spinal cord injury may experience spinal shock immediately after the trauma. Spinal shock is a condition in which the patient temporarily loses all spinal reflexes below the level of the injury. The patient may become bradycardic and hypotensive. The sympathetic motor neurons exiting the spinal cord from T1 to L2 cannot stimulate the patient's heart to increase its rate or strength of contraction. These same neurons are unable to stimulate vasoconstriction and the patient's systolic blood pressure can drop, decreasing blood flow and putting the patient into shock. Loss of sympathetic motor stimulation to the sweat glands makes it difficult for patients to sweat and release heat produced by the body and may cause fever. The patient may have flaccid paralysis, anesthesia, and absent bowel and bladder control. Male patients may develop priapism. This altered state may persist for several weeks.

- *Treatment:* the initial evaluation and management of TSCI patients focuses on the ABCDs (airway, breathing, circulation, and disability). Unstable injuries are immobilized and the extent of the patient's injuries is evaluated. Patients with bradycardia may require pacing and atropine. Hypotensive patients may require intravenous fluids and vasopressors. All patients with TSCI should be screened for bladder distension. Methylprednisolone 30 mg/kg followed by 5.4 mg/(kg h) over 23 hours is the only treatment that has been suggested to improve clinical outcomes in patients with non-penetrating TSCI. The evidence is limited and use is debated. If given to patients within 8 hours of primary SCI, treatment with glucocorticoids is thought to reduce cord edema, prevent potassium depletion, and promote neurologic recovery. Treatment with glucocorticoids is a treatment option, not a treatment standard.

- *Definitive therapy:* all patients with TSCI should have complete spinal imaging. They require neurosurgical consultation to evaluate the need for decompression and stabilization. The application of traction with skull tongs or a halo headpiece should be decided in consultation with a neurosurgeon. Early surgery is indicated in patients who fail to maintain reduction or continue to have compression despite reduction. It is also indicated in patients who have bony encroachment despite reduction. Early surgery is required in patients who have incomplete sensorimotor loss and failure of closed reduction. Acute TSCI patients require ICU admission for cardiovascular and respiratory monitoring. Patients should receive deep venous thrombosis and stress ulcer prophylaxis, pain control, and early physiotherapy.

Clinical course

The keys to this patient's diagnosis are the careful attention to history, recognition of an abnormal neurologic exam, and radiographic findings.

Historical clues	Physical findings	Ancillary studies
• Fall from height	• Cervical spine pain and deformity	• CT scan showing C5-C6 fracture-dislocation
• Neck pain	• Abnormal neurologic exam	
• Numbness of extremities	• Spinal shock	

CT scan performed upon arrival demonstrated a fracture-dislocation at the C5–C6 vertebra. The patient was transferred to the intensive care unit after the neurosurgeon immobilized his neck using skull tongs. Surgical decompression and stabilization of the cervical spine was performed the following evening. Weakness of the patient's diaphragm and chest wall muscles led to difficulty breathing and the patient was intubated. The patient failed extubation and tracheostomy was performed on his tenth hospital day. The patient had no change in his arm strength or sensation but developed marked spasms and exaggerated lower-extremity deep tendon reflexes. The patient's urinary incontinence was controlled by placement of a Foley catheter. When he no longer required assisted ventilation, the patient was transferred to a long-term care facility.

Further reading

Dawodu ST. Spinal cord injury: definition, epidemiology, pathophysiology. www.Emedicine.com. February, 2007.

Baron BJ, Scalea TM. Spinal cord injuries. In Tintinalli JE, Kelen GD, Stapczynski JS, et al., eds., *Tintinalli's Emergency Medicine: A Comprehensive Study Guide*, 6th edition. New York: McGraw-Hill, 2004, pp. 1569–82.

Tator CH. Update on the pathophysiology and pathology of acute spinal cord injury. *Brain Pathol* 1995;5:407.

American Academy of Emergency Medicine. Position statement: steroids in acute spinal cord injury. Available at: www.aaem.org/positionstatements.

Chief complaint: eye, ear, nose, and throat complaints

Sandra Maruszak, Alexandra L. Chomut, Luke T. Day, Martin O'Malley,
Christopher Brook, Dan Pauze, Wendy DeMartino, Rebecca Jeanmonod,
Tim Barcomb, Michelle P. Tomassi

Case #1

HPI

A 56-year-old female reports sudden onset of pain in her left jaw while chewing nuts, approximately 2 hours ago. She states her dentist mentioned the filling in her left molar showed a small crack during her last visit and had recommended a crown. She localizes the pain to this tooth. She reports that drinking cold liquids and chewing on the affected side increase the pain. She denies any difficulty swallowing. She tried taking acetaminophen, but experienced little relief from the pain. She has not noted any bleeding from the tooth and states she is otherwise healthy and has no other complaints.

Past medical history

The patient states she has no medical problems and denies any surgeries.

Medications

She does not regularly take any medications, but reports taking 1000 mg of acetaminophen after the incident today.

Allergies

She has no known drug allergies.

Physical exam

- *Vital signs:* the patient's temperature is 36.4°C, her heart rate is 86 bpm, her blood pressure is 138/81, her respiratory rate is 14, and her room air oxygen saturation is 99%.
- *General:* she is a pleasant, cooperative female who appears uncomfortable.
- *Head and neck:* there are no signs of trauma. The patient's oropharynx is patent with no erythema or edema. She has moist mucous membranes. She has multiple large fillings in

Case Studies in Emergency Medicine, ed. R. Jeanmonod, M. Tomassi and D. Mayer.
Published by Cambridge University Press © Cambridge University Press 2010.

her molars but no erythema, lacerations, or edema noted. Bite alignment is normal. Her left lower first molar (#19) is tender to tapping with a tongue blade. A fracture extending from the lingual to the buccal surface with exposed dentin is observed but no bleeding is noted. There are no skin changes to the face or jaw.

Questions for thought

- What is the appropriate treatment for this patient?
- What would be worrisome physical findings in a dental pain patient?
- What would be worrisome comorbidities in a dental pain patient?

Diagnosis

Dental fracture.

Discussion

- *Epidemiology:* dental trauma is common in children. The maxillary central incisors are most commonly injured in falls and collisions. Adults frequently have stress fractures, which are more common in the molars. Risk increases with age, the presence of extensive restoration, and parafunctional habits, such as teeth-grinding.
- *Pathophysiology:* the crown is the visible portion of the tooth and is covered by white enamel. Dentin underlies the enamel and is creamy yellow in color. The inner portion of the tooth contains pulp, nerves, and blood vessels. The primary function of the pulp is to make dentin.

    Dental fractures are commonly classified by the Ellis classification system. Ellis class I fractures involve only the enamel. Ellis class II involve the dentin, and class III fractures expose pulp.
- *Presentation:* patients with Ellis class I fractures may have sharp edges along the fracture line that can be irritating to the tongue or mucosa. Ellis class II fractures account for 70% of fractures. Patients frequently experience sensitivity to hot and cold stimuli. In addition, the creamy yellow dentin will be visible. Ellis class III fractures will reveal bleeding from the pulp. If the tooth is wiped dry with sterile gauze, blood or redness should be seen, identifying the fracture as a class III.
- *Diagnosis:* panoramic radiographs (Panorex) can help assess fractures but are not available in all emergency departments. If the fracture was associated with trauma, additional imaging, such as facial CT may be warranted.
- *Treatment:* Ellis class I fractures can be filed, smoothing sharp edges for patient comfort. Class II fractures need to be covered to help prevent pulpal necrosis (although the pulp is not directly exposed in a class II fracture, depending on the amount of dentin lost, the pulp may be contaminated). A glass ionomer dental cement or calcium hydroxide paste, covered with aluminum foil, is the most common treatment to prevent contamination and provide pain relief. Current studies are finding success using topical application of 2-octyl cyanoacrylate (Dermabond) to glue tooth fragments together until the patient can undergo definitive treatment. Patients will need pain medication and, depending

upon how quickly they can be seen by the dentist, may require antibiotics. Oral penicillin 500 mg 4 times daily or clindamycin 300 mg 4 times daily can be taken for uncomplicated infections. Oral pain medications, soft diet, and ice packs to the affected cheek may reduce pain. In patients with significant secondary infection, evidenced by sinusitis, severe trismus, or skin changes, admission may be warranted. Other at-risk populations are those who are immunosupressed from medications, malignancies, or diabetes.

- *Definitive therapy:* patients with Ellis class II or III fractures need to be directed to a dentist for definitive care. Tooth vitality is greatest with rapid treatment by a dentist and referral within 24 hours is recommended.

Clinical course

This patient's diagnosis was evident based on her history and physical exam.

Historical clues	Physical findings
• Previous dental work	• Dental fracture visualized
• History of dental crack	• No secondary infection
• Pain after chewing on nuts	

The patient's tooth was covered with calcium hydroxide paste and aluminum foil and the patient was discharged home with a scheduled follow-up to her dentist the next day. Ultimately, the tooth was crowned without further complications.

Further reading

Hile LM, Linklater DR. Use of 2-octyl cyanoacrylate for the repair of a fractured molar tooth. *Ann Emerg Med* 2006;**47**(5).

Sullivan DD. Initial care for fractures, luxations, and avulsions: prompt recognition and swift, appropriate – and often simple – action can improve the prognosis of many dental injuries. *J Am Acad Physician Assist* 2002;**15**(9):48(6).

Auerback P. *Wilderness Emergencies*, 5th edition, Philadelphia, PA: Mosby Elsevier, 2007.

Tintinalli JE, Kelen DG, Stapczynski JS, eds. *Emergency Medicine: A Comprehensive Study Guide*. New York: McGraw-Hill, 2004.

Rodriguez D, Sarlani E. Decision making for the patient who presents with acute dental pain. *AACN Clin Issues* 2005;**16**(3):359–72.

Ceallaigh PO, Ekanaykaee K, Beirne CJ, Patton DW. Diagnosis and management of common maxillofacial injuries in the emergency department. Part 5 dentoalveolar injuries. *Emerg Med J* 2006;**24**:429–30.

Case #2

History

A 44-year-old man presents to the ED complaining of double vision especially when he looks up. He first noticed it yesterday. He also says that the left side of his face has "felt funny." He explains that last week he was hit in the eye with a baseball when his 10-year-old son and he were playing catch together. He had not been paying attention and the ball hit him straight in the face. The patient states that he immediately put an ice pack on it and his wife took him to the urgent care center, where his eye began to swell. The physician at the urgent care center told him to take ibuprofen to decrease the swelling and keep ice on it and that in a few days the swelling would go down. The patient did just that and stated that the swelling "really started to come down" in the last few days. This is when he noticed the double vision. He has not noted a change in his visual acuity. He denies loss of consciousness, headache, eye pain, or discharge or bleeding from the eye.

Past medical history

The patient has a history of anxiety and seasonal allergies but is otherwise healthy. The patient quit smoking 10 years ago and has a 10 pack-year history.

Medications

The patient takes alprazolam and ranitidine as needed.

Allergies

The patient has no known drug allergies.

Physical exam and ancillary studies

- *Vital signs:* the patient's temperature is 36.8°C, his heart rate is 72 bpm, his blood pressure is 135/86, his respiratory rate is 12, and his room air oxygen saturation is 98%.
- *General:* he is awake and alert, in no acute distress, sitting comfortably.
- *Head and neck:* on head exam, the patient has a left periorbital ecchymosis. He also has enophthalmos and depression of his left globe. There is some left orbital crepitus. He has decreased extraocular movement of the left eye especially in the upward direction. His pupils are equally round and reactive to light with normal corneal reflexes. The patient has decreased sensation over the left cheek. All other cranial nerves are intact. His neck is atraumatic with a midline trachea.

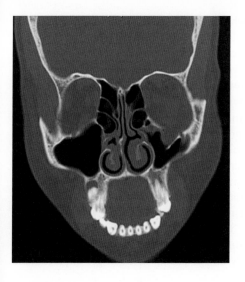

Figure 6.1. This CT shows a coronal section of the patient's face. On the left, there is an inferior orbital wall fracture with herniation of orbital contents, probably including the inferior rectus muscle. Image courtesy of Dr. Edward Wladis, used with permission.

- *Cardiovascular:* the patient's heart has a regular rate and rhythm, with no murmurs appreciated.
- *Lungs:* his lungs are clear bilaterally.
- *Extremities and skin:* he has no other signs of trauma.
- *Radiographs:* a representative cut from the patient's facial CT is shown in Figure 6.1.

Questions for thought

- What in the history would make this a likely diagnosis?
- What are other injuries that could present similarly?
- What diagnostic tools can you use to determine the extent of the injury?
- How should you manage this patient?
- Does anyone else need to be consulted?
- What are potential complications of this type of injury?

Diagnosis

Orbital floor "blowout" fracture.

Discussion

- *Epidemiology:* this is the most common simple fracture of the orbit. Males are nearly four times more likely than females to have this type of injury. The most common causes are due to assault, motor vehicle accidents, and sports injuries. This type of injury is less common in children because of differences in face shape and increased amounts of subcutaneous fat.

- *Pathophysiology*: blowout fractures occur when a force strikes the lid and globe causing retropulsion of the orbital contents. This leads to an increase in intraorbital pressure
  resulting in orbital floor rupture, as this is the thinnest orbital wall. Orbital contents can
  be displaced inferiorly into the maxillary sinus. Although orbital floor blowouts are by far
  the most common, medial orbital wall blowout (ethmoid bone) as well as the zygomatic
  and orbital apex blowouts have been documented.
- *Presentation*: our patient's presentation is common for patients with blowout fracture as a
  result of injury or trauma. Patients typically present with decreased visual acuity, diplopia
  especially on upward gaze and restricted ocular movement. Enophthalmos or proptosis
  due to swelling may be identified. Patients may also note altered sensation in the infraor-
  bital nerve distribution. Periorbital edema and ecchymosis are likely and orbital crepitus
  may be present. Patients may present immediately or a few days to a week after the initial
  injury after the swelling has gone down when they first notice diplopia, decreased visual
  acuity or restricted ocular movement. The "white eyed" fracture (medial wall blowout
  with entrapment of eye muscles) is more common in the pediatric population because
  the flexible orbital floor makes it more likely for the orbital tissue to get displaced and
  trapped.
- *Diagnosis*: imaging must be done to accurately diagnose a blowout fracture and determine whether other structures are involved. The Caldwell frontal view and Water's view
  of the orbital floors on X-ray are the most useful plain-film views. An AP view can also
  be done. CT scans can give physicians and surgeons a more detailed picture of the injury
  incurred and delineate whether there is any involvement of surrounding structures, especially entrapment of the inferior rectus, as this is an indication for surgery. Forced duc-
  tions can also be performed to evaluate the inferior rectus muscle. A complete eye exam
  should be done in the ED as nearly one-third of patients with blowout fractures will suffer
  ocular damage including abrasion, hyphema, retinal tear, or lens dislocation.
- *Treatment*: most fractures do not require surgical repair. Immediate surgery is indicated
  if there is entrapment of the inferior rectus muscle, early enophthalmos or a "white-eyed"
  blowout fracture. If there is no entrapment in a patient with diplopia, surgical repair is
  indicated if the diplopis is still present after 2 weeks. If there is no entrapment, the patient
  may be referred to ophthalmology, plastic surgery, or otolaryngology within 2 weeks.
  Approximately half of these patients will not require any surgical treatment. When the
  swelling decreases the injury can be better evaluated. All patients with blowout fracture
  should be referred to ophthalmology for a full dilated ophthalmologic exam to rule out
  eye injury. Patients should be put on oral antibiotics (cephalexin), and oral steroids to
  decrease inflammation and minimize fibrosis. A nasal spray should be given and patients
  should be advised not to blow their nose as the increase in pressure may cause contents
  from the sinuses to extrude into the orbit.
- *Definitive therapy*: the indications and timing of surgical repair are highly debated. If
  exophthalmos or diplopia persists after 2 weeks, surgery is indicated. Surgical repair using
  silicon, titanium mesh, Teflon or medphor is used to repair the orbital floor.

Clinical course

The keys to this patient's diagnosis are careful attention to the history, physical exam, and
radiologic studies.

Historical clues	Physical findings	Radiologic studies
• Recent history of orbital trauma	• Periorbital ecchymosis	• Head CT with axial and coronal 2.0 mm cuts demonstrate left inferior rectus entrapment
• History of periorbital edema	• Limited ocular movement	
• Worsening symptoms with decreased swelling	• Enophthalmos and depression	
• Facial paresthesia	• Orbital crepitus	

This man was diagnosed with blowout fracture with inferior rectus entrapment and was referred to oculoplastics and underwent surgical fracture repair. The surgery was performed through the conjunctiva. He did not have any complications with the surgery, no eyelid retraction, bruising or ectropion; however, he continued to have left-side facial paresthesia for another 6 months before it completely resolved. Two weeks after surgery he returned to the ophthalmologist for follow-up, where his exam was normal. His diplopia resolved, and his ocular movements and visual acuity were within normal limits.

Further reading

Burnstine MA. Clinical recommendations for repair of isolated orbital floor fractures: an evidence-based analysis. *Ophthalmology* 2002;**109**(7):1207–10.

Jordan DR, et al. Intervention within days for some orbital floor fractures: the white-eyed blowout. *Ophthal Plast Reconstr Surg* 1998;**14**(6):379–90.

Mitchell J. Chapter 238. Ocular emergencies. In *Tintinalli's Emergency Medicine*. New York: McGraw-Hill, 2004.

Sharma V, et al. A review of epidemiology, clinical presentations and management of blowout fractures. *All India Opthalmological Society Conference Proceedings: Orbit/Plastic Surgery Session*, 2006, p. 406.

Case #3

History

A 24-year-old male is brought into the ED by the ambulance from the local prison for the chief complaint of jaw pain. He is accompanied into the ED by two Department of Corrections officers, who state that he had been in an altercation with a fellow inmate. He had been pushed to the floor, striking his chin on the ground (interestingly, the other inmate is in another examination room with multiple facial lacerations). Since that time he has been able to talk only in muffled, but intelligible, sentences. Through writing, he states that he is not having trouble breathing or swallowing. He states that he did not lose consciousness. He reports that his vision is normal and that he has no pain on eye movements. His face has no numbness or weakness. He feels his teeth are not meeting normally.

Past medical history

According to the medical records from the prison, the patient is in good health, with no significant past medical or social history. He does not know when he last received a tetanus booster.

Medications

The patient takes no medications.

Allergies

The patient has no known drug allergies.

Physical exam and ancillary studies

- *Vital signs:* the patient's temperature is 36.4°C, his pulse is 90 bpm, his respiratory rate is 16, his blood pressure is 136/100, his oxygen saturation is 98% on room air, and his pain is rated 8/10.
- *General:* he is an awake and alert, well-developed, well-nourished male resting in bed in slight distress secondary to pain.
- *Head and neck:* the patient has blood leaking from the corner of his mouth. There is edema surrounding the angle of his right jaw. He has pain on palpation bilaterally under the corners of his jaw, right greater than left. The patient's skull and facial bones are grossly normal to palpation bilaterally. His mandible has crepitus and pain to palpation at the symphysis and right angle. There is no condylar tenderness. His mouth fills with blood without obvious source after suctioning. There is no facial elongation. There is no movement or instability with facial "rocking." He has no epistaxis. There is no rhinorrhea or otorrhea. On inserting a tongue blade between the patient's teeth and asking him to hold it tightly by biting, he is unable to hold it firmly and complains of pain.

- *Cardiovascular:* the patient has a regular rate and rhythm.
- *Lungs:* his lungs are clear to auscultation bilaterally.
- *Abdomen:* the patient has no abdominal tenderness. His bowel sounds are normal.
- *Extremities and skin:* there is no pain or midline tenderness along the length of his spine. There are abrasions and bruising over the dorsal surfaces of both hands and forearms.
- *Neurologic:* the patient is awake, alert, and oriented, with a Glasgow coma scale of 15. His cranial nerves are grossly intact. His vision is 20/30 bilaterally. His pupils are equally round and reactive to light. The patient is unable to masticate normally. He cannot smile or frown, but can open and close his eyelids and wrinkle his forehead.
- *Radiographs:* the patient's panorax mandible X-ray reveals a simple, non-displaced fracture midline at the the mental symphysis, and a comminuted, displaced fracture at the right mandibular angle. CT of his head and face demonstrates no other injuries.

Questions for thought

- For what other serious injuries do you need to evaluate in this patient?
- What is the initial approach to the patient with facial and skull injuries?
- What is the radiographic approach to a patient with this presentation?
- What is the disposition and treatment of this patient?
- How do you deal with patients who are victims of assault, and how do you ensure safety of the patient and staff in a closed environment such as the ED?

Diagnosis

Mandibular fracture.

Discussion

- *Epidemiology:* although the mandible is the strongest of the facial bones, it is also the second most commonly fractured, with only nasal bone injuries occurring more frequently. Physical assaults and falls onto the point of the jaw are the most common causes. The epidemiology of facial fractures differs depending on environment; whereas in urban areas assault is more common, in rural settings motor vehicle crashes and sporting injuries predominate. As assault is a common cause of facial and head trauma, if there is any suspicion (i.e. mechanism not consistent with injury) the practitioner should attempt to sensitively determine the true cause of the injuries, including questions about assault and domestic violence. If there is the slightest concern for child or elder abuse, it is mandated that the police and social services be contacted by the physician.
- *Pathophysiology:* the ring shape of the mandible lends itself to fractures at multiple points along the bone, as a force at one point will cause a torque stress along the entire jawline. Thus, more than 50% of such fractures are multiple. A mandibular fracture may occasionally be a clinical diagnosis, made without radiographs. However, if there is significant mechanism, the possibility of other facial, skull, and cervical fractures should be considered. In many cases, radiographs will need to be ordered to exclude these other injuries.

- *Presentation:* the history of blunt trauma to the jaw or face along with mandibular pain and the complaint of malocclusion (where the teeth feel like they "don't fit together right") is specific for mandibular fractures. Other clinical signs include bruising at the angle of the jaw (pathognomonic), deformity, facial "widening," crepitus, lower lip numbness, point tenderness to palpation, open or "step-off" fractures, blood in the mouth, and dental trauma including missing teeth. In evaluating any patient with head and face trauma the absolute first priority is to ensure that the patient has a patent airway, is well ventilated, and does not have any other life-threatening injuries, as the mechanism of facial fractures is often significant enough to cause other injuries. For example, in the fractured jaw the resulting *flail mandible* allows the tongue to collapse into the back of the throat and obstruct it, or loose teeth and blood could be swallowed and aspirated. Other concerns in the patient with this injury include mandibular dislocations, facial fractures (maxillary, orbital, or nasal), skull fractures, and intracranial and ophthalmologic injuries.

  Once assured that airway and breathing are patent, life-threatening injuries are stabilized, and the cervical spine is cleared clinically or radiographically, common facial fractures should be evaluated by history and physical exam. The skull and face should be examined for any asymmetry, crepitus, depressions, ecchymosis, pain, or facial elongation. Nasal fractures are the most common, and are a clinical diagnosis. Edema, tenderness, deformity, and epistaxis confirm the diagnosis, and radiographs are unnecessary unless there is concern about the adjacent orbit. One catastrophic injury which needs to be ruled out is a maxillary or *Le Fort* fracture, in which part or all of the midface bones separate from their mooring to the skull, leading to facial instability, airway compromise and possible central nervous system injury. This fracture should be considered when the face appears "elongated" and the bones of the roof of the mouth can be "rocked" up and down. Check the nose and ears for any sign of cerebrospinal fluid leaks. The famous "Battles Sign" and "Racoon Eyes," significant for basilar skull fractures, are relatively late findings, and not sensitive enough for an urgent diagnosis.

- *Diagnosis:* in making the diagnosis, the most specific complaint is of malocclusion in the setting of trauma. In the physical exam, the examiner should perform a tongue-blade test, in which a wooden tongue depressor is placed between the patient's clenched teeth, and twisted. In the patient without a fracture the blade will twist and break. However, a patient with a fractured jaw will immediately open the mouth to avoid the pain. This test is 95% sensitive and 65% specific for mandibular fractures. Plain films will demonstrate maxillofacial and mandibular injury. The dental panoramic view offers the best plain-film view of the mandible, but is often bypassed in favor of CT scan, which may be more readily available. CT scans are standard in evaluating and ruling out concomitant orbital, nasal and maxillary fractures.

- *Treatment:* in treating the patient with a suspected mandibular fracture, airway, breathing, and circulation take priority. Suction the mouth if blood or loose teeth are present. Simple maneuvers such as a chin lift (in the patient without concern for cervical injury) or jaw thrust (in the patient with suspected c-spine involvement) are sufficient. The practitioner can place a temporizing device such as a nasopharyngeal airway (avoid in mid-face trauma for fear of penetrating the central nervous system), or physically pull the tongue out of the back of the throat with a piece of gauze. If concern for the airway persists rapidly prepare for intubation, with materials for a surgical cricothyroidotomy on hand should it be unsuccessful.

The patient should receive proper analgesia. Some patients will have improved pain control with a Barton bandage, which is simply an Ace bandage wrapped around the head to splint the jaw in a position of comfort. Antibiotics are given to all patients prophylactically to prevent infections due to anaerobic oral flora; options include penicillin G, amoxicillin or clindamycin. Supportive care is generally sufficient. Disposition is based on the severity and number of fractures. Isolated mandibular fractures can be referred to an outpatient otolaryngologist, maxillofacial surgeon, and/or dentist. Patients with comorbidities or difficult-to-control pain will need to be admitted to the hospital.

Clinical course

The approach to this patient's care included an attentive approach to his history and physical examination, which were pathognomonic for an isolated mandible fracture.

Historical clues	Physical exam	Ancillary studies
• History of fall onto point of jaw	• Pain and crepitus to palpation at right angle of jaw	• Panorax with mandibular fracture
• Complaint of malocclusion	• Positive Tongue Blade Test	• No other injuries identified on CT
• No difficulty breathing, changes in vision, or extraocular pain		

The patient was treated with 10 mg of intravenous morphine, which decreased his pain to a 3/10. He was treated with 600 mg of clindamycin IV. He was given a tetanus booster; this is standard of practice in any patient with an open wound who does not know their immunization status. Otolaryngology was consulted and admitted the patient for surgical reduction and fixation. The wounds on his hands and forearms, secondary to covering his head during the assault, were cleaned and bandaged.

The patient was accompanied by two Department of Corrections officers and was cooperative throughout the encounter. However, due to the presence in the ED of another person involved in the altercation, hospital security was brought in to ensure departmental safety. This approach is often necessary when multiple patients involved in accidents or fights come into the ED at the same time, and not only ensures the security of ED physicians, staff, and students, but also ensures the safety of patients from each other, should tempers flare again.

It is important to remember that you will encounter all types of patients in the emergency department, from all socioeconomic and cultural backgrounds. Some will be difficult, some will be docile, some will be heartening, some will be saddening. It is the mark of a true practitioner of the craft to be able to treat all patients with dignity and respect, assuming nothing about the circumstance that brought them into the ED. This diversity of patients and pathologies is what makes the ED such a fascinating place, and should be embraced. Besides, after taking care of this patient, we were lucky enough to be able to walk down the hall and suture his assailant's facial lacerations, and he was nice enough to ask whether the other patient was doing ok!

Further reading

Tintanelli's Emergency Medicine, 6th edition. New York: McGraw-Hill, 2004.

Case #4

History

A 28-year-old male presents to the ED complaining of redness, tearing, and mild decrease in vision in his right eye. The patient reports that about 24 hours prior he was sharpening a chain-saw blade using a grinder. The patient states that while he was grinding the blade the grinder kicked back and he felt a sensation of "something hitting my eye." He tried to flush his eyes with some contact lens solution he had, and the eye "seemed better for a while." He states today his vision seems a little more blurry and he thinks he may still have something in his eye. He has some mild photophobia, mild blurring of his vision in the right eye, and he notes significant redness to his eye. On review of systems the patient reports that he has started to experience some increasing nausea since arrival.

Past medical history

The patient had his appendix out when he was 22 years old. He is otherwise healthy.

Medications

The patient is not taking any medications currently.

Allergies

The patient has no known drug allergies.

Physical exam and ancillary studies

- *Vital signs:* the patient's temperature is 36.2°C, his heart rate is 75 bpm, his blood pressure is 119/70, his respiratory rate is 15, and his room air oxygen saturation is 100%.
- *General:* the patient is awake and alert. He is squinting his right eye in the ED lights.
- *Head and neck:* the patient's right pupil is mildly sluggish on reactivity testing. He has a normal, round, and reactive left pupil. There is no relative afferent pupillary defect. There is no hyphema seen on exam. With fluorescein application there appears to be a linear area of staining in the nasal aspect of the cornea. The pupil appears slightly irregular.
- *Vision:* the patient's acuity is 20/400 in his right eye, 20/20 in his left eye without corrective lenses.
- *Radiographs:* a representative cut from the patient's facial CT is shown in Figure 6.2.

Questions for thought

- What are the initial tools you would use to evaluate this patient?
- What are the appropriate initial actions to take to stabilize this patient?

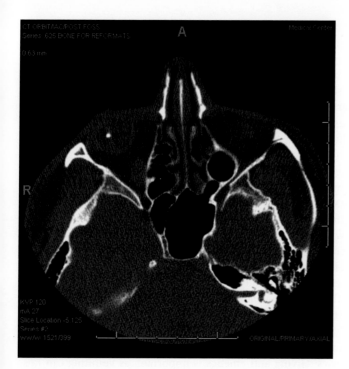

Figure 6.2. This CT scan shows a metallic foreign body in the posterior segment of the patient's right eye.

- Once the preliminary diagnosis has been made what other tests should be ordered?
- What other questions might you want to ask?
- What medications should be avoided in this patient?
- How does one urgently treat this condition in ED?
- What is definitive treatment of this condition?
- Why is this patient's vision decreased?

Diagnosis

Penetrating globe injury to right eye.

Discussion

- *Epidemiology:* any time a patient describes an eye injury sustained during activities such as striking metal on metal, high-speed grinding, or other activities that may produce high-velocity projectiles, there is a significant risk of penetrating or lacerating globe trauma and this type of injury should always be suspected and considered.
- *Pathophysiology:* a small shard or piece of the material being worked with enters the globe at high speed. Small metallic foreign bodies may violate the globe with minimal disruption of the external parenchyma, making a high index of suspicion critical to the diagnosis.

- *Presentation:* an irregular or peaked pupil can indicate penetrating or perforating injury. The pupil may be peaked toward the location of the globe wound. The presence of 360° subconjunctival hemorrhage should also raise suspicion of a full-thickness ocular injury, and the physician should be careful not to place any pressure on the eye. In cases where there are obvious signs of significant globe trauma, it may be best to obtain imaging studies before attempting to pry open a swollen lid to assess the globe.
- *Diagnosis:* if the diagnosis is in question, the primary issues that should raise suspicion of a more serious injury include decreased vision, an abnormally shaped pupil, and hyphema. Additionally, the history of high-speed grinding is suspicious for a possible retained intraocular foreign body. It is important to document the patient's visual acuity in both eyes and attempt assessment of pinhole vision in any eye when the acuity is less than 20/20. When the vision is decreased and a perforated globe is suspected, further exam should be deferred until consultation with an ophthalmologist is obtained. Further examination in this case will probably need to be carried out in an operating room, so it is important to give the patient nothing by mouth until assessment is completed.
- *Further workup:* the current diagnostic study of choice is CT of the orbits. When ordering a CT for ocular injuries an optimal study includes axial and coronal views with thin (1–1.5 mm) cuts through the orbits. This should include axial and direct coronal views or coronal reconstructions. It is felt that with modern CT scanners wooden foreign bodies can be assessed adequately, as well.
- *Treatment:* broad-spectrum antibiotics and pain management are important first steps to treatment of these injuries. Giving anti-emetics is important, as vomiting can raise intraocular pressure. The provider should immediately place a metal or plastic shield over the eye and instruct the patient not to touch the eye.
- *Definitive therapy:* in this particular case, the most appropriate ED actions are to avoid any pressure on the eye, shield the eye, place the patient on bed rest, avoid Valsalva maneuvers, and obtain urgent consultation with an ophthalmologist. This case presents a surgical emergency and further exam, exploration, and treatment are best carried out in an operating room setting.

Clinical course

The patient's diagnosis was suspected based on careful attention to his history and physical exam, and was confirmed with imaging studies.

Historical clues	Physical findings	Ancillary studies
• High-velocity metal grinding mechanism	• Decreased visual acuity	• CT demonstrating ocular foreign body
• Decreased visual acuity	• Irregular pupil	
• Eye pain	• Decreased pupillary reactivity	
• Nausea	• Fluorescein uptake in a linear distribution consistent with corneal laceration	

The patient was given broad-spectrum antibiotics, analgesics, and anti-emetics in the ED. Ophthalmology was consulted. The patient was taken to the operating room for further examination and foreign body removal. The patient remained in the hospital for several days. On follow-up, he continues to have decreased vision in his right eye, but it is much improved as compared to the time of his initial visit. He now wears goggles when working with machinery.

Further reading

Kuhn F, Pieramici D. *Ocular Trauma: Principles and Practice*. Thieme, 2002.

Chern KC. *Emergency Ophthalmology: a Rapid Treatment Guide*. New York: McGraw-Hill, 2002.

Case #5

History

An 8-year-old African-American boy is brought in to the emergency department in the early hours of Monday morning. His parents explain that he started developing right ear pain on Friday, which was similar to prior ear infections. They thought it could wait to see the pediatrician until Monday morning, but during the night he started complaining of severe pain in his right ear and they noticed a "rash" behind the ear. He did not sleep and his fever climbed throughout the night, so they decided to bring him in this morning.

Past medical history

The patient was born full-term and is up to date with all of his immunizations. He has had multiple ear infections in the past, but they have all resolved with antibiotics. He also has a history of diabetes mellitus type 1.

Medications

The patient is taking insulin for his diabetes, but no other prescribed medications. He was given the "normal dose" of acetaminophen at home just prior to coming to the ED.

Allergies

The patient is allergic to penicillin as per his mother, who says that he got a rash when he was given amoxicillin for a prior ear infection.

Physical exam and ancillary studies

- *Vital signs:* the patient's temperature is 39.7°C, his heart rate is 130 bpm, his blood pressure is 85/52, his respiratory rate is 30, and his room air oxygen saturation is 100%.
- *General:* the patient is awake and alert, and in moderate distress. He is crying and holding his hand over his right ear while leaning against his mother.
- *Head and neck:* his pupils are equally round and reactive to light, with intact cranial nerves. The patient's mucous membranes are dry, and his neck is supple. His left tympanic membrane is clear to otoscopic examination, and right tympanic membrane is bulging and appears to have purulent fluid behind it. The patient has a tender 2×3 cm area of erythema and fluctuance posterior to the right auricle overlying the mastoid bone.
- *Cardiovascular:* the patient has a regular tachycardia without rubs or murmurs.
- *Lungs:* he is breathing regularly, and his lungs are clear to auscultation bilaterally.
- *Extremities and skin:* the patient's extremity exam is unremarkable, and his skin is warm to the touch.
- *Pertinent abnormal labs:* the patient's complete blood count is remarkable for a white blood cell count of 15 500, with 75% neutrophils, 19% lymphocytes, and 4% bands.

Questions for thought

- What are the appropriate initial actions to take with this patient?
- How can a definitive diagnosis be made?
- How does one treat this condition in the emergency department?
- What are some of the complications of this disease?

Diagnosis

Mastoiditis with subperiosteal abscess.

Discussion

- *Epidemiology:* acute otitis media (AOM) is a common entity in the pediatric population and is often seen in the ED. It is estimated that almost every child suffers from one case of AOM in his lifetime, although some children are more prone to developing recurrent infections. Risk factors for AOM include exposure to other children at a child care facility, exposure to second-hand smoke, and structural abnormalities of the ear canal and middle ear. The most commonly isolated organisms in AOM are *Streptococcus pneumoniae*, *Moraxella catarrhalis*, and *Haemophilus influenzae*. Other pathogens often isolated in chronic otitis media include *Staphylococcus aureus*, *Pseudomonas aueruginosa*, and *Proteus mirabilis*. High rates of antibiotic resistance have been documented in most species, and resistance should be considered when initiating antibiotic therapy. Mastoiditis is rare in the antibiotic era, but it is still one of the more common complications of otitis media and presents a serious risk to the health of the patient.
- *Pathophysiology:* AOM often occurs in children after an upper respiratory tract infection as a direct result of eustachian tube dysfunction. Organisms from the nasopharynx take advantage of this dysfunction, colonizing the middle ear, and causing infection and inflammation. Usually, infection of the middle ear resolves on its own without antimicrobial therapy, and many medical experts adhere to a watchful waiting policy in older patients. However, in a small percentage of cases, infection can spread directly into the mastoid air cells, which are connected with the tympanic cavity, leading to accumulation of pus and the necrosis of the mastoid bone (termed coalescence). If the infection worsens, it can lead to abscess formation within the subperiosteal space, causing fluctuance posterior to the auricle, and it can also initiate the development of an abscess in the occipital region (Citelli's abscess) or the neck (Bezold's abscess). Other important complications of AOM include meningitis, brain abscess, facial nerve paralysis, and labyrinthitis.
- *Presentation:* the typical patient with mastoiditis is a pediatric patient presenting with a history of middle ear infection. The patient will often have a fever, signs of otalgia, including tugging on their ears, and possibly a history of recurrent ear infections. As in this case, physical examination of this patient may reveal posterior spread of the infection into the mastoid bone, with swelling, erythema, and tenderness in the overlying tissue. The presence of fluctuance indicates development of a subperiosteal abscess, which can spread further into the occipital region and the neck. Otoscopic inspection of the ear canal and

tympanic membrane may reveal erythema or dullness of the membrane, the presence of a middle ear effusion, or fullness of the posterior ear canal.

- *Treatment:* all patients with mastoiditis should be started on intravenous antibiotics that cover for the common AOM pathogens, and this should be begun as soon as possible. These patients should then be admitted to the hospital for observation and management by an otolaryngologist.
- *Definitive therapy:* definitive therapy for mastoiditis varies, and can range from conservative management with only IV antibiotics to surgical intervention. Typically children are admitted and tried on conservative management, and, if they do not improve rapidly, are treated with a cortical mastoidectomy. Patients with more severe disease, indicated by coalescence of the infection and necrosis of the mastoid, are treated with complete mastoidectomy and myringotomy.

Clinical course

The keys to this patient's diagnosis are careful attention to his history, physical exam, and ancillary studies.

Historical clues	Physical findings	Ancillary studies
• Chronic ear infections	• Bulging TM, middle ear effusion	• Elevated WBC with left shift
• High fever	• Tender, fluctuant area posterior to the auricle	
• Ear pain	• Warm skin	
• "Rash" behind the patient's ear		

The patient was suspected of having mastoiditis based on his history and physical exam findings. He underwent CT of his head and neck, which supported his clinical diagnosis by showing fluid in his mastoid air cells and evidence of subperiosteal abscess. Upon confirmation of the diagnosis, the practitioner started IV cefuroxime and admitted the patient to the otolaryngology department. The patient was monitored for 24 hours, but did not show signs of improvement, so a cortical mastoidectomy was performed. After surgery, he was continued on antibiotics, and the infection resolved without further complications.

Further reading

Stone CK, Humpries RL, eds. *Current Diagnosis and Treatment: Emergency Medicine*, 6th edition. New York: McGraw-Hill, 2008.

Lalwani AK. *Current Diagnosis & Treatment in Otolaryngology – Head & Neck Surgery*, 2nd edition. New York: McGraw-Hill, 2008.

Agrawal S, Husein M, MacRae D. Complications of otitis media: an evolving state. *J Otolaryngol* 2005;**34**(Suppl 1):S33.

Eskin B. Should children with otitis media be treated with antibiotics? *Ann Emerg Med* 2004;**44**:537.

Case #6

History

A 68-year-old female on warfarin for atrial fibrillation presents to the ED with 3 hours of a continuous nosebleed. The patient states that she has been bleeding mostly from her right nostril with only scant amounts from her left nostril. She has a minimal amount of blood going down her throat. She has held pressure but is unable to completely stop the bleeding. She has no lightheadedness, weakness, fatigue, or chest pain. She has been on warfarin for several years and has had no recent change in her medication, with an INR last week measured at 2.1. She denies any history of trauma or prior epistaxis.

Past medical history

The patient has atrial fibrillation, hypertension, hyperlipidemia, and coronary artery disease.

Medications

Her medications include a baby aspirin, warfarin, atenolol, and atorvastatin.

Allergies

The patient has no known drug allergies.

Physical exam and ancillary studies

- *Vital signs:* the patient's temperature is 36.2°C, her heart rate is 86 bpm, her blood pressure is 152/92, her respiratory rate is 18, and her room air oxygen saturation is 97%.
- *General:* the patient is awake and alert, interactive and pleasant.
- *Head and neck:* she is holding a small cloth over her right nare. Upon removal there is a small amount of oozing from that nare. She has no blood or friable tissue in the left nare and no active bleeding seen in the posterior pharynx. There is no conjunctival pallor. The patient's sclerae are anicteric. Her cranial nerves have normal function.
- *Cardiovascular:* the patient has an irregular rhythm. She has strong distal pulses. There is no clubbing or cyanosis.
- *Extremities and skin:* she has trace bilateral edema, with no clubbing or cyanosis. Her capillary refill is less than 2 seconds distally. Her skin is warm and dry without any purpura or petechiae.
- *Pertinent labs:* the patient's labs are remarkable for an INR of 2.2 and a hematocrit of 40%. The remainder are normal.

Questions for thought

- What are the appropriate initial actions to take to stabilize this patient?
- Once stable, what are other diagnostic tools you can use to make a diagnosis?
- How does one urgently treat this condition in the emergency department?
- What are some definitive treatments of this condition?
- What are some of the potential complications of treating this patient?

Diagnosis

Anterior epistaxis.

Discussion

- *Epidemiology:* epistaxis is a very common complaint encountered in the ED setting. It is seen most commonly in children under 10 and adults older than 50.
- *Pathophysiology:* epistaxis is typically divided into two anatomical distributions, anterior and posterior bleeding. Anterior bleeds are by far the more common and originate most commonly along the nasal septum along a branch of arteries known as Kiesselbach's plexus and less commonly along the inferior turbinate. Posterior bleeds originate from the posterior aspect of the sphenopalatine artery. Nasal irritation, trauma and local infections are the most common causes of bleeding. Several conditions may contribute as well, such as iatrogenic coagulopathies or bleeding disorders, vascular malformations, tumors, nasal steroids, and alcohol use. Foreign body must always be considered, especially in the infant and toddler.
- *Presentation:* most cases of epistaxis are controlled at home and only a minority present to the ED. Patients may present after bleeding for a few minutes or for hours. Bleeding may be coming from one nostril or both and may be entering the throat. Patients with prolonged or massive epistaxis may present with signs of anemia and even hemodynamic instability. Delineation of an anterior versus posterior bleed is imperative. Anterior bleeds, such as in this patient, typically occur from one nare and have minimal amount of blood seen in the posterior pharynx. Posterior bleeds may protrude from both nares and often exhibit continued bleeding down into the posterior pharynx even when packed anteriorly. Obtaining hematocrit levels and markers of coagulation is not necessary unless clinically indicated by prolonged bleeding, symptoms or signs of anemia, or anticoagulant use.
- *Treatment:* treatment includes stopping, localizing, and then eradicating the bleed. Contributing conditions such as coagulopathies need to be addressed. Initial arrest of the bleed can often be performed with pressure by squeezing the nares together and leaning the head forward. Should this not work, cotton pledgets soaked with viscous lidocaine and a vasoconstrictor such as oxymetazoline can be placed into the nares to create hemostasis. After 30 min, these can be removed to further delineate the site of the bleed. If there is a small and discrete lesion readily identified, chemical cautery can be attempted, typically with silver nitrate sticks. Extensive or bilateral septal cautery should be avoided as it may

lead to skin necrosis or septal perforation. Should there be a more brisk bleed, immediate tamponade may be necessary with nasal tampons, Vaseline gauze or epistaxis-specific balloon catheters. The opposite nare may also need to be packed to create a counteracting pressure. A posterior source should be considered when anterior packing does not resolve the epistaxis. Posterior tamponade can be done with a Foley catheter, or, if available, a specialized balloon catheter. It may need to be performed in conjunction with anterior packing to stop the bleed. Massive epistaxis may require airway intervention and fluid or blood product administration to ensure hemodynamic stability.

- *Definitive therapy:* most patients with controlled bleeding, such as in this patient, can be safely sent home with otolaryngology follow-up in 1 to 2 days. At that point a more definitive examination can take place to exclude possible tumors, vascular malformations, or other contributing causes. Should there be persistent or uncontrollable bleeding, urgent consultation with an otolarnygologist is warranted. Sometimes patients require urgent operative intervention or angiographic embolization. Most posterior bleeds which have been packed require hospitalization for observation. For those patients who do go home with packing, systemic antibiotics may be prescribed for prophylaxis against possible toxic shock syndrome although this is of unproven benefit.

Clinical course

The keys to this patient's diagnosis are careful attention to her history, physical exam, and ancillary studies.

Historical clues	Physical findings	Ancillary studies
• On warfarin	• No posterior pharyngeal bleeding	• Elevated INR
• Only one nare involved	• One nare involvement	
• No prior history		
• No recent trauma		

This patient's exam was consistent with an anterior nose bleed. This diagnosis is entirely clinical. It was believed that her warfarin was contributing to the bleeding, so labs were checked in the ED. Her right nare was packed initially with cotton pledgets which were soaked in viscous lidocaine and oxymetazoline. Removal of the pledgets after 30 minutes revealed a large area of excoriation with only very mild active bleeding along the septal wall. The patient was then packed with a balloon tamponade and observed. No further bleeding was observed. Because the patient was not supertherapeutic on her warfarin and because the bleeding was easily controlled, there was no need for urgent reversal of her coagulopathy. She was sent home to follow up with an otolarnygologist and had no further recurrence.

Further reading

Douglas R, Wormald P. Update on epistaxis. *Curr Opin Otolaryngol Head Neck Surg* 2007;**15**:180–3.

Leong S, Roe R, et al. No frills management of epistaxis. *Emerg Med J* 2005;**22**:470–2.

Pallin D, Chng Y, et al. Epidemiology of epistaxis in US emergency departments, 1992 to 2001. *Ann Emerg Med* 2005;**46**(1):77–81.

Case #7

History

A 42-year-old female who has had a right-sided sore throat for the last week presents to the ED. She states that the pain is getting steadily worse, and she's starting to have difficulty opening her mouth all the way. The patient has not had a runny nose or cough. She denies any fevers, nausea, vomiting, or difficulty swallowing. She has no shortness of breath. She works as a nurse and therefore has numerous sick contacts.

Past medical history

The patient has a history of poorly controlled seizures. She also has a remote history of pulmonary embolus. She gives a history of frequent sore throats, with a previous history of having an abscess "somewhere in my mouth."

Medications

The patient takes carbemazepine, warfarin, trazadone, and levetiracetam.

Allergies

This patient has no known drug allergies.

Physical exam and ancillary studies

- *Vital signs:* the patient's temperature is 37.2°C, her heart rate is 90 bpm, her respiratory rate is 20, her blood pressure is 150/85, and her room air oxygen saturation is 98%.
- *General:* she is awake and alert, and non-toxic-appearing. There is no respiratory distress.
- *Head and neck:* the patient's head is normocephalic and atraumatic. Her pupils are equal, round, and reactive to light. She has moist oral mucosa. She has some mild trismus. Her trachea is midline. The patient's tympanic membranes are clear. She has an enlarged and erythematous right peritonsillar area. There are no exudates. However, the area is hard and very tender to palpation. Her uvula is slightly deviated to the left.
- *Cardiovascular:* the patient's heart has a regular rate and rhythm. There are no murmurs, rubs, or gallops.
- *Lungs:* her lungs are clear to auscultation bilaterally, without wheezes, rales, or rhonchi.
- *Abdomen:* the patient's abdomen is soft, non-tender, and non-distended, with normal bowel sounds.
- *Extremities and skin:* the patient has no petechiae or other lesions. Her skin is warm and dry.

Questions for thought

- What is the cause of this patient's pain?
- How do these patients usually present?
- What is the appropriate ED therapy for this patient?
- What are some complications of this process?

Diagnosis

Right peritonsillar abscess.

Discussion

- *Epidemiology:* peritonsillar abscess is the most common deep space infection in the head and neck, with approximately 45 000 cases annually. It consists of a collection of purulent material between the tonsillar capsule and superior constrictor and palatopharyngeus muscles. Pharyngitis is often the inciting event and an abscess can occur even after treatment with antibiotics. Risk factors for abscess formation include chronic tonsillitis, multiple trials of antibiotics and previous abscess. It is most commonly seen in 20–30 year-olds. There is equal male to female incidence ratio. Although primarily unilateral, it may be bilateral. Identification of organisms is not necessary for treatment, but typically aerobic and anaerobic flora are grown out from cultures.

- *Pathophysiology:* peritonsillar abscesses typically start as superficial infections and spread to become deep infections. Abscesses primarily form at the superior pole on the tonsils after an episode of tonsillitis; however, the exact mechanism is not known. The most common aerobic pathogen is *Streptococcus*, while the most common anaerobic pathogen is *Prevotella* and *Peptostreptococcus*. Complications include airway obstruction, rupture of abscess with aspiration of the contents, cavernous sinus thrombosis, epiglottitis, septicemia, endocarditis, retropharyngeal abscess, and mediastinitis.

- *Presentation:* symptoms usually begin 3–5 days prior to evaluation and include fever, malaise, "hot potato" voice, sore throat, odynophagia, dysphagia, otalgia, and neck pain. Sometimes, however, patients have more chronic infections, and present with pain only, as with our patient. Physical examination signs include trismus, inferior and medial displacement of tonsils, tonsillar erythema or exudate, localized fluctuance, contralateral deflection of swollen uvula, palatal edema, tender cervical lymphadenopathy, drooling, tachycardia, and dehydration. The diagnosis is typically clinical, although soft tissue X-ray of the neck may be helpful to rule out other pathology. If unsure, CT with intravenous contrast or ultrasound of the tonsil may confirm the diagnosis, but this is usually not necessary.

- *Treatment:* needle aspiration, incision and drainage, and tonsillectomy are treatment choices. Tonsillectomy is usually delayed until the abscess is healed to prevent surgical complications. Needle aspiration is the least invasive and effectively treats 85% of patients, but is somewhat controversial, as incision and drainage has a higher success rate. If aspiration is negative then a CT should be done to rule out parapharyngeal or retropharyngeal space disease. Antibiotic therapy should follow these procedures. Appropriate antibiotics include penicillin or clindamycin for patients with penicillin allergies. Due to streptococcus resistance, metronidazole may be added to penicillin. Some studies also suggest the use of steroids to help with pain control and trismus. Close follow-up with otolaryngology is important if there is no improvement noted 24 hours after the procedure.

Clinical course

The keys to this patient's diagnosis are her history and physical exam.

Historical clues	Physical findings
• Throat pain	• Peritonsillar fullness
• Difficulty with mouth opening	• Peritonsillar tenderness
• History of prior abscess	• Trismus
	• Uvula deviation

The patient was suspected of having a chronic peritonsillar abscess because of her physical exam findings. She had a paucity of systemic complaints, which if present are more suggestive of an acute infection. She underwent needle aspiration of her peritonsillar space with an 18 gauge needle. Eight milliliters of pus were aspirated, confirming her diagnosis. She was given a dose of dexamethasone and clindamycin in the ED, and was sent home on a 7 day course of antibiotics. She was seen for a recheck at 24 hours by the otolaryngology department, as reaccumulation of pus sometimes occurs after needle aspiration of peritonsillar abscesses. She was doing well at that time and had an uncomplicated course.

Further reading

Chow A. Peripharyngeal fascial "space" infections. Up-To-Date. September 16, 2007.

Mehta N. Peritonsillar abscess. Emedicine. Topic 417. May 16, 2007.

Lamkin RH, Portt J. An outpatient medical treatment protocol for peritonsillar abscess. *Ear Nose Throat J* 2006;**85**:658.

Case # 8

History

A 2-year-old girl presents to the ED with her mother. Her mother states that the patient has had a congested nose for the last day or so. She had not thought much of it, since "everyone in the family" has had a cold, but the little girl began to have foul-smelling drainage from one nostril. Unlike everyone else in the family, the child has not had a cough, fever, or sore throat. She has been eating and drinking well. She complains only that her nose hurts.

Past medical history

The patient is healthy. She was a term newborn, and is up to date on her immunizations.

Medications

The patient takes no medications.

Allergies

The patient is allergic to penicillins.

Family history

The patient's parents and grandparents are healthy.

Social history

The child lives at home with her parents, an older brother, and a younger sister. She is not in daycare.

Physical exam and ancillary studies

- *Vital signs:* the patient's vital signs are as follows: temperature 36.7°C, heart rate 113 bpm, blood pressure 90/60, respiratory rate 20, room air oxygen saturation 100%.
- *General:* the patient is awake, alert, and appropriate. She is in no distress.
- *Head and neck:* the patient's pupils are equally round and reactive. Her tympanic membranes are normal bilaterally. She has foul-smelling discharge from her left nostril. On nasal exam, you see a blue bead in the nostril. There is nothing on the other side. The patient's oropharynx is without lesions, and her mucous membranes are moist.
- *Cardiovascular:* her heart is regular, without murmurs. She has good capillary refill in her extremities.
- *Lungs:* the patient's lungs are clear and equal, with no stridor or wheezing.
- *Abdomen:* the patient's abdomen is soft without apparent tenderness. There are no masses or organomegaly.
- *Neurologic:* the patient's neurologic exam is normal.

Questions for thought

- What is the definitive treatment for this patient?
- What is the likelihood you will succeed in treating her?
- What are important steps to take in determining how best to treat the patient?

Diagnosis

Nasal foreign body.

Discussion

- *Epidemiology:* the ear and the nose are two of the most common sites to encounter foreign bodies. The patients who present with these problems are most frequently children less than 5 years of age and the mentally ill. Other sites of foreign bodies in the mentally ill are the rectum, vagina, and urethra, as well as ingested foreign bodies.
- *Presentation:* patients with nasal foreign bodies can present in a variety of ways. The most common way patients present is entirely asymptomatic. Typically, this is because the parent witnesses the event or the child tells the parent about it. Less commonly, patients will present with unilateral nasal drainage, halitosis, pain, and sinusitis. In some cases, particularly in the case of button batteries in the nose, patients can present with bony erosion and skin changes. It is important to remember that patients may have more than one foreign body, so when seeing a patient with a foreign body in one nostril or ear, it is imperative to always check the other side for other foreign bodies.
- *Treatment:* the treatment for a nasal foreign body is removal. This can be accomplished in a number of ways. If the object is almost obstructing the nostril and is smooth and round, positive pressure (by either blowing into the patient's mouth with an Ambu bag or by blowing into the patient's other nostril with a piece of tubing) may dislodge the object. This has a success rate of about 80%. Objects can also be removed with forceps or right angles. If the object is not obstructing, one can pass a small Foley catheter beyond the object, blow up the balloon, and draw the object out. If there is much secondary swelling, as in the case of an object that has been present for a few days or weeks, it is often helpful to place oxymetazoline in the nose to reduce swelling and bleeding. After the object is removed, it is important to reassess the site of the object to make sure there is no tissue damage and no second foreign body higher up. The overall success rate for ED removal of nasal foreign bodies is at least 67%. If a foreign body cannot be removed in the ED, the patient should be sent to otolaryngology, or otolaryngology should see the patient in the ED. Particularly in the case of button batteries, the foreign body should be removed as soon as possible to prevent tissue destruction. The best success is usually obtained on the first attempt, so your first attempt should be your best attempt.

Clinical course

The keys to this patient's diagnosis are careful attention to history and physical exam.

Historical clues	Physical findings
• Nasal pain	• Unilateral purulent drainage
• Nasal drainage	• Absence of other infectious signs
• Patient age	• Foreign body visualized on exam

The patient was noted to have a foreign body in her nose on exam. A single attempt at air insufflation with an Ambu bag was unsuccessful at dislodging the bead, perhaps because the hole in the bead prevented a good seal. An attempt was made with a right angle, but the bead was pushed deeper and was not able to be grasped with the angle or with forceps. Oxymetazoline was sprayed into the child's nose, and a small Foley catheter was passed beyond the bead. The provider blew up the Foley balloon and extracted the bead. On reinspection, there were no other foreign bodies. The mother was educated on age-appropriate toys. They were discharged to follow up with her pediatrician for her next well-child visit.

Further reading

Backlin S. Positive-pressure technique for nasal foreign body removal in children. *Ann Emerg Med* 1995;**25**:554–5.

Botma M, Bader R, Kubba H. 'A parent's kiss': evaluating an unusual method for removing nasal foreign bodies in children. *J Laryngol Otol* 2000;**114**(8):598–600.

Brown L, Denmark TK, et al. Procedural sedation use in the ED: management of pediatric ear and nose foreign bodies. *Am J Emerg Med* 2004;**22**:310–14.

Case #9

History

A 49-year-old man presents to the ED early in the morning complaining of difficulty breathing. He states it started with a progressively worsening sore throat that began approximately 16 hours ago culminating with the sensation that his throat was closing upon awakening this morning. He describes the sensation of oxygen hunger and states the pain in his throat is now "10 out of 10" in severity. The dyspnea is worse when he lies down. His voice is a higher pitch than usual. His voice change is also progressively worse over the past day and he tells you his voice was "muffled" when he went to bed last night. He describes severe throat pain with swallowing or any manipulation of his anterior neck. He denies any trauma or foreign body in the airway. He also denies any recent illnesses, cough, or fever. He has no other complaints. He took 600 mg of ibuprofen 1 hour prior to presentation for the throat pain.

Past medical history

The patient has a history of hepatitis C, kidney stones, chronic alcohol use, and dental pain. He has smoked one pack of cigarettes per day for 20 years. He works as a carpenter. He is unclear about his immunization history.

Medications

In addition to the ibuprofen, the patient uses topical benzocaine when needed for severe dental pain.

Allergies

The patient is allergic to penicillin.

Physical exam and ancillary studies

- *Vital signs:* the patient's temperature is 37.0°C, his heart rate is 121 bpm, his blood pressure is 141/84 mmHg, his respiratory rate is 20, and his room air oxygen saturation is 97%.
- *General:* he is awake and alert. He is an ill-appearing, unkempt man sitting up in the hospital bed speaking in partial sentences.
- *Head and neck:* the patient's pupils are equally round and reactive to light, and his cranial nerves are intact. The patient's mucous membranes are moist. Only the patient's superior posterior oropharynx is adequately visualized as he is unable to fully open his mouth without severe pain. What can be seen is remarkable for pronounced erythema and injection. Any palpation of his anterior neck causes severe pain disproportionate to the clinical exam. No masses are appreciated. He has full range of motion of the neck with a midline trachea. Cervical lymphadenopathy is present.

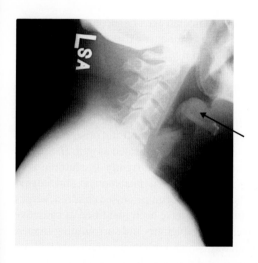

Figure 6.3. This soft tissue X-ray of the neck shows an enlarged epiglottis (thumb sign) and narrowing of the airway.

- *Cardiovascular:* on auscultation, the patient has a regular tachycardia without murmurs, rubs, or gallops. His peripheral pulses are intact.
- *Lungs:* the patient's lungs are decreased throughout, with bibasilar rales and scattered wheezes but no stridor.
- *Extremities and skin:* he has no evidence of edema, clubbing, or cyanosis.
- *Pertinent labs:* the patient's white blood cell count is 7.6 and his platelets are 59. All other labs are normal or negative.
- *Radiographs:* the patient's chest X-ray was normal. His lateral soft tissue neck X-ray is shown in Figure 6.3.

Questions for thought

- What are the appropriate initial actions to take to stabilize this patient?
- What abnormalities can be seen on the patient's X-ray that can help determine the diagnosis?
- What other diagnostic tools could be used to confirm the diagnosis?
- What is definitive treatment of this condition?
- Why does he have the feeling that his throat is closing?
- What service should be consulted for definitive management of his condition?

Diagnosis

Epiglottitis.

Discussion

- *Epidemiology:* the epidemiology of epiglottitis has changed considerably since the introduction of the *Haemophilus influenzae* vaccine in the 1980s. The incidence of epiglottitis in children has declined dramatically since the vaccine gained more widespread use in the early 1990s. This has increased the median age of epiglottitis from approximately 3 years of age prior to the introduction of the vaccine to a median age of onset moving towards adolescence and adulthood today. A slight male predominance exists and, in adults, the disease has been associated with other comorbid conditions such as hypertension and diabetes mellitus. Incidentally, the incidence in adults was reported in one study to be slowly rising since the vaccine's initiation from 0.88 to 3.1 per 100 000 from the early to late 1990s.

- *Pathophysiology:* epiglottitis is an inflammation of the epiglottis and surrounding tissues that is usually caused by bacterial infection, although viral infection and other inflammatory reactions (i.e. thermal or chemical injuries) have been implicated as well. *H. influenzae* is believed to be responsible for less than 25% of cases currently. In children who have received the vaccine, *Streptococcus pyogenes, Streptococcus pneumoniae*, and *Staphylococcus aureus* are the more common culprits. In immunocompromised children, herpes simplex, varicella, pseudomonas, and candida species have been identified as causative microbials as well. As the inflammation envelops the epiglottis and surrounding tissues, the local edema leads to obstruction of the airway, which inhibits inspiration but allows for expiration. It is a rapidly progressive disease and can quickly evolve into bacteremia if untreated.

- *Presentation:* this presentation is typical for epiglottitis. Patients with epiglottitis typically present after 12–24 hours of worsening odynophagia and dyspnea. Patients often have a toxic appearance, and rapid airway obstruction mandates the emergency physician be prepared to establish a definitive airway as soon as the diagnosis is suspected. This patient had other classic symptoms including tachycardia, adenopathy, and exquisite tenderness to minimal palpation of the anterior neck. Other common symptoms not seen in this patient but commonly seen include soft inspiratory stridor, fever, and drooling. The muffled voice, classically described as "hot potato," is another common feature. Dyspnea is usually worse in the supine position and patients are typically seen sitting up, leaning forward with a hyperextended neck that forces the chin forward, maximizing airway diameter. Cough is usually absent in patients with epiglottitis, helping to distinguish it from croup.

- *Treatment:* epiglottitis can be a rapidly progressive emergency and initial management should be directed toward maintenance of a patent airway if compromise is suspected. The patient should be observed closely in the emergency department with a pulse oximeter, cardiac monitor and, as stated above, should not be left unattended even for imaging if more than mildly ill. The patient should be left sitting up and started on humidified oxygen.

- Intravenous antimicrobial therapy should be initiated early and the emergency physician will not have the results of epiglottis or blood cultures to guide therapy. First-line agents are cephalosporins, specifically cefuroxime or ceftriaxone. Alternative choices include ampicillin-sulbactam, piperacillin-tazobactam, or TMP-SMX. In a penicillin-allergic patient or in an area with highly penicillin-resistant pneumococci, clindamycin or vancomycin should be started. Steroids are often added to reduce airway edema and inflammation.

- *Definitive management:* once the diagnosis of epiglottitis is suspected, a consultation with the otolaryngologist is necessary to arrange for admission. Some patients will need to go to the operating room for a definitive airway and others may need admission to the intensive care unit.

Clinical course

The keys to this patient's diagnosis are careful attention to his history, physical exam, and ancillary studies.

Historical clues	Physical findings	Ancillary studies
• Acute-onset odynophagia	• Ill-appearing	• Normal or near normal laboratory workup
• Progressive dyspnea	• Dyspnea improved with sitting up	• Lateral neck X-ray with edematous epiglottis ("thumb sign")
• Voice change	• Tachycardia	
• Severe throat pain	• Exquisite anterior neck tenderness	
	• Erythematous oropharynx	
	• Muffled voice	

This man was recognized to have epiglottitis based on his clinical presentation and X-ray. Epiglottitis can be diagnosed based on history, clinical examination, and radiographic findings, as in this case, or by direct visualization of the epiglottis using laryngoscopy. Visualization of the epiglottis using a tongue depressor is contraindicated and there have been case reports of cardiopulmonary arrest occurring in children with moderate to severe symptoms when this was attempted.

In this case, the X-ray showed a "thumb sign," which is a classic finding on an inspiratory soft tissue lateral neck film in a patient with epiglottitis. The thumb sign represents a markedly edematous (the shape of a thumb) epiglottis. The epiglottis usually appears long and thin. In addition, the hypopharynx is often dilated as a result of the obstructed upper airway.

The patient was placed on a cardiac monitor, pulse oximeter, and had humidified oxygen started. He was given a normal saline bolus through a peripheral IV and was given dexamethasone and morphine intravenously. As he was penicillin-allergic, the decision was made to start him on clindamycin. The otolaryngology team was asked to see the patient and he was admitted to their service. A CT of the neck was ordered which confirmed the diagnosis. The patient improved on the above therapy and was discharged home following a 3 day hospital stay.

Further reading

Progress toward elimination of Haemophilus influenzae type b invasive disease among infants and children–United States, 1998–2000. *MMWR Morb Mortal Wkly Rep* 2002;**51**:234.

Tintinalli J, Kelen G, Stapczynski S. *Emergency Medicine: a Comprehensive Study Guide*, 6th edition. New York: McGraw-Hill, 2004.

Chang, YL, Lo, SH, Wang, PC, Shu, YH. Adult acute epiglottitis: experiences in a Taiwanese setting. *Otolaryngol Head Neck Surg* 2005;**132**:689.

Berger, G, Landau, T, Berger, S, et al. The rising incidence of adult acute epiglottitis and epiglottic abscess. *Am J Otolaryngol* 2003;**24**:374.

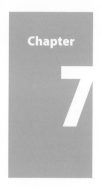

Chief complaint: pelvic discomfort

Devin Minior, Donald Jeanmonod, Wendy Woolley, Mara McErlean, Sahar Amery, Deno Gualtieri, Warner Wang, Taylor Spencer, Ana Margarita Hernandez-Silen

Case #1

History

A 19-year-old male college student presents to the emergency department with a 90-minute history of left testicular pain. The patient notes that he was taking a shower when the sudden onset of pain began in his left testicle. The pain was characterized as sharp and constant, localized to the proximal head of the testicle near the epididymis, with some relief when in a prone, crawling position. The patient denies any previous history of testicular pain, denies any history of sexually transmitted diseases (STDs), and denies any current penile lesions or discharge. On arrival to the ED, the patient has some nausea but denies vomiting. He denies fevers, chills, abdominal pain, or change in urinary or bowel habits.

Past medical history

The patient has a childhood history of asthma, but has not had an asthma exacerbation in over 6 years. He denies any history of tobacco use. The patient is in a monogamous relationship and denies any history of STDs.

Medications

The patient takes no medications.

Allergies

The patient has an allergy to amoxicillin.

Physical exam and ancillary studies

- *Vital signs:* the patient has a temperature of 36.7°C, his heart rate is 83 bpm, his blood pressure is 144/74, his respiratory rate is 12, and his room air oxygen saturation is 100%.
- *General:* the patient is awake and alert, but in clear discomfort.

Case Studies in Emergency Medicine, ed. R. Jeanmonod, M. Tomassi and D. Mayer.
Published by Cambridge University Press © Cambridge University Press 2010.

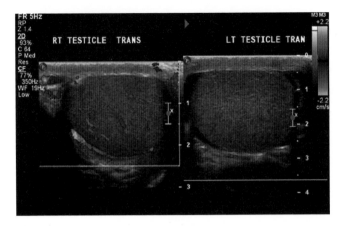

Figure 7.1. The patient's testicular ultrasound shows testicles which are symmetric in size and homogeneous in echogenicity. There is a moderate left hydrocele. The left testicle measures 3.1 × 2.9 × 2.4 cm, the right testicle measures 3.2 × 1.7 × 1.7 cm. On Doppler interrogation, there is no flow identified to the left testicle, consistent with testicular torsion.

- *Head and neck:* his pupils are equally round and reactive to light; cranial nerves are intact. The patient's mucous membranes are dry. His neck is supple with a midline trachea.
- *Cardiovascular:* the patient's heart has regular rate and rhythm with no murmurs, rubs, or gallops.
- *Lungs:* his lungs are clear to auscultation bilaterally, otherwise unremarkable.
- *Extremities and skin:* there is no clubbing, cyanosis, or edema. The patient's skin is warm and dry, with appropriate capillary refill.
- *Genitals:* the patient has normal genitalia with no appreciated lesions, erythema, or penile discharge. His proximal left testicle and epididymis are exquisitely tender, but not swollen or enlarged. There are no lumps or lesions noted on the remainder of bilateral testicular examination. The patient has loss of his cremasteric reflex on the left.
- *Pertinent abnormal labs:* the patient's complete blood count, basic metabolic panel, and urine studies are within normal limits.

Questions for thought

- What are the appropriate initial actions to take to stabilize this patient?
- Once stable, what are other diagnostic tools you can use to make a diagnosis?
- How does one urgently treat this condition in the emergency department?
- What is definitive treatment of this condition?

Diagnosis

Left testicular torsion.

Discussion

- *Epidemiology:* testicular torsion involves the left testicle more often than the right. The incidence in males younger than 25 is approximately 1 in 4000. Since testicular torsion is a true emergency, it must be rapidly differentiated from other complaints of testicular pain such as epididymitis, orchitis, hydrocele, and acute appendicitis. In adolescents, torsion is the leading cause of testicle loss, and thus demands immediate diagnosis and management in the ED. Most testicular torsion occurs in males younger than 30 with a peak age of 14 years, although it may occur at any age. A smaller peak also occurs in neonates due to the undescended position of their testicles.

- *Pathophysiology:* the tunica vaginalis envelops the testicle in the scrotal sac, preventing significant mobility of the testicle within the scrotum. In approximately 12% of males, a congenital abnormality known as the bell clapper deformity is usually bilateral and results in a high attachment of the tunica vaginalis. In these males, the testicle can rotate freely and twist on the spermatic cord within the tunica vaginalis. This causes venous occlusion, engorgement, and arterial ischemia which can in turn lead to infarction of the affected testicle if not urgently managed. It has been shown that the testicle must torse 720° before arterial blood flow is compromised enough to cause infarction.

- *Presentation:* history most often includes a sudden onset of severe unilateral scrotal pain, although less frequently the pain may be gradual in onset. Up to 50% of patients may report a previous history of intermittent testicular pain that has spontaneously resolved. Eliciting factors include physical activity, sexual activity, or trauma. Testicular torsion may also develop during sleep due to unilateral cremaster muscle contraction. Accompanying complaints may include nausea, vomiting, abdominal pain, inguinal canal pain, fever, and urinary frequency. Young boys who present with nonspecific abdominal pain must have testicular torsion included in their differential diagnosis. On physical exam, the involved testicle may be hyperemic, firm, tender, and elevated in position relative to the other testicle. There may also be edema and enlargement of the testicle or scrotum. Ipsilateral cremasteric reflex may be absent and Prehn's sign may be negative (no relief of pain on manual elevation of the affected testicle).

- *Diagnosis:* given the urgent nature of testicular torsion, diagnosis is made clinically. Prompt diagnosis, immediate urologic referral, and definitive treatment to salvage the testicle are of utmost importance. Detorsion within 6 hours has a salvage rate of 100%, but this rate is reduced to 20% at 12 hours, and 0% at 24 hours. If the patient presents to the ED soon after pain has started and the clinical presentation is equivocal, color Doppler ultrasonography may be used to assess arterial blood flow to the testicle. Ultrasound may also provide information about scrotal anatomy and other testicular disorders. Color Doppler has a sensitivity of 80–90%, specificity of 75–95%, and accuracy of 97% in the diagnosis of testicular torsion. Radionucleotide scan of the testicles may also have some value in assessing testicular blood flow and identifying other pathology.

- *Treatment:* early diagnosis and prompt urologic referral are the mainstays of treatment for successful salvage of the affected testicle. In the ED, appropriate pain medication should be administered. Emergency physicians may try to detorse the testicle at the bedside. Manual detorsion involves twisting the testicle outward in an "open book" fashion, by rotating the testicle 180° in a medial to lateral direction. Since the testicle is often torsed 720°, it may need to be rotated 2–3 times for complete detorsion. The endpoint of successful manual detorsion is pain relief (sometimes accompanied by resolution of testicular hyperemia), and is successful in 30–70% of patients.

- *Definitive therapy:* the urgent nature of testicular torsion and high incidence of repeat episodes in patients with a congenital deformity of the tunica vaginalis will demand definitive treatment. This involves surgical exploration, detorsion, and preemptive bilateral orchiopexy by urology.

Clinical course

The keys to this patient's diagnosis and treatment are careful attention to his history, physical exam, prompt attempts at manual detorsion, and urologic consultation.

Historical clues	Physical findings	Ancillary studies
• Sudden onset of unilateral testicular pain	• An exquisitely tender testicle not relieved by elevation	• Color Doppler ultrasonography of bilateral testicles demonstrating little to no vascular flow on the left
• History of similar episodes	• Loss of cremasteric reflex on affected side	

This male was recognized to have testicular torsion based on clinical presentation and confirmation with color Doppler ultrasonography. The patient was given analgesia in the ED. Manual detorsion was attempted at the bedside, but was unsuccessful in relieving the patient's discomfort. Given the urgent nature of the presentation, the patient was immediately sent for color Doppler ultrasonography and prompt urologic consultation was sought. Soon after consultation, the patient was taken to the operating room for surgical detorsion of the left testicle and bilateral orchiopexy.

Case #2

History

A 34-year-old female presents to the emergency department with a chief complaint of left lower quadrant pain. The patient reports that the pain has been waxing and waning over the course of approximately $2\frac{1}{2}$ weeks. She describes the pain as sharp, seemingly having no exacerbating or alleviating component. The patient had presented to the emergency department 12 days previously with a similar complaint. At that visit the patient had also had intermittent vaginal bleeding which has since ceased. The patient was found to be pregnant at that visit and had a quantitative βHCG of 352. She was further evaluated with a transabdominal and transvaginal pelvic ultrasound, which did not demonstrate an intrauterine pregnancy. The patient was referred to follow up with the gynecology service. The patient reports that she had followed up with her gynecologist and reports that she had repeat blood work performed, but does not know what that showed. The patient states that she became concerned when the pain became more acute today.

Past medical history

The patient is G_4P_{1021}. She has had one spontaneous vaginal delivery and two surgical terminations of pregnancy. The patient has a history of irregular menses and believes that her last menstrual period was approximately 5–6 months ago. She also states that she was diagnosed and treated for a urinary tract infection approximately 2 months ago. The patient has a history of sarcoidosis. She reports smoking approximately one pack of cigarettes daily.

Medications

The patient is supposed to be taking Prozac and prenatal vitamins, but is noncompliant.

Allergies

The patient has no known drug allergies.

Physical exam and ancillary studies

- *Vital signs:* the patient's temperature is 36.7°C, her heart rate is 102 bpm, her blood pressure is 117/64, her respiratory rate is 16, and her room air oxygen saturation is 100%.
- *General:* the patient is awake, alert, and oriented, sitting up in bed. She is non-toxic in appearance.
- *Head and neck:* her head is normocephalic and atraumatic. The patient's mucous membranes are moist.
- *Cardiovascular:* the patient has borderline tachycardia without murmurs or rubs. Her bilateral femoral pulses are palpable.

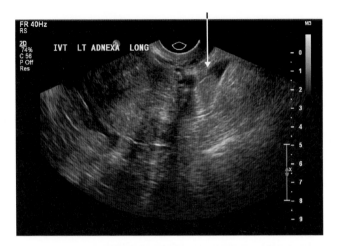

Figure 7.2. The patient's ultrasound demonstrates a complex left adnexal mass, which with a positive pregnancy test and no identifiable intrauterine pregnancy is suspicious for ectopic pregnancy.

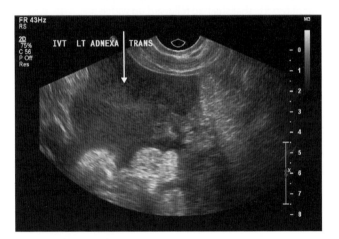

Figure 7.3. The patient's ultrasound demonstrates a large amount of free fluid in the pelvis.

- *Lungs:* the patient's lungs are clear to auscultation bilaterally without wheezes, rales, or rhonchi.
- *Abdomen:* her abdomen is obese, with normoactive bowel sounds. The patient is markedly tender to palpation in the left lower quadrant without rebound tenderness or guarding.
- *Pelvic:* the patient has normal external genitalia. Her cervical os is closed without discharge in the vaginal vault. There is no cervical motion tenderness. Left adnexal tenderness without appreciable mass is noted.
- *Extremities and skin:* there is no clubbing, cyanosis, or edema. The patient's skin is warm and dry with good capillary refill.
- *Pertinent abnormal labs:* the patient's hemoglobin and hematocrit are 10.1 and 30.2 respectively, which are down from 12 and 36.3 measured 12 days prior. Her type and screen reveal that she is blood type B negative. The patient's quantitative βHCG is 707 mIU/mL, which is up from 352 mIU/mL 12 days ago.
- *Imaging studies:* the patient had bedside ultrasound performed using a transvaginal approach, shown in Figures 7.2 and 7.3.

Questions for thought

- What is the differential diagnosis for this patient?
- What further diagnostic tools can you use to make the diagnosis?
- What would be the current expected βHCG given the value of 352 mIU/mL 12 days prior to presentation?
- At what βHCG would you expect to see an intrauterine pregnancy by transvaginal ultrasound? By transabdominal ultrasound?
- What are risk factors for this condition?
- What actions should be considered in the emergency department?
- What is definitive treatment of this condition?

Diagnosis

Ruptured ectopic pregnancy.

Discussion

- *Epidemiology:* the frequency of ectopic pregnancy has been increasing in the past several decades from an incidence of 0.5% of pregnancies being ectopic in the 1970s to 2% of pregnancies being ectopic in the mid-1990s. However, with improved medical diagnostics and treatments, the death rate has fallen from 35 deaths per 10 000 ectopic pregnancies in the 1970s to 4 deaths per 10 000 in the mid 1990s. Ectopic pregnancy is most commonly diagnosed between 6 and 10 weeks gestational age. Six to sixteen percent of first-trimester pregnancies presenting to the emergency department with complaints of pain or bleeding will be an ectopic pregnancy. If the patient has both these complaints, the incidence of ectopic pregnancy climbs to approximately 39% and will increase to 54% if the patient also has a risk factor for ectopic pregnancy.
- *Pathophysiology:* most ectopic pregnancies implant in the fallopian tube, with 80% in the ampulla, 12% in the isthmus, 5% in the fimbria, and 2% in the interstitial region. Situations that alter the architecture of the fallopian tube, thus blocking the usual transit of the fertilized ovum, constitute the greatest risk factors for ectopic pregnancy. A history of previous tubal surgery conveys a 21-fold risk, a history of previous ectopic pregnancy conveys a 7–13-fold risk, pelvic inflammatory disease increases risk 4-fold, and fertility assistance increases risk 3-fold. Other risk factors include smoking, IUD use, and advanced maternal age.
- *Presentation:* the most common presenting symptom of ectopic pregnancy is pelvic pain, which has been reported to be present in 90–97% of cases. About 79% of patients will have vaginal bleeding and about 54% of patients will be found to have a tender adnexal mass. The classic triad of pelvic pain, vaginal bleeding, and tender adnexal mass is present in 45% of women with ectopic pregnancy. Other symptoms will include GI symptoms and abdominal tenderness.
- *Diagnosis:* as with most disease processes, history and physical examination are not sufficiently sensitive or specific to make a diagnosis. The diagnostic modality of choice is the ultrasound, which is correlated to the level of the βHCG. The initial goal of

ultrasound is to demonstrate an intrauterine pregnancy, because the presence of an intrauterine pregnancy on ultrasound significantly decreases the chance of there being an ectopic pregnancy. This is because the incidence of a heterotopic pregnancy, which is the simultaneous existence of an intrauterine pregnancy and an ectopic pregnancy, is estimated to be approximately 1 in 7000 pregnancies. The incidence of heterotopic pregnancy increases to about 1 in 200 pregnancies if the patient is using modern reproductive technology. An intrauterine pregnancy should be reliably demonstrable on transvaginal ultrasound with a βHCG of 1500–1800 mIU/mL. Therefore, if an intrauterine pregnancy is not demonstrated, it should be assumed to be ectopic. With a βHCG of ≥ 1500 mIU/mL, transvaginal ultrasound has a reported sensitivity and specificity of 67–100% and 90–100%, respectively. Even if the βHCG is less than the discriminatory threshold, ultrasound should be performed to identify findings of ectopic pregnancy (since ectopic pregnancy, due to its abnormal site of implantation, can reach demonstrable size while producing lower levels of βHCG).

Other tests used in the diagnosis of ectopic pregnancy include following serial βHCG levels which should double every 2 days. A pregnancy can be considered "abnormal" if the βHCG does not increase by 66% in 2 days. That said, 15% of normal pregnancies will have a βHCG that does not increase by 66% in 2 days. Another test sometimes used in the evaluation of ectopic pregnancy is a single progesterone level. If it is greater than 25 ng/mL, there is a 97% chance of normal pregnancy. If the progesterone level is less than 5 ng/mL, the pregnancy is abnormal. This leaves an indeterminate range of 5–25 ng/mL.

- *Treatment:* treatment depends on the findings of the ultrasound and the βHCG level. If the patient has a quantitative βHCG of less than 1500 mIU/mL and an ultrasound that demonstrates an empty uterus, the patient should be followed with serial βHCG levels until a level of 1500 mIU/mL is reached or it is determined that the pregnancy is abnormal. If the βHCG is greater than 1500 mIU/mL and no pregnancy is demonstrated on ultrasound, then one should assume that there is an ectopic pregnancy. Options to treat include methotrexate therapy versus laparoscopy.

Clinical course

In order to make the diagnosis of ectopic pregnancy, one must first identify the woman of childbearing age presenting with abdominal pain or vaginal bleeding as being pregnant. One should assume that all pregnancies are ectopic pregnancies until proven otherwise.

Historical clues	Physical findings	Ancillary studies
• Pregnancy	• Lower quadrant abdominal pain	• Abnormal rise in βHCG
• Abdominal pain	• Left adnexal tenderness	• Ultrasound demonstrating complex left adnexal mass
• Vaginal bleeding		• Ultrasound demonstrating free fluid

In the setting of pregnancy, without demonstrable intrauterine pregnancy and a moderate amount of free fluid in the pelvis, this patient was clinically diagnosed with a ruptured ectopic pregnancy. Of note was the drop in the patient's hematocrit from the previous visit. The obstetrics and gynecology service was consulted and the patient was taken urgently to the operating room, where she underwent partial salpingectomy. The patient recovered uneventfully in the hospital and was discharged with instructions to take iron supplementation.

Further reading

Goldstein SR. Early pregnancy: normal and abnormal. *Semin Reprod Med* 2008;**26**:277–83.

Morin L, Van Den Hof MC. SOGC clinical practice guidelines. Ultrasound evaluation of first trimester pregnancy complications. Number 161, June 2005. *Int J Gynaecol Obstet* 2006;**93**:77–81.

Dighe M, Cuevas C, Moshiri M, Dubinsky T, Dogra VS. Sonography in first trimester bleeding. *J Clin Ultrasound* 2008;**36**:352–66.

Mol F, Mol BW, Ankum WM, Van Der Veen F, Hajenius PJ. Current evidence on surgery, systemic methotrexate and expectant management in the treatment of tubal ectopic pregnancy: a systematic review and meta-analysis. *Hum Reprod Update* 2008;**14**:309–19.

Case #3

History

A 14-year-old female presents with a complaint of severe right-sided lower abdominal pain. She reports that about 45 minutes prior to arrival the pain woke her from sleep and has been constant. She has been unable to find a position of comfort and is reporting 10/10 right-sided pain. The patient states that the pain is sharp in nature, radiates into her right pelvic area, and is associated with nausea and vomiting. She denies fevers or chills. She reports that she has never had pain like this before.

Past medical history

The patient has no medical problems. Her last menstrual period was 3 months ago. Her menarche was at age 12 and she reports that her periods are usually regular although associated with severe cramping pain that is unlike the pain she has today.

Medications

The patient takes no medications.

Allergies

The patient is allergic to sulfa and penicillin, which both cause her to develop a rash.

Physical exam and ancillary studies

- *Vital signs:* the patient's temperature is 36.9°C, her heart rate is 86 bpm, her blood pressure is 112/72, her respiratory rate is 16, and her room air oxygen saturation is 96%.
- *General:* the patient is awake, alert, and non-toxic in appearance. She is in no acute distress, but appears markedly uncomfortable.
- *Head and neck:* her head is normocephalic and atraumatic. The patient's mucous membranes are moist.
- *Cardiovascular:* the patient's heart has regular rhythm with normal S1 and S2 sounds. There are no murmurs appreciated. The patient has 2+ palpable peripheral pulses throughout.
- *Respiratory:* the patient's lungs are clear to auscultation with adequate air entry in all fields. There are no rales, rhonchi, or wheezes.
- *Musculoskeletal:* no deformities are noted. The patient has right costovertebral tenderness to percussion.
- *Abdominal:* the patient has voluntary guarding. She is tender to palpation in the right lower quadrant and suprapubic region, without any rebound or rigidity.
- *Skin:* the patient's skin is warm and dry, without rashes or lesions.

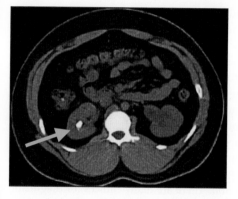

Figure 7.4. The patient's noncontrast CT of the abdomen and pelvis demonstrates a single minimally obstructing calculus within the lower pole of the right kidney, resulting in mild right hydronephrosis.

- *Pertinent abnormal labs:* the patient's urine dip shows 1+ protein and 1+ blood. Her urinalysis shows 5–10 RBCs and no bacteria. The patient's pregnancy test is negative. Her blood work is relevant for a white count of 12.4.
- *Imaging studies:* a representative cut from the patient's CT is shown in Figure 7.4.

Questions for thought

- What differential diagnoses should be considered for this patient?
- What initial actions should be taken?
- What other diagnostic modalities could be considered?
- What is the appropriate ED management of this patient?
- What should the patient's disposition be?

Diagnosis

Urolithiasis.

Discussion

- *Epidemiology:* kidney stones are one of the most common and painful disorders of the urinary tract. One in 20 people develop a kidney stone at some point in their life. Stones occur most commonly in males in the third to fifth decade of life. They are more common in whites than blacks. Children under 16 years of age account for approximately 10% of kidney stones.
- *Pathophysiology:* kidney stones result from crystal particles which consolidate and separate from the urine. They are most commonly calcium-based and combined with either oxalate or phosphate, but they can also be composed of uric acid, cystine, and struvite. As a result, diseases characterized by elevated levels of calcium such as hyperparathyroidism and hypercalciuria predispose to urolithiasis. There are many other conditions that increase the risk for stone formation including genetics, chronic disease, infection, medication use, gout, surgery, and dehydration. In addition, those who have a history of kidney stones are more prone to develop stones in the future.
- *Presentation:* urinary tract stones are often asymptomatic, until there is some degree of obstruction. The ureteral distension caused by the obstruction leads to severe episodic

pain that is typically very acute in onset and occurs at rest. The rapid development of symptoms helps to differentiate stone disease from other diagnoses. Patients are often unable to find a position of comfort and may be writhing or pacing the exam room. The pain will often radiate from the flank into the groin area. Patients typically complain of nausea and vomiting, and may experience gross hematuria.

- *Diagnosis:* the diagnosis of urinary tract stones is often made based on history and physical examination. Findings of fever, hemodynamic instability, peritoneal signs, or abdominal masses should be sought to help exclude other diagnoses that can mimic stone disease in presentation. A urinalysis should be performed and should include a urine pregnancy test in women of childbearing age. Hematuria, whether microscopic or gross, should raise the suspicion of urolithiasis. Laboratory studies can be useful to ascertain whether the stone obstruction has affected renal function. There are many choices for diagnostic imaging, but noncontrast CT scan is the preferred modality. Other options include ultrasonography, intravenous pyelogram (IVP), and plain radiographs. Although not required for all patients, imaging in the ED helps to confirm the presence of a stone and exclude alternate diagnoses.

- *Treatment:* emergency department treatment is directed towards adequate pain control and hydration. Intravenous opioids in conjunction with nonsteroidal anti-inflammatory medications work synergistically to achieve analgesia. Symptomatic relief of nausea and vomiting may require the use of anti-emetic medications. If there is any concern for infection, antibiotics with appropriate Gram-negative coverage should be initiated.

- *Disposition:* small, distal ureteral stones have a high likelihood of spontaneous passage that will not require intervention beyond analgesia and hydration. Larger stones (>6 mm), irregularly shaped stones, and proximal obstructing stones have a lower spontaneous passage rate and will require urologic intervention. In most cases, patients can be discharged when there is no evidence of obstruction and the pain is controlled with oral analgesics. These patients should follow up with urology for evaluation and prophylactic management for future stones.

Clinical course

The keys to this patient's diagnosis and treatment are careful attention to her history and physical exam. Definitive diagnosis is made with noncontrast CT of the abdomen and pelvis.

Historical clues	Physical findings	Ancillary studies
• Sudden onset of symptoms	• Patient unable to find comfortable position	• Urinalysis demonstrating presence of blood
• Flank pain radiating to groin	• Ipsilateral costovertebral angle tenderness	• Stone on noncontrast CT of the abdomen and pelvis
• Gross hematuria		

This patient was treated with ketorolac, ondansetron, and IV fluid with resolution of her symptoms. She was found to have an additional stone in her distal ureter without any signs of infection, and was appropriately discharged from the emergency department. She was given a prescription for oral analgesics. The patient was provided a urinary strainer to collect any passed stone material for evaluation. She was instructed to follow up with her pediatrician for evaluation and urology referral. The patient was also advised to return to the ED for fever, vomiting, or uncontrolled pain.

Further reading

Engineer R, Peacock WF. Chapter 96. Urologic stone disease. In Tintanelli JE, et al., eds., *Emergency Medicine: A Comprehensive Study Guide*, 6th edition New York: McGraw-Hill, 2004.

Teichman JM. Clinical practice. Acute renal colic from ureteral calculus. *N Engl J Med* 2004;**350**:684–93.

Case #4

History

An 86-year-old woman is found on the floor at home. Her family states that she lives alone and is usually very independent. The patient was last seen in her normal state of health 12 hours prior. At that time, she told her daughter that she was not feeling well and that she was planning to go to bed early. When the patient did not answer the telephone the following morning, her daughter went to the house and found her mother lying on the floor in the bedroom. It did not appear that the patient had gone to bed the night before. She was found to be incontinent of urine. The patient was unable to stand because of pain in her right pelvis, so EMS was called for assessment and transportation to the ED.

Past medical history

The patient has a history of hypertension.

Medications

The patient takes lisinopril on a daily basis.

Allergies

The patient has no known drug allergies.

Physical exam and ancillary studies

- *Vital signs:* the patient's temperature is 38.4°C, her heart rate is 138 bpm, her blood pressure is 88/51, her respiratory rate is 24, and her room air oxygen saturation is 97%.
- *General:* the patient is awake, alert, and complaining of right hip and pelvis pain.
- *Head and neck:* there are no signs of trauma. The patient's pupils are equally round and reactive to light. Her mucous membranes are dry. Her neck is supple with a midline trachea and no tenderness to palpation.
- *Cardiovascular:* the patient's heart has a regular rate and rhythm, without rub or gallop.
- *Lungs:* the patient's lungs are decreased throughout all fields, with bibasilar crackles.
- *Abdomen:* abdominal exam is benign.
- *Extremities and skin:* the patient's right leg is shortened and externally rotated. There is tenderness over the right hip and the patient has pain with any movement at the affected hip. There is trace bilateral edema and delayed capillary refill, but no clubbing or calf tenderness.
- *Neurologic:* the patient is alert to self, but not to date or place. Her cranial nerves are intact. She has intact strength in the feet and normal sensation.
- *Pertinent abnormal labs:* the patient's white blood cell count is 17.8 and her CPK is 340, but the remaining blood work (including cardiac markers) is within normal limits. Her

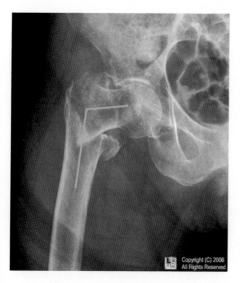

Figure 7.5. The patient's right hip plain film confirms a comminuted intertrochanteric fracture with varus deformity (line) of the femoral shaft.

urinalysis by catheter specimen is positive for blood, leukocyte esterase, nitrites, and ketones. It has a specific gravity of 1.030 and 30–50 WBCs per high-powered field.

- *EKG:* the patient's EKG shows sinus rhythm with no acute ischemic changes.
- *CXR:* there are no acute abnormalities.

Questions for thought

- What are the appropriate initial actions to take for this patient?
- What additional imaging studies are appropriate?
- Which medications should be used?
- What should be the patient's disposition?

Diagnosis

Right hip fracture, urosepsis, and dehydration.

Discussion

- *Epidemiology:* hip fracture is common in the elderly population. An estimated 350 000 hip fractures occur annually and this is expected to increase as the population ages. Ninety percent of hip fractures occur in patients 65 and older. Three-quarters of hip fractures occur in women (most often white) because of their higher incidence of osteoporosis. Other risk factors for hip fractures include sedentary life style, alcohol use, thin body habitus, dementia, and specific medications (including psychotropic medications and chronic steroids). Hip fractures are rare in the young and healthy and usually occur as the result of significant trauma, whereas hip fractures in the elderly are generally the result of a fall from a standing position.
- *Pathophysiology:* the hip consists of a ball and socket joint, composed of the acetabulum and the proximal femur. The thick capsule and strong ligamentous support around the

joint make dislocation unusual, particularly in young people. The blood supply to the joint is primarily along the femoral neck, therefore the location of the fracture predicts the likelihood of disruption in blood supply to the femoral head. Fractures that imperil the blood supply are generally fixed with a prosthetic femoral head. Those in which the blood supply is secure are repaired with fixation screws or plates. Fractures of the acetabulum itself are uncommon.

- *Presentation:* elderly patients with hip fracture will present with hip pain and inability to bear weight after a seemingly minor fall. The affected leg is often shortened and externally rotated because of the now unopposed muscle forces on the distal fragment. There will be tenderness to palpation over the hip joint and pain with attempts to perform passive range of motion at the hip. Any presentation should prompt an evaluation for the cause of the fall itself, including syncope, infection, or stroke. In addition, all patients should be evaluated for other complications sustained as a result of the fall, such as intracranial hemorrhage, pressure skin breakdown, or rhabdomyolysis.
- *Diagnosis:* diagnosis is made by plain films. A chest film is often included to rule out comorbid conditions and to clear the patient for the anticipated surgical procedure. Evaluation for other acute illnesses or injuries is based on the history, but may include EKG, cardiac enzymes, evaluation for infection, or CT scan of the head. Patients with persistent pain and inability to bear weight should be assumed to have an occult fracture. This should be ascertained with CT scan or nuclear bone scan imaging.
- *Treatment:* ED treatment should be directed at pain control and therapy for any comorbidities or concomitant injuries. Orthopedic consultation is necessary to expedite evaluation and surgical repair. Patients will require admission.
- *Definitive therapy:* definitive therapy is usually based on surgical repair through open reduction and internal fixation (ORIF). Most patients will require inpatient rehabilitation for ambulation training before being able to return home.

Clinical course

The keys to this patient's diagnosis and treatment are attention to her history and, in particular, her physical exam. Prompt diagnosis and treatment are crucial.

Historical clues	Physical findings	Ancillary studies
• Fall from a standing position	• Shortened, externally rotated lower extremity	• Fracture evident on plain films
• Inability to bear weight due to pain and joint instability	• Pain with movement at the right hip	

This patient was diagnosed with an intertrochanteric fracture of the right hip. In addition, she was found to have urosepsis, dehydration, and mild rhabdomyolysis. She was treated with analgesics, antibiotics, antipyretics, and IV fluids. She was taken to the operating room for ORIF on the following day, where she had an Austin Moore prosthesis placed. Her sensorium returned to baseline and she remained alert and appropriate for the duration of her hospitalization. She was transferred to a rehabilitation center on the sixth hospital day.

Further reading

Orwig DL, Chan J, Magaziner J. Hip fracture and its consequences: differences between men and women. *Orthop Clin North Am* 2006;**37**(4):611–22.

Parker M, Johansen A. Hip fracture. *BMJ* 2006;**333**(7557):27–30.

Wilkins CH, Birge SJ. Prevention of osteoporotic fractures in the elderly. *Am J Med* 2005;**118**(11):1190–5.

Case #5

History

A 64-year-old white female presents to the ED complaining of pelvic pain which has progressively worsened since earlier today. She has been having intermittent pelvic pain with no other associated symptoms over the course of the past month. Her bowel movements have been regular, but at times her stools have been "pellet" shaped. Earlier today, the patient began having worsening abdominal cramping and left lower quadrant (LLQ) pain. She also reports chills and subjective fever with loss of appetite. She denies vomiting, nausea, or bloody stools. She denies any weight loss and states that generally she is in good health.

Past medical history

The patient had a left ankle fracture 10 years ago with surgical fixation. She had a colonoscopy 4 years ago which showed several diverticula, but was otherwise normal. She does not smoke, drink, or use illicit drugs. Her mother has diabetes. Her father died of colon cancer in his sixties.

Medications

The patient takes no medications.

Allergies

She has no known drug allergies.

Physical exam and ancillary studies

- *Vital signs:* the patient's temperature is 38.1°C, her heart rate is 108 bpm, her blood pressure is 110/70, her respiratory rate is 20, and her room air oxygen saturation is 98%.
- *General:* the patient is awake and oriented. She looks to be in mild distress from abdominal pain.
- *Head and neck:* her pupils are equally round and reactive to light, and her cranial nerves are intact. She has mildly dry mucous membranes. Her neck is supple with no adenopathy. She has no jugular venous distension.
- *Cardiovascular:* the patient has a regular tachycardia, with no murmurs, rubs, or gallops.
- *Lungs:* her lungs are clear to auscultation bilaterally.
- *Abdomen:* the patient has tenderness in her left lower quadrant on palpation. She has some voluntary guarding, but no rebound. Her bowel sounds are decreased. Her rectal exam is guaiac-negative.
- *Extremities and skin:* the patient has no edema, cyanosis, or clubbing.

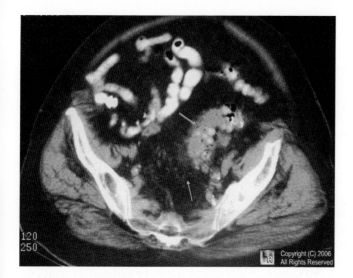

Figure 7.6. This CT of the abdomen and pelvis shows a thickened sigmoid colon (upper arrow) with some pericolic fluid accumulation (lower arrow).

- *Pertinent labs:* the patient's complete blood count reveals a white blood cell count of 12.8 and a hematocrit of 39%. Her chemistries and liver function tests are normal.
- *Radiographs:* the patient's chest radiograph is normal. A representative cut from her abdominal and pelvis CT is shown in Figure 7.6.

Questions for thought

- What are the appropriate steps to take to treat this patient in the ED?
- What must be initially avoided in this patient?
- How do you treat recurrent attacks of this problem?

Diagnosis

Diverticulitis.

Discussion

- *Pathophysiology and epidemiology:* the cause of diverticulitis is probably mechanical obstruction due to retention of undigested food residues and bacteria in the diverticula, forming a hard mass called a fecalith. Eventually, these diverticula may undergo microperforation from increased pressure and local infection, leading to intramural or extracolonic inflammation. Diverticulitis is more common in men than women. It is more likely to occur in the left colon than in the right colon. Left-sided diverticula are more likely to become inflamed, whereas right-sided diverticula are more likely to bleed.
- *Presentation:* acute diverticulitis is a disease of variable severity. It is characterized by intermittent crampy left lower quadrant abdominal pain, fever, chills, leukocytosis, and

259

alteration of bowel habits. Patients may have signs of peritoneal irritation. Some patients may have a palpable abdominal mass present from an inflammatory phlegmon, most typically in the left lower quadrant. Constipation may be noted prior to onset of illness, or the inflammation around the colon may cause constipation after painful symptoms have begun.

- *Diagnosis:* CT scan is the safest and most cost-effective method for definitive diagnosis. During the acute phase, colonoscopy and sigmoidoscopy should not be done and are contraindicated for 4–6 weeks due to risk of colonic perforation. In patients with a history of diverticulitis and symptoms consistent with diverticulitis who do not have an acute abdomen, diagnosis may be made on a clinical basis. In these settings, patients may be treated without CT scanning.
- *Treatment:* treatment should cover both aerobic and anaerobic Gram-negative organisms. The clinician may treat mild diverticulitis in stable patients without peritoneal signs with outpatient metronidazole plus either ciprofloxacin or trimethoprim/sulfamethoxazole. These patients should have close follow-up with their primary care doctor. For patients with peritoneal signs, treatment includes admission to the hospital. These people should be placed on bowel rest, given IV hydration, and provided with IV antibiotics to cover for aerobic and anaerobic Gram-negative organisms. It is important to provide analgesia to patients in pain.

Patients with recurrent episodes (two or more) of diverticulitis will need surgical consultation with resection of the affected area. Patients over the age of 50 should undergo colonoscopy after the acute event has resolved to rule out a colonic malignancy.

Clinical course

The keys to this patient's diagnosis are careful attention to her history, exam, and ancillary studies.

Historical clues	Physical findings	Ancillary studies
• Intermittent abdominal pain	• Left lower quadrant tenderness	• Elevated white blood cell count
• Left lower quadrant pain	• Guarding	• CT scan with colonic and pericolonic inflammation
• Recent constipation	• Tachycardia	
• Recent colonoscopy with diverticula	• Low-grade fever	

The emergency clinician recognized that the patient probably had diverticulitis, and treated her with fentanyl for pain and piperacillin/tazobactam to cover for colonic bacteria. The patient's CT showed she had colonic inflammation, and the patient was admitted to the hospital under the surgical service for further management. After 3 days of therapy, her symptoms improved and the patient was discharged home to finish her antibiotic course as oral therapy. Four months later, the patient had a recurrent episode, and ultimately had a resection of her sigmoid colon to prevent further problems. Her post-operative course was uneventful.

Further reading

Angott BE, Bross RJ, Still CD. Overview and treatment of diverticular disease. *J Am Osteopath Assoc* 2001;**101**(4 Suppl Pt 1):S19–21.

Bogardus ST Jr. What do we know about diverticular disease? A brief overview. *J Clin Gastroenterol* 2006;**40** Suppl 3:S108–11.

Case #6

History

A 21-year-old female presents to the ED with lower pelvic pain and back pain first noted several hours ago. The pain varies from cramp-like to sharp and does not radiate. She admits to some vaginal spotting, discharge, and a positive home pregnancy test. Her last menstrual period was 4–5 weeks ago. She has some nausea with the pain and vomited once today but has been able to eat and drink. She has no fevers, chills, dysuria, urinary frequency, diarrhea, or constipation.

Past medical history

The patent denies any past illnesses or surgeries. She has had one prior pregnancy which was aborted. She was treated 1 year ago for a sexually transmitted disease.

Medications

The patient takes birth control pills.

Allergies

The patient has no known drug allergies.

Social history

The patient is single, admits to occasional alcohol intake, denies smoking, and denies drug use. She is sexually active with multiple partners.

Physical exam and ancillary studies

- *Vital signs:* the patient's vital signs are as follows: temperature 35.9°C, heart rate 75 bpm, blood pressure 96/51 mmHg, respiratory rate 18, room air oxygen saturation 99%, and pain of 8/10.
- *General:* the patient is awake, alert, and lying on her side with knees drawn to her abdomen.
- *Cardiovascular:* the patient's heart is auscultated at a regular rate without murmur, rub, or gallop. Her radial and dorsalis pedis pulses are palpated as 2+.
- *Lungs:* the patient has normal non-labored respiration. The lungs are auscultated to have good air entry without wheezes, rhonchi, or rales.
- *Abdomen:* the lower abdomen is markedly tender suprapubically without other areas of tenderness. Voluntary guarding is noted over the suprapubic area without rigidity or rebound. McBurney's point is non-tender. The uterus is below the pelvic rim. There are no masses or abdominal defects. Percussion over the costovertebral angles does not produce pain.

- *Extremities and skin:* the patient has warm and dry skin without rash. She has no clubbing, cyanosis, or edema.
- *Pelvic:* the perineum, vulva, and labia are non-tender and without rashes or skin lesions. The vaginal vault contains a scant amount of blood without clot or tissue. The cervix is non-parous and without lesions. Bimanual exam finds a cervix that is exquisitely tender. The patient's uterus is of normal size without masses, and there are no adenexal masses or pain.
- *Pertinent labs:* the patient's quantitative HCG is less than 2, her hematocrit is 33, her white blood cell count is 9, and her urinalysis is negative. Gonococcal and chlamydia cervical swabs are taken and the results are pending.
- *Ultrasound:* pelvic ED bedside ultrasound shows an empty uterus with a small amount of free fluid.

Questions for thought

- What is the differential diagnosis for a woman presenting with pelvic pain?
- What is the appropriate workup for women with pelvic pain?
- What is the appropriate ED treatment for this patient?
- What other testing should the patient have?

Diagnosis

Pelvic inflammatory disease (PID).

Discussion

- *Epidemiology:* PID is a disease of women in their reproductive years, often between 15–25. The true incidence of PID is unavailable, with data ranging from 140 000 to 2.5 million visits per year. Well-documented risk factors for disease include multiple sexual partners, non-use of barrier contraception, and younger age. Other risk factors may include a lower socio-economic status, recent IUD placement, and douching.
- *Pathophysiology:* PID is a polymicrobial disease caused by ascension of the bacteria from the lower genital tract to the upper tract involving the uterus, fallopian tubes, adenexa, and in severe cases the peritoneum. In most cases the causative organism is *C. trachomatis* (in 20–40% of cases) and *N. gonorrhoeae* (in 30–80% of cases); however, lower genital tract bacteria have been demonstrated in up to 30% of cases. It is the resultant inflammation that causes long-term morbidity such as chronic pelvic pain and increased risk for ectopic pregnancy. In severe cases, Fitz-Hugh-Curtis syndrome can develop. This syndrome is characterized by violin-like strings of adhesions to the liver and right upper quadrant pain. Another complication of PID is tubo-ovarian abscess.
- *Presentation:* the presentation of PID can vary greatly from asymptomatic to septic shock. The most common complaint is pelvic or lower abdominal pain which is often dull or cramping. The classically described "chandelier sign" (severe pain with cervical motion) may be noted but is not required to be present on exam. In most cases, the pain duration should be less than 2 weeks and will often begin within several days after the end

of the menstrual cycle. Vaginal discharge is present in approximately 75% of cases and vaginal bleeding in 30–40% of cases. Laboratory studies for leukocytes, erythrocyte sedimentation rate, C-reactive protein, or leukocytes on vaginal smear can be used but are not required for diagnosis.

- *Treatment:* the CDC recommends empiric treatment for all sexually active young women or women otherwise at risk for STDs complaining of pelvic pain and tenderness either at the cervix, uterus, or adenexa on exam if no other explanation for the pain can be found. Treatment should cover both gonorrhea and chlamydia. The CDC recommends two parenteral treatment options: doxycycline plus an extended-spectrum cephalosporin, or clindamycin plus gentamycin. For patients who are well enough for outpatient treatment, the usual therapy is ceftriaxone one time and doxycycline for 14 days, given orally.

    Sexually transmitted diseases are reported to the department of public health. Depending on where the patient lives, there are different notification options for the patient's sexual partners.

Clinical course

The keys to the patient's diagnosis are careful attention to her history, physical exam, and ancillary studies.

Historical clues	Physical findings	Ancillary studies
• Sexually active with multiple partners	• Cervical motion tenderness	• Negative pregnancy test, ruling out other etiologies
• Pelvic pain		
• History of sexually transmitted disease		

In this patient, the treatment course was altered by report of the positive home pregnancy test causing concern for ectopic pregnancy. With the HCG result as well as ultrasound to rule out ectopic pregnancy, the diagnosis of PID became apparent. The small amount of free fluid in the pelvis was either physiologic or may have been caused by PID. Before reliable imaging, PID was diagnosed by aspiration of blood or pus in the cul-de-sac. This patient and most with PID lacked lab findings or fever but did meet the criteria of pelvic pain and had the classic cervical tenderness on exam. Given the morbidity of untreated disease, it is better to treat than not. In addition to antibiotics, proper treatment of PID or other STDs should include both cultures as well as recommendations for outpatient HIV testing and education or information about safer sexual practices.

Further reading

Workowski KA, Berman SM. Sexually Transmitted Diseases Treatment Guidelines, 2006. *MMWR* 2006;**55**(RR-11).

Update to CDC's Sexually Transmitted Diseases Treatment Guidelines, 2006: fluoroquinolones no longer recommended for treatment of gonococcal infections. *MMWR* 2007;**56**(14):332–6.

Trigg BG, Kerndt PR, Aynalem G. Sexually transmitted infections and pelvic inflammatory disease in women. *Med Clin N Am* 2008;**92**:1083–113.

Lareau SM, Beigi RH. Pelvic inflammatory disease and tubo-ovarian abscess. *Infect Dis Clin N Am* 2008;**22**:693–708.

Case #7

History

A 53-year-old man presents to the ED with complaint of pelvic pain and nausea that has become progressively worse over the past few days. He vomited once this morning. Further questioning reveals that the patient recently underwent thoracic surgery for a chronic right pleural effusion and that he has been on pain medicines since surgery. He has not had a bowel movement for the last 6 days and states that he has not passed gas for 2 days. He reports abdominal cramping that is so bad, he cannot lay still. He has not had any fevers in the post-operative period.

Past medical history

The patient has insulin-dependent diabetes mellitus, end-stage renal disease on peritoneal dialysis, cardiomyopathy, chronic right pleural effusion, hypertension, hepatitis C, and metabolic brain injury secondary to hypoglycemic coma.

Past surgical history

The patient has had peritoneal dialysis catheter placement, history of hemodialysis access creation, and right-sided decortication with parietal pleurectomy 2 weeks ago.

Medications

The patient takes omeprazole, minoxidil, amlodipine, candesartan, clonidine, oxcarbazepine, metoclopramide, calcitriol, polyethylene glycol 3350, docusate sodium, calcium acetate, insulin glargine, and sliding-scale insulin aspart.

Allergies

The patient has no known allergies.

Physical exam and ancillary studies

- *Vitals signs:* the patient's temperature is 36.1°C, his blood pressure is 106/84, his pulse is 63, his respiratory rate is 20, his oxygen saturation is 93% on 2 liters nasal cannula.
- *General appearance:* the patient appears to be in mild distress, very uncomfortable, constantly shifting positions. He is alert and oriented.
- *Head and neck:* the patient's head is normocephalic and atraumatic. Pupils are equal, round, and reactive to light. Mucous membranes are dry.
- *Lungs:* the patient's lungs are clear bilaterally.
- *Cardiovascular:* the patient's heart has regular rate and rhythm. He has 2+ peripheral pulses without edema.

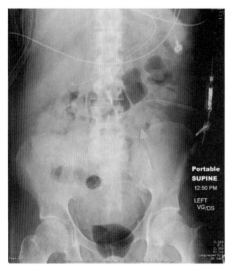

Figure 7.7. The patient's abdominal X-ray shows colonic distension secondary to stool retention (arrow). This is consistent with fecal impaction.

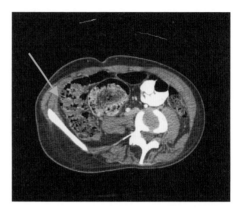

Figure 7.8. The patient's computed tomography shows significant fecal impaction (arrow).

- *Abdomen:* the patient's abdomen is soft and mildly distended. He is diffusely tender, but has no focal point of tenderness. There is no rebound or involuntary guarding. The patient has hypoactive, normal-pitched bowel sounds.
- *Rectal:* the patient has solid brown stool in his rectum, which is negative for fecal occult blood. He has normal anal sphincter tone. There are no palpable masses.
- *Pertinent labs:* the patient's sodium is 151, chloride is 126, bicarbonate is 17, and creatinine is 7.2.

Questions for thought

- What steps should be taken immediately during the initial evaluation of the patient?
- Which service(s) should be consulted?
- What are the causes of this condition?
- What are the initial treatment options?
- What treatments are ineffective?
- What is the definitive treatment course for this condition?

Diagnosis

Fecal impaction.

Discussion

- *Epidemiology:* it is estimated that chronic constipation has a prevalence of 10–20%. The incidence increases in the elderly.

Table 7.1. Etiology of chronic constipation

Neurogenic	Non-neurogenic	Drugs
Diabetes mellitus	Electrolyte imbalance (hypokalemia)	Analgesics
Spinal cord injury	Hypothyroidism	Anticholinergics
Multiple sclerosis	Myotonic dystrophy	• Antihistamines
Hirschsprung disease	Panhypopituitarism	• Antidepressants
Chagas disease	Idiopathic constipation	• Antipsychotics
Pseudo-obstruction	Normal-transit constipation	Cationic agents
Autonomic neuropathy	Slow-transit constipation	• Iron
Irritable bowel syndrome		• Aluminum (antacids)
		Neurally-active
		• Antihypertensives
		• Calcium-channel blockers
		• 5HT3 antagonists

- *Pathophysiology:* constipation and fecal impaction are common gastrointestinal complaints, which have varied etiologies (see Table 7.1). In the general population, a frequent cause is medication side effect, most notably narcotics.
- *Presentation:* patient presentation depends on the extent of constipation and fecal impaction. Most patients will report abdominal pain with cramping and decreased frequency of bowel movements from their baseline. Dehydration may also accompany the patient's abdominal complaints. Nausea, vomiting, and lack of flatus should alert the clinician to the possibility of an intestinal obstruction.
- *Diagnosis:* the patient's physical examination is key to making the diagnosis of fecal impaction. Abdominal distention, diffuse tenderness to palpation, and hypoactive bowel sounds are the typical findings. A rectal exam should be performed to determine whether the patient has fecal impaction, evidenced by hard stool in the rectal vault. Additionally, it is important to determine whether the patient has a positive fecal occult blood test, as this may suggest presence of colonic malignancy.
- Laboratory studies should be obtained to evaluate for electrolyte imbalance as both a possible cause and a result of the fecal impaction.
- Radiographic studies include plain radiographs of the abdomen. Findings of colonic distention with significant stool retention are consistent with fecal impaction.
- *Treatment:* initial treatment algorithm in the ED includes fluid resuscitation, placement of urinary catheter to evaluate adequacy of resuscitation, and nasogastric tube decompression as indicated by exam and radiographic findings. A surgical consultation is frequently necessary for definitive treatment.
- *Definitive treatment:* definitive management frequently requires manual fragmentation and enemas to soften the stool and provide lubrication. Serial abdominal X-rays are necessary to monitor treatment progress. If disimpaction is unsuccessful, a Gastrografin enema (usually performed by a radiologist under fluoroscopy) may be successful, especially with proximal impactions. If unsuccessful, decompression via sigmoidoscopy or colonoscopy may be attempted. Once disimpaction is achieved, the patient is placed on a bowel regimen to achieve at least one bowel movement every other day. Promotility agents are frequently ineffective (metoclopramide, erythromycin). Further workup to complete the patient's evaluation (such as endoscopy, manometry, and transit studies) can be performed as an outpatient.

Clinical course

The initial evaluation starts with a careful history and physical exam to elucidate likely causes of the patient's complaints.

Historical clues	Physical findings	Ancillary studies
• Diabetic	• Abdominal distention	• Labs suggestive of hemoconcentration
• Renal failure	• Crampy visceral pain	• Electrolyte abnormalities (especially K^+)
• Recent history of narcotic use	• Hypoactive bowel sounds	• Abdominal X-ray/CT with colonic distention and stool retention
• Lower abdominal pain	• Hard stool in rectal vault	
• Lack of bowel movements and flatus		

A thorough history and physical exam suggested that the cause of the patient's fecal impaction was multi-factorial, with the use of narcotics in the post-operative period being a significant contributing cause. Following initial evaluation, two large-bore peripheral IV lines were established. Fluid resuscitation was initiated for dehydration. A CT of the abdomen and pelvis was performed as well, with significant fecal impaction identified. A surgical consultation was requested and the patient was admitted for disimpaction. Multiple initial attempts at manual disimpaction and enemas were unsuccessful. The patient subsequently had a Gastrografin enema performed, which was successful. A lactulose-based bowel regimen was initiated to keep the patient stooling. The patient was subsequently discharged with instructions for gastroenterology follow-up for further evaluation and colonoscopy.

Case #8

History

A 3-year-old female presents to the emergency department with her mother, who states that her child "keeps saying her stomach hurts" and pointing to her pelvis. The mother says the patient has had similar complaints intermittently over the past 3 months. She states her child is less playful and seems ill even between episodes of pain, but the mother is unable to identify any other specific symptoms. The child has had no fevers or chills, no vomiting, no diarrhea or constipation. Although the patient normally stays with a neighbor during the day, the mother has stayed home from work with the child during these episodes. The patient was previously seen by her pediatrician during these episodes of pain. The workup by the pediatrician revealed no clear source, and she was diagnosed with "functional abdominal pain."

The mother states that she has monitored the child's meals and activities, but has not identified any triggers. After the last episode 1 week ago, the pelvis pain had seemed to improve without any specific treatment, and the mother was able to return to work. However, the child's pain has returned over the past 3 days and she has been more anxious, tearful, and withdrawn. The only other symptom the mother identifies is a diaper rash, which she found after the child returned from the neighbor's today. The patient's mother says the neighbor does not change the child's diaper enough, which has been a recurrent problem.

Past medical history

The mother states her daughter has no significant past medical history and her vaccines are up to date. Development is moderately delayed for age, including difficulties with toilet training and speech.

Medications

The patient takes no medications.

Allergies

The patient has no known drug allergies.

Physical exam and ancillary studies

- *Vital signs:* the patient's temperature is 37.7°C rectally. Her heart rate is 118 bpm as she cries. She is breathing at 20 breaths per minute with an oxygen saturation of 99% on room air.
- *General:* the patient is a withdrawn female who becomes quite agitated and tearful when she is touched or examined.

- *Head and neck:* the head is normocephalic and atraumatic. Pupils are equal and round, and mucous membranes are moist. There are no abnormalities identified.
- *Cardiovascular:* S1 and S2 are auscultated with a regular rate and rhythm. There are no clicks, rubs, or murmurs appreciated, but the patient is mildly tachycardic.
- *Lungs:* the patient's lungs are clear to auscultation bilaterally without wheezes, rhonchi, or rales. It is difficult to fully assess the lungs, however, as the child cries throughout the exam.
- *Abdomen:* the patient's abdomen is soft, non-distended, but diffusely tender even to light touch. Normal active bowel sounds are appreciated. The patient voluntarily guards.
- *GU:* the patient has normally developed external female genitalia. Her perineum is erythematous primarily along the labia majora, with sparing of the skin folds. There is no weeping or skin drainage identified.
- *Neurological:* no neurological deficits or abnormalities are identified. The patient moves all her extremities freely.
- *Pertinent labs:* the patient's complete blood count, comprehensive metabolic panel, and urinalysis are entirely within normal limits.
- *Imaging:* the patient's abdominal plain films are read as negative, with no evidence of obstruction or constipation. Her abdominal ultrasound shows no evidence of appendicitis, intussusception, or ovarian pathology.

Questions for thought

- What differential diagnosis must be considered in the setting of an otherwise negative workup?
- Why is this patient at a higher risk for this condition?
- What further testing is needed?
- Which service(s) should be consulted?
- What are the initial treatment options?

Diagnosis

Abdominal pain associated with child abuse.

Discussion

- *Epidemiology:* the Third National Incidence Study of Child Abuse and Neglect (NIS-3) provides a broad definition for sexual abuse, including intrusion, genital molestation, exposure, inappropriate fondling, and unspecified sexual molestation.

  According to the Center for Disease Control's *Child Maltreatment*, 3.3 million reports of alleged child abuse and neglect affecting about 6 million children produced 905 000 substantiated cases in 2006. Child Protective Services (CPS) estimates that there are between 1.2 and 1.9 substantiated victims of sexual abuse per thousand every year. Approximately 2000 children are victims of fatal abuse each year. Between 90 and 280 per thousand adults surveyed experienced some form of sexual abuse or assault in their childhood. Interestingly, research has shown a national decline in physical and sexual abuse since the mid 1990s.

- *Pathophysiology:* females are at a higher risk of sexual abuse than males, particularly those from low-income families. Economically disadvantaged children are also more often victims of other forms of crime, violence, and abuse. Men perpetrate most sexual abuse and sex crimes. Child sex offenders tend to be juveniles or young adults under the age of 30 who have been sexually abused themselves. Ninety percent of sexual abuse and sex crimes are committed by perpetrators who know their victims. Acquaintances are the most common offenders, followed by family members, and then strangers.

- *Presentation:* an estimated 15% of children diagnosed with sexual abuse present with behavioral disturbances and complaints not related to the genitourinary tract.

- *Diagnosis:* the large majority of child sex abuse cases leave no physical evidence. This is most commonly a result of the less invasive forms of sexual abuse employed by astute perpetrators, such as fondling, frotteurism, oral–genital contact, or exploitation. Nonspecific findings may be present, including erythema, rashes, and irritation in the genitals or rectum, but these must be correlated with the known history, observed behaviors, and other indications of abuse. Vague complaints such as abdominal or pelvic pain or behavioral disturbances may also be suggestive, and in the face of an otherwise comprehensive negative workup should prompt the consideration of abuse. Unfortunately, substantiating the diagnosis of sexual abuse, however probable, is often very challenging and difficult.

  More obvious findings of abuse may include the presence of sexually transmitted infections or significant genitorectal trauma (such as hematomas, fissures, changes in rectal tone, or disruption of the prepubertal female hymen). If indicated, cultures of the throat, vagina, or rectum may identify exposure. Serologic tests for syphilis or HIV should be considered. Counseling should precede any such tests. Nongenital physical injuries, such as grip marks on the forearms, are rare. However, other conditions may falsely mimic sexual abuse, including lichen sclerosis, dermatitis, vaginitis, congenital dermal melanocytosis (Mongolian spots), Crohn's disease, osteogenesis imperfecta, or accidental trauma. Clinicians must be able to distinguish among these possibilities.

  A forensic exam (which typically includes collection of clothing and trace evidence, fingernail scrapings, wet mounts, and skin swabs based on Wood's lamp examination) should be completed to more definitively diagnose abuse. If a child has had exposure to semen within the past 72 hours, this may be detected by exam using markers such as acid phosphatase.

- *Treatment:* if the clinical suspicion for sexual abuse is high, the child should be treated with post-exposure prophylaxis against chlamydia, gonorrhea, and HIV. In postmenarcheal female patients, the possibility of pregnancy can be treated with oral contraception. Appropriate wound care should be employed for any identified trauma. Clinicians are mandated reporters, therefore involvement of the police, Child Protective Services, social work, and counseling services should be sought. If a child is not safe at home, alternative arrangements must be made for the child from the emergency department, rather than allowing the child to be discharged to an unsafe environment.

- *Definitive therapy:* the legal system may become involved in cases of sexual abuse against children. This requires well-documented medical records, since recollection alone may be inadequate. Mental health professionals should be available to evaluate and treat the acute stress reaction. Long-term mental health involvement may be indicated due to concerns about posttraumatic stress disorder (PTSD). Both child and family require emotional support, and efforts should be made to prevent future exposures to abuse.

Clinical course

Child abuse can be an elusive diagnosis and is often missed. It should always be considered in the differential diagnosis, particularly when there is no other explanation for the child's symptoms and the history is unreliable (changing stories or implausible scenarios).

Historical clues	Physical findings	Ancillary studies
• Developmental and behavioral delays	• Anxious, tearful	• Forensic exam
• Recurrent unexplained pain	• Disproportionate pain	• Sexually transmitted disease testing
• Concerning contact identified	• Nonspecific exam without clear organic etiology	• Testing to rule out other sources of pain
• Holes in the patient's history	• Perineal trauma	

Due to the concerns raised by the exam, the hospital's social worker and Child Protective Services were contacted. In discussion with the child's mother, she realized that the redness in her daughter's groin would heal whenever the child stayed home, but came back regularly while at the neighbor's house. The mother came to acknowledge that this might represent abuse. A sexual assault forensic examination was completed, including skin swabs of the affected area. There was no evidence of sexually transmitted diseases.

Investigation by Child Protective Services revealed that the family's neighbor was a known pedophile. They discovered that the pedophile had a pattern of frotteurizing his victims and he admitted to doing the same to the patient. Although the evidence collected from the sexual assault forensic exam did not produce any DNA evidence, the District Attorney was able to pursue legal action based on the medical records and the pedophile's admission.

The child and her family reached out to a counselor. There was gradual improvement in the patient's pelvic pain, although her development delays persisted.

Further reading

Crimes Against Children Research Center. Retrieved December 10, 2008, from www.unh.edu/ccrc.

Giardino AP, Giardino ER. Child abuse & neglect: sexual abuse. Retrieved December 10, 2008, from eMedicine.com.

Kellogg N and the Committee on Child Abuse and Neglect. The evaluation of sexual abuse in children. *Pediatrics* 2005;**116**(2):506–12.

Berkowitz CD. Chapter 297. Child abuse and neglect. In Tintanalli JE, Kelen GD, Stapczynski JS, eds., *Emergency Medicine: A Comprehensive Study Guide*. Nerw York: McGraw-Hill: 2004, pp. 1847–50.

Sirotnak AP, Krugman RD, Chiesa A. Chapter 7. Child abuse & neglect. In Hay WW, Levin, MJ, Sondheimer, JM, Deterding RR, eds., *Current Pediatric Diagnosis and Treatment*. New York: McGraw-Hill, 2009.

US Department of Health and Human Services, Administration on Children, Youth and Families. *Child Maltreatment 2006* (Washington DC: US Government Printing Office, 2008). Retrieved December 10, 2008, from CDC.gov.

Case #9

History

A 25-year-old G_0 woman presents to the ED complaining of acute onset of severe stabbing right lower quadrant pelvic pain. The pain radiates to her right groin, and is 10/10. The pain improves when she stays still. The patient also complains of a low-grade fever and nausea, with vomiting three times today. The patient denies any similar symptoms in the past.

Past medical history

The patient suffers from environmental allergies.

Past ob/gyn history

The patient is currently undergoing hormonal treatment for infertility. As part of her infertility workup, a diagnostic pelvic laparoscopy was recently performed which revealed a right ovarian cyst. The patient has no history of sexual transmitted infections. She has a history of normal Pap smears. The patient's last menstrual period was 2 weeks ago. She has smoked one pack of cigarettes per day for the last 8 years. She denies alcohol and illicit drug use.

Medications

The patient's medications include prenatal vitamins, folic acid, and clomiphene citrate.

Allergies

The patient has no known drug allergies.

Physical exam and ancillary studies

- *Vital signs:* the patient's temperature is 37.8°C, her heart rate is 110 bpm, her blood pressure is 118/61, her respiratory rate is 20, and her room air oxygen saturation is 98%.
- *General:* the patient is awake, alert, and in acute distress.
- *Head and neck:* her pupils are equally round and reactive to light, her cranial nerves are intact. The patient's mucous membranes are dry. Her neck is supple.
- *Cardiovascular:* the patient's heart has regular rate and rhythm. She is tachycardic. There are no murmurs, rubs, or gallops appreciated.
- *Lungs:* the patient's lungs are clear to auscultation bilaterally.
- *Abdomen:* her bowel sounds are decreased in all four quadrants. She is tender to palpation in the right lower quadrant, with positive voluntary guarding and positive rebound.
- *Sterile speculum exam:* the patient has grossly normal female external genitalia. There is no vaginal bleeding or discharge. The patient has a nulliparous cervix, with no grossly apparent lesions.

- *Bimanual vaginal exam:* the patient has a small anteverted uterus. There is a right adnexal mass, which is tender to palpation. The patient's left adnexa has no appreciable mass or tenderness to palpation.
- *Extremities and skin:* the patient has no edema, clubbing, or calf tenderness. She has good capillary refill. The patient has a masculine hair distribution pattern.
- *Pertinent abnormal labs:* the patient's labs are relevant for a white blood cell count of 14.2 with left shift, hematocrit of 10.5, and hemoglobin of 31.5. Her urine pregnancy test is negative.
- *Transvaginal ultrasound with Doppler:* there are multiple left ovarian simple cysts; the largest one is $0.7 \times 0.8 \times 0.6$ cm. The patient's right ovary is enlarged at $8 \times 7.6 \times 10$ cm with multiple simple cysts, the largest one measuring $4 \times 5.5 \times 3$ cm. Doppler ultrasound reveals adequate arterial and venous waveforms in the left ovary, but diminished in the right ovary. There is a moderate amount of free fluid within the posterior cul-de-sac. The patient has an anteverted uterus, which is normal in size and measures $8.6 \times 3.4 \times 4.9$ cm. The endometrial echogenic complex (EEC) is within normal thickness limits at 6 mm.

Questions for thought

- What are the appropriate initial actions to take?
- What other diagnostic tools can be employed?
- How does one urgently treat this condition in the ED?
- What is the definitive treatment?

Diagnosis

Ovarian torsion.

Discussion

- *Epidemiology:* ovarian torsion is the fifth most common gynecological emergency. It affects patients of all ages, but 80% of cases occur in females under the age of 50. Pregnancy and ovarian hyperstimulation during fertility treatment pose increased risk for torsion.
- *Pathophysiology:* ovarian torsion occurs when an abnormally enlarged ovary torses (or twists) on itself. It typically results from masses (cysts or tumors) that are greater than 4 cm, although ovarian torsion is also possible with smaller masses. Torsions are most commonly adnexal, in that they affect both the ovary and the ipsilateral fallopian tube. Upwards of 60% of torsions are right-sided. Torsions in young females are most often adnexal and not caused by ovarian pathology. They tend to involve a normal ovary and either a lengthy fallopian tube or a shortened mesosalpinx (portion of the broad ligament that stretches along the underside of the fallopian tube to the ovary). In early pregnancy, the ovary is prone to torsion from enlarged corpus luteum cysts. The multiple theca lutein cysts which form as a result of ovulation induction for infertility treatment pose an even

greater risk of torsion. Patients with ovarian torsion normally have lymphatic, venous out-flow, and arterial inflow compromise. The arterial supply is not usually as compromised as the venous supply, due to the increased muscular tone of arteries. The progression of ovarian torsion begins with ischemia, which then leads to necrosis, followed by infarction, local hemorrhage, and peritonitis.

- *Presentation:* the clinical presentation of ovarian torsion is variable. Patients usually present with lower pelvic pain, which may be sudden in onset and sharp in nature. It can radiate to the back, flank, or groin. Nausea and vomiting may or may not be present. Fever may develop as a sign of necrosis.
- *Diagnosis:* ovarian torsion should be considered in all female patients with lower abdominal or pelvic pain and a known ovarian mass. If the diagnosis of ovarian torsion is in question, the best study to obtain is transvaginal ultrasound with color flow Doppler imaging. CT and MRI can detect ovarian lesions, but have limited ability in diagnosing torsion. Definitive diagnosis is based upon surgical findings.
- *Treatment:* the treatment for ovarian torsion is operative evaluation of the organ to determine its viability. The standard of care, if feasible, is detorsion and salvage of the affected adnexum, with resection of the causative mass.
- *Definitive therapy:* definitive management of ovarian torsion is oophoropexy if the affected ovary is viable, and oophorectomy if it is not.

Clinical course

The keys to this patient's diagnosis are careful attention to her history, physical exam, and ancillary studies.

Historical clues	Physical findings	Ancillary studies
• Young female	• Tachycardia	• Leukocytosis
• Acute-onset lower abdominal pain	• Low-grade fever	• Negative pregnancy test
• Nausea and vomiting	• Abdominal pain with peritoneal irritation	• Bilateral ovarian cysts, with right ovarian enlargement and diminished arterial and venous flow on Doppler ultrasound
• Known ovarian cyst		
• Undergoing fertility treatment	• Right adnexal mass	

This woman was diagnosed with ovarian torsion based on her presentation, negative pregnancy test, and transvaginal ultrasound findings. Two large-bore IVs were placed and she was immediately brought to the operating room. On laparoscopy, the patient's right ovary was noted to be enlarged and torsed, with marked vascular engorgement. Once the ovary was successfully detorsed, a cystectomy was performed. Anatomy was restored and the organ was salvaged.

Further reading

Stenchever MA, Droegemueller W, Herbst AL, Mishell D. *Comprehensive Gynecology*, 4th edition Philadelphia, PA: Mosby, 2001, pp. 519–20.

Anders, JF, Powell, EC. Urgency of evaluation and outcome of acute ovarian torsion in pediatric patients. *Arch Pediatr Adolesc Med* 2005;**159**:532.

Pansky, M, Smorgick, N, Herman, A, et al. Torsion of normal adnexa in postmenarchal women and risk of recurrence. *Obstet Gynecol* 2007;**109**:355.

Bayer, AI, Wiskind, AK. Adnexal torsion: can the adnexa be saved?. *Am J Obstet Gynecol* 1994;**171**:1506.

Case #10

History

A 30-year-old woman G_1P_{0010} presents to the ED complaining of pelvic pain that started some years ago. The pain is located bilaterally in her pelvic area and gets worse with menstruation. She states that her menses have been heavier over the last 6 months and she has experienced intense pain with intercourse over the last couple of weeks. The patient denies any fever, nausea, diarrhea, urinary symptoms, or vaginal discharge.

Past medical history

The patient suffers from chronic pelvic pain and chronic fatigue syndrome.

Past ob/gyn history

The patient has been trying to get pregnant for the last 2 years. She has an irregular menstrual cycle. Her last menstrual period began yesterday. She has no history of sexually transmitted infections and she has had normal Pap smears. She has had one pregnancy, for which she had a medical elective termination.

Medications

The patient's medications include prenatal vitamins and folic acid.

Allergies

The patient has no known drug allergies.

Physical exam and ancillary studies

- *Vital signs:* the patient's temperature is 37.0°C, her heart rate is 76 bpm, her blood pressure is 112/70, her respiratory rate is 18, and her room air oxygen saturation is 99%.
- *General:* the patient is awake, alert, and in no acute distress.
- *Head and neck:* her pupils are equally round and reactive to light, her cranial nerves intact. The patient's mucous membranes are dry. Her neck is supple.
- *Cardiovascular:* the patient's heart has regular rate and rhythm, with no murmurs, rubs, or gallops.
- *Lungs:* her lungs are clear to auscultation bilaterally.
- *Abdomen:* her bowel sounds are normoactive in all four quadrants. She is tender to palpation in her bilateral lower quadrants, with positive voluntary guarding and negative rebound. No masses are palpated.
- *Sterile speculum exam:* the patient has grossly normal female external genitalia. There is no vaginal bleeding or discharge. She has a nulliparous cervix, with no grossly apparent lesions.

- *Bimanual vaginal exam:* the patient has a small anteverted uterus, which is slightly tender to mobilization. There is tenderness to palpation of the uterosacral ligaments bilaterally. Multiple small nodules are palpated in the cul-de-sac. No adnexal masses are appreciated and there is no adnexal tenderness to palpation.
- *Extremities and skin:* there is no edema, clubbing, or calf tenderness. The patient has good capillary refill. She has masculine hair distribution pattern.
- *Pertinent abnormal labs:* the patient's urine pregnancy test is negative. All other laboratory exams are within normal limits.
- *Transvaginal ultrasound with Doppler:* there is a moderate amount of free fluid within the posterior cul-de-sac. The patient's anteverted uterus is normal in size, measuring $8.6 \times 3.4 \times 4.9$ cm. Her endometrial echogenic complex (EEC) is within normal limits at 6 mm. The patient's right and left ovaries are normal in size, with no masses, and good arterial and venous flow.

Questions for thought

- What is the pathogenesis of this condition?
- What are the pathognomonic physical exam findings?
- What further imaging modalities should be used in this patient?
- What is definitive treatment?

Diagnosis
Endometriosis.

Discussion
- *Epidemiology:* endometriosis is characterized by the presence of endometrial glands and stroma outside the endometrial cavity and uterine musculature. It affects women of reproductive age, primarily ages 25–35. The incidence is estimated to be between 5 and 20%, although it is difficult to ascertain given that a large proportion of patients are asymptomatic. Approximately 30–40% of women with endometriosis are infertile. The incidence is higher in women belonging to a higher socioeconomic level, possibly due to their delay in pregnancy (which is thought to increase the risk of endometriosis).
- *Pathophysiology:* endometriosis is not well understood. There are different theories proposed to explain its pathogenesis. One of them is retrograde menstruation, where there is menstrual flow through the fallopian tubes towards the pelvis, and subsequent implantation of the endometrial glands and stroma. Another theory is based on direct transplantation, in which there is direct seeding of the endometrium (at the time of a cesarean section, for instance). A third theory hypothesizes that endometriosis occurs as a result of dissemination through lymph and blood vessels. Finally, the coelomic metaplasia theory holds that peritoneal epithelium can transform into endometrial tissue, potentially in response to irritation or inflammation from refluxed menstrual blood.
- *Presentation:* patients usually present with chronic lower abdominal pain that worsens with menses and/or ovulation. Dysmenorrhea, intense dyspareunia, cyclical bladder

or bowel symptoms, abnormal menstrual bleeding, chronic fatigue, and infertility are characteristic.

- *Diagnosis:* endometriosis should be considered in all female patients who report chronic lower abdominal pain that worsens with menses and who have palpable nodules on their uterosacral ligaments. Transvaginal ultrasound is helpful in identifying any endometriomas, but not useful in determining the extent of disease. A definitive diagnosis is based upon surgical findings (superficial "powder burn" or gunshot lesions on the ovaries, serosal surfaces, and peritoneum).
- *Treatment:* the treatment of endometriosis should be directed at improving the patient's quality of life and future fertility. Treatment usually starts medically with GnRH analogs, oral contraceptive pills, progestins, danazol, and aromatase inhibitors. Surgical excision of the lesions is recommended when symptoms are severe or they have failed to resolve with medical therapy.
- *Definitive therapy:* hysterectomy and bilateral salpingo-oophorectomy constitute definitive treatment for endometriosis and are typically performed when all other treatments have failed.

Clinical course

The keys to this patient's diagnosis are careful attention to her history, physical exam, and ancillary studies.

Historical clues	Physical findings	Ancillary studies
• Female in reproductive age	• Abdominal pain with no peritoneal irritation	• Negative pregnancy test
• Chronic lower abdominal pain exacerbated by menses	• Nodularity in the cul-de-sac	• Normal transvaginal ultrasound
• Infertility	• Tenderness with uterine mobilization and palpation of the uterosacral ligaments	
• Dyspareunia		
• Irregular menses		

This woman was thought to have endometriosis based on her presentation, negative pregnancy test, and normal transvaginal ultrasound. She was seen and evaluated by the gynecology service. The patient's pain was controlled in the emergency department and she was discharged home with appropriate oral pain medications. She was instructed to follow up with gynecology to schedule an outpatient laparoscopy to visualize her pelvic organs and potentially excise any endometriotic lesions.

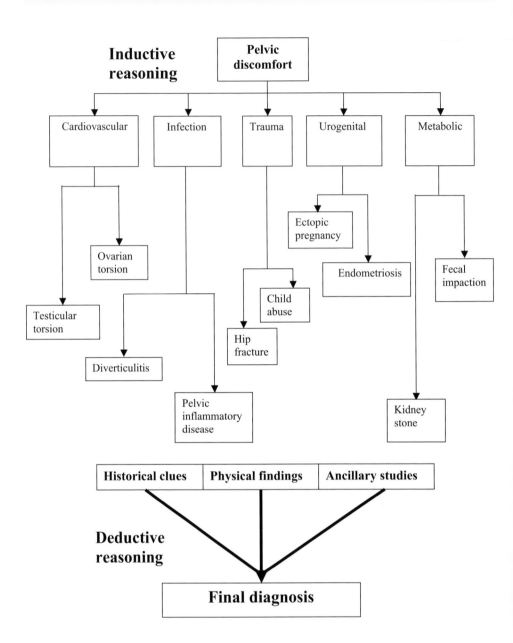

Chapter 8

Chief complaint: headache

Christopher Brook, Rebecca Jeanmonod, Mara McErlean, Rose M. Domingo,
Chamé C. Blackburn, Adam Lloyd, Rena M. Rovere, Margaret Goldon Denio,
Susan M. Rhee, Tyler J. Kenning, Jeffrey K. Claus

Case #1

History

> A 68-year-old Caucasian female presents to the ED with 3 weeks of worsening
> headache and an intermittent low-grade fever. Her headache is localized to the
> right forehead, and a complete history reveals intermittent loss of vision in the
> right eye during the last week. She also feels "sore" in her neck and shoulders, and
> although she has no other specific complaints, describes herself as "just feeling a
> bit under the weather."

Past medical history

The patient's history is significant for coronary artery disease, chronic obstructive pulmonary
disease, controlled hypertension, and hyperlipidemia. She underwent angioplasty 3 years
prior for angina, and has been symptom-free since. The patient denies alcohol consumption
and quit smoking within the last year, but has a 35 pack-year history.

Medications

The patient's medications include atenolol, lisinopril, atorvastatin, fluticasone, albuterol
inhaler, and a baby aspirin daily.

Allergies

The patient has no known drug allergies

Physical exam and ancillary studies

- *Vital signs:* the patient's temperature is 38.2°C, her heart rate is 86 bpm, her blood pressure
  is 118/71, her respiratory rate is 16, and her room air oxygen saturation is 95%.
- *General:* the patient is awake, alert, oriented, and in no acute distress.

Case Studies in Emergency Medicine, ed. R. Jeanmonod, M. Tomassi and D. Mayer.
Published by Cambridge University Press © Cambridge University Press 2010.

- *Head and neck:* her pupils are equally round and reactive to light. She has no photophobia, and her cranial nerves are intact. The patient's right forehead is tender over the temporal artery with a small palpable nodule. Palpation of the nodule reproduces the patient's headache. Her neck is supple and non-tender.
- *Cardiovascular:* the patient's heart has a regular rate and rhythm, without gallops, rubs, or murmurs. She has weak upper extremity pulses.
- *Lungs:* her lungs are mildly decreased throughout, but otherwise are clear to auscultation.
- *Pertinent labs:* the patient's complete blood count is remarkable for a white blood cell count of 8.8 and a hematocrit of 40.6%. Her erythrocyte sedimentation rate is 98 mm/h. Her remaining labs are normal or negative.

Questions for thought

- What diagnostic tests other than erythrocyte sedimentation rate can be used to measure inflammation?
- What part of her history is worrisome for ischemic disease?
- How does one treat this condition in the emergency department?
- What other symptoms might you expect with this disease?
- Does a negative erythrocyte sedimentation rate rule out temporal arteritis?

Diagnosis

Temporal arteritis (giant cell arteritis)

Discussion

- *Epidemiology:* temporal arteritis is an uncommon disease, with an estimated prevalence of less than 1% of the population. It is almost unheard of in patients younger than 50 years of age, but there is an increase in prevalence as the population ages. It is more common in people of Scandinavian descent, but epidemiologic data are lacking in many parts of the world.
- *Pathophysiology:* patients with temporal arteritis have inflammation of both their large- and small-diameter arteries. The pathogenesis probably involves an autoimmune reaction against the vessels, and typically involves extracranial branches of the carotid arteries, such as the temporal and the ophthalmic artery. Other possible manifestations include involvement of the aorta and its major branches, increasing the risk of thoracic aneurysm. Progressive inflammation in the arteries can lead to ischemia and claudication in the distal structures.
- *Presentation:* patients with temporal arteritis usually present with a headache, although not necessarily localized to the region of the temporal artery. Other important historical and physical exam findings are tenderness or abnormalities of the temporal artery, jaw claudication, visual symptoms (including monocular loss of vision and diplopia), and polymyalgia rheumatica, which has been associated with temporal arteritis. Many patients also present with constitutional symptoms including fever, fatigue, and weight loss. Because this condition does not present with a consistent constellation of symptoms,

clinical suspicion should be aroused with involvement of any of the extracranial branches of the carotid artery, especially in conjunction with systemic symptoms or polymyalgia rheumatica. If temporal arteritis is suspected the best tests available in the emergency room are markers of systemic inflammation. Erythrocyte sedimentation rate is the standard lab test ordered to measure this, and a value less than 50 mm/h is a strong predictor against the presence of temporal arteritis, although a negative test does not completely rule out the disease. Therefore, strong clinical suspicion in the presence of an erythrocyte sedimentation rate less than 50 mm/h should be followed up with a temporal artery biopsy. C-reactive protein has also been evaluated as a method of determining systemic inflammation and should be utilized if available. Definitive diagnosis of temporal arteritis requires a surgical biopsy and evaluation by a pathologist.

- *Treatment:* treatment of a patient with temporal arteritis involves systemic anti-inflammatory agents such as glucocorticoids. The typical starting therapy is a daily dosage of 40–60 mg of prednisone or its equivalent. For patients with visual loss or more severe symptoms some experts recommend higher doses. Because the disease is vascular in nature and ischemic damage can occur, antiplatelet therapy in the form of a daily 81 mg aspirin is also indicated. Therapy should be initiated and the patient should be admitted for a temporal artery biopsy if clinical suspicion is still high after evaluation.

- *Definitive therapy:* because of the risk of vision loss, treatment is necessary and extended tapering of glucocorticoids is the therapy of choice. For patients who are steroid-resistant or cannot tolerate steroids, immunomodulatory therapy and antibiologics have been used with some success. In the presence of visual symptoms, higher doses of IV steroids are warranted.

Clinical course

The keys to this patient's diagnosis are careful attention to her history, physical exam, and ancillary studies.

Historical clues	Physical findings	Ancillary studies
• Headache	• Tender temporal region	• Elevated erythrocyte sedimentation rate
• Visual abnormalities	• Low-grade fever	
• History of fatigue	• Supple neck	
• Aching upper extremity muscles consistent with polymyalgia rheumatica	• Poor peripheral pulses	

The provider caring for this patient recognized the classic presentation of temporal arteritis, and ordered the correct study. Based upon the elevated erythrocyte sedimentation rate and her symptoms, the patient was started on prednisone and continued on her antiplatelet therapy. She was admitted to the hospital for a temporal artery biopsy, and the pathology department made the final diagnosis of giant cell arteritis. The patient received a full course of steroids. Her visual symptoms did not return, and she had no further complications.

Further reading

Imboden J, et al. *Current Rheumatology Diagnosis and Treatment*, 2nd edition. New York: McGraw-Hill, 2007.

Pipitone N, Salvarani C. Improving therapeutic options for patients with giant cell arteritis. *Curr Opin Rheumatol* 2008;**20**(1):17–22.

Smetana GW, Shmerling RH. Does this patient have temporal arteritis? *JAMA* 2002;**287**(1):92–101. Review.

Lawrence RC, et al. Estimates of the prevalence of arthritis and selected musculoskeletal disorders in the United States. *Arthritis Rheum* 1999;**42**(2):396.

Case #2

History

A 46-year-old man presents to the ED with a headache. The patient has had a headache for the last week to 10 days. It has been getting steadily worse. It is a constant ache, present over his entire head but worst in his occipital area. Today, while the patient was at work at a dry cleaning establishment, the patient had an episode of confusion and syncope, so he was sent here by his employer. All history is from the patient's boss, as the patient seems somewhat sleepy and confused. His boss does not know whether the patient has any medical problems. The patient denies medical problems.

Past medical history

The patient has no known past medical history.

Medications

It is unknown whether the patient takes any medications.

Allergies

The patient has no known drug allergies.

Social history

The patient has been working at the same dry cleaning establishment for the last 8 months. He is not known to be a smoker or drinker. The patient denies drug use. Per his employer, the patient moved to the United States from Haiti 7 years ago.

Physical exam and ancillary studies

- *Vital signs:* the patient's vital signs show a temperature of 37.4°C, a heart rate of 124 bpm, a respiratory rate of 20, a blood pressure of 95/65, and a room air oxygen saturation of 97%.
- *General:* the patient is confused. He is able to state his name and recognizes his employer, but he seems sleepy and nods off when not stimulated.
- *Head and neck:* the patient's mucous membranes are moist. His neck is supple, although he seems uncomfortable when his neck is ranged. His sclerae are non-icteric.
- *Cardiovascular:* the patient's heart is regularly tachycardic, without murmurs, rubs, or gallops.
- *Lungs:* the patient is in no respiratory distress. His lungs are clear and equal.
- *Abdomen:* the patient is very thin. His abdomen is soft and non-tender, with no organomegaly.

- *Extremities and skin:* the patient's distal extremities are cool with poor capillary refill. He is not diaphoretic. He has no rashes.
- *Neurologic:* his pupils are equal, round, and reactive to light. The patient is sleepy and not compliant with exam. He does follow some commands and does not appear to have a focal neurologic deficit.
- *Pertinent labs:* the patient's glucose level is 95. His complete blood count is remarkable for a white blood cell count of 2.8, with 10% lymphocytes. The patient's other laboratory values are all within normal limits.
- *EKG:* the patient's EKG shows sinus tachycardia, with no ischemic changes.
- *Radiographs:* the patient's chest X-ray shows no evidence of cardiomegaly or pneumonia. His head CT is read as normal.

Questions for thought

- What are the appropriate initial actions to take to stabilize this patient?
- What is the differential diagnosis for this patient?
- What is the appropriate treatment to initiate in the ED in this patient?
- What is his prognosis?

Diagnosis

Cryptococcal meningitis.

Discussion

- *Epidemiology:* cryptococcus is a relatively uncommon form of meningitis, after viral and bacterial meningitides; however, it is the most common fungal cause. Although the true incidence is unknown, it is known that the disease most commonly affects those who are immunosuppressed, whether from medications or underlying medical conditions. Cryptococcal meningitis is one of the AIDS-defining illnesses in those with HIV disease, and is uncommon with CD4 counts above 100. In the United States, the incidence of the disease is falling because of antiretroviral therapy and aggressive treatment. In developing nations, however, this disease is a common cause of mortality.
- *Pathophysiology:* cryptococcal meningitis occurs from hematogenous seeding of the meninges. The pathogen enters the body via a pulmonary route, becomes blood-borne, and is carried to the brain. Once the meninges are involved, the organism grows with relatively little inhibition, as the cerebrospinal fluid lacks antibodies and white blood cells to help fight infection. The organism infects the brain, as well. Therefore, this entity would more accurately be described as a meningoencephalitis.
- *Presentation:* patients with HIV-associated *Cryptococcus* typically present over the course of 1–2 weeks. Many have fever and headache, although patients can have very non-specific complaints, such as malaise and fatigue. About 25% of patients will present with altered mental status. They may also have findings related to pulmonary involvement, such as tachypnea or cough, or findings related to systemic disease, such as rash. Rarely, the disease can present fulminantly, with rapid deterioration and death. Even in those

who present with a more indolent course, the mortality of cryptococcal meningitis is about 10% with appropriate treatment. It is universally fatal in those who are not treated. Patients presenting with altered mental status or with low cerebrospinal fluid white blood cell counts have a worse prognosis.

- *Treatment:* in the ED, treatment generally consists of antifungal therapy. Currently, amphotericin B and flucytosine is the regimen of choice. Since at presentation the provider often does not know the cause of the patient's meningitis, the patient usually also receives antibiotic coverage of bacterial causes of meningitis. In patients such as this one, airway support and circulatory support with IV fluids and pressors are critical.

- *Definitive therapy:* definitive therapy in the cryptococcal meningitis patient is appropriate antifungal therapy. In addition, a large percentage of these patients will have very high opening pressures on lumbar punctures. These patients may require repeated spinal taps or placement of a ventriculoperitoneal shunt to reduce intracranial pressure. Long term, patients with AIDS-associated cryptococcal meningitis require prophylaxis to prevent recurrence.

Clinical course

The keys to this patient's diagnosis are careful attention to history, physical exam, and the use of ancillary studies to rule out other pathology.

Historical clues	Physical findings	Ancillary studies
• Immigrant from Haiti	• Slim build	• Low white blood cell count
• Indolent headache	• Low blood pressure	• Low percentage of lymphocytes
• Altered mental status		• Unremarkable head CT
		• Negative toxicology panels

Upon presentation, the patient's diagnosis was not clear. The provider was concerned about a toxicologic cause of altered mental status, as the patient was exposed to many chemicals at the dry cleaning establishment. The provider was also concerned about an infectious process, since the patient had tachycardia, hypotension, and a low white blood cell count. Therefore, broad-spectrum antibiotic therapy was initiated prior to the patient's head CT. Shortly after return from the radiology suite, the patient had a deterioration in status requiring intubation. Repeat vital signs at that time showed him to have a fever of 38.9°C.

After intubation, the patient underwent lumbar puncture. His opening pressure was very high, such that his spinal fluid overflowed the top of the manometer. The fluid studies showed a white count of 23 and no red cells. The fluid was sent for Gram stain and culture, which is the definitive test for diagnosing cryptococcal meningitis. On microscopy, the lab technician was able to identify *Cryptococcus* and the patient was initiated on antifungal therapy.

The patient was admitted to the intensive care unit, where he had daily lumbar punctures for 3 days. He continued to deteriorate despite adequate therapy and died on hospital day 4. While in the hospital, he was diagnosed with AIDS. It is unknown whether the patient had any knowledge of his HIV status.

Further reading

Jarvis JN, Harrison TS. HIV-associated cryptococcal meningitis. *AIDS* 2007;**21**:2119.

Cox GM, Perfect JR. Cryptococcus neoformans var neoformans and gattii and Trichosporon species. In Edward LA, ed., *Topley and Wilson's Microbiology and Microbial Infections*, 9th edition. London: Arnold, 1997.

Saag MS, Powderly WG, Cloud GA, et al. Comparison of amphotericin B with fluconazole in the treatment of acute AIDS-associated cryptococcal meningitis. *N Engl J Med* 1992;**326**:83.

Case #3

History

A 47-year-old male construction foreman presents to the ED with a sudden severe headache. His co-workers state that he was arguing over the telephone with a supplier when he let out a cry and fell to the floor. The co-workers noticed no seizure activity and the patient did not experience bladder or bowel incontinence. On EMS arrival, the patient was somnolent but arousable and complained of a headache that began at the base of his skull. He states that this headache is dissimilar from his prior migraine headaches.

Past medical history

The patient has a past medical history of infrequent migraines.

Medications

The patient takes butalbital with acetaminophen as needed for migraines.

Allergies

The patient has no known drug allergies.

Physical exam and ancillary studies

- *Vital signs:* the patient's temperature is 37°C, his heart rate is 72 bpm, his respiratory rate is 16, his blood pressure is 170/100, and his oxygen saturation is 97% on room air.
- *General:* the patient is a somnolent middle-aged male who easily wakens to voice.
- *Head and neck:* the patient's pupils are round and reactive. His gag reflex is present. The patient complains of pain with any attempt to flex the neck.
- *Cardiovascular:* the patient's heart has a regular rate and rhythm, with no murmurs, rubs, or gallops.
- *Lungs:* the patient's lungs are clear to auscultation bilaterally without wheezes, rales, or rhonchi.
- *Extremities:* the patient has good perfusion, with no clubbing, cyanosis, or edema.
- *Neurologic:* the patient is somnolent but easily arousable. No focal deficit.
- *Pertinent labs:* blood counts, chemistries, and coagulation factors are within normal limits.
- *EKG:* the patient's EKG shows sinus rhythm with nonspecific ST and T wave changes.
- *Imaging studies:* a cut from the patient's head CT is shown in Figure 8.1.

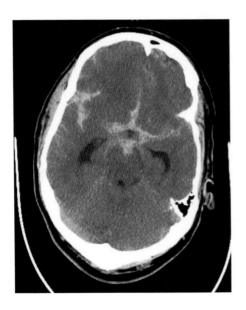

Figure 8.1. The patient's noncontrast cranial CT shows an acute subarachnoid hemorrhage.

Questions for thought

- What are the appropriate initial actions to take to stabilize this patient?
- Once stable, what are other diagnostic tools you can use to make a diagnosis?
- What medications should be avoided in this patient?
- How does one urgently treat this condition in the emergency department?
- What is definitive treatment of this condition?

Diagnosis

Subarachnoid hemorrhage (SAH).

Discussion

- *Epidemiology:* SAH accounts for approximately 8% of all acute stroke syndromes. Although also associated with trauma, the most serious of SAHs are the result of rupture of saccular aneurysms around the base of the brain. Women are slightly more affected than men and the average age of onset is 50. There is significant morbidity associated with spontaneous SAH, with 10% resulting in sudden death. Forty percent of patients will die in the first week. Blacks have a higher incidence of SAH than whites. Correlations have been found with hypertension, hyperlipidemia, collagen vascular diseases, and family history.
- *Pathophysiology:* aneurysms occur at bifurcations of vessels within the Circle of Willis at the base of the brain. Over 80% of SAHs are caused by saccular aneurysms. Other congenital or acquired vascular anomalies account for the remainder. In a minority of patients, no aneurysm can be identified.

- *Presentation:* patients complain of sudden onset of headache that is classically described as a "thunderclap," originating at the base of the skull. Seizure is common, as is photophobia, nausea, and vomiting. Patients may have focal neurologic deficit or may have signs of brain herniation. "Sentinel" headaches from minor bleeding or expansion of aneurysm size are reported. The incidence of vasospasm and recurrent hemorrhage is high, with worsened prognosis associated with advanced age, coma at presentation, re-bleed, and vasospasm.
- *Diagnosis:* diagnosis is usually made by CT scan without contrast, which shows most SAHs. Patients with very suggestive histories should undergo lumbar puncture to evaluate for signs of hemorrhage if the head CT is normal. CTA will often be diagnostic. MRA may also be used.
- *Treatment:* treatment begins with supportive therapy and control of the blood pressure. Calcium-channel blockers are typically titrated intravenously to allow for rapid adjustments in therapy. Ventilatory support is provided as necessitated by decreased levels of consciousness and inability to maintain airway.
- *Definitive therapy:* definitive therapy includes operative repair or endovascular coiling of aneurysm. The ability to utilize an endovascular approach is determined by the size and location of the aneurysm.

Clinical course

The keys to this diagnosis are the sudden onset of severe headache, somnolence, and neck stiffness noted on exam.

Historical clues	Physical findings	Ancillary studies
• Sudden onset	• Hypertension	• CT scan
• Severe pain	• Somnolence	
• Location of headache	• Neck stiffness	
• Change from prior headache pattern		

This 47-year-old male presented with sudden, severe headache that was different from his prior history of migraine headaches. His initial hypertension was thought to be due to pain and was not specifically addressed. Subsequent blood pressure readings were over 200 mmHg systolic. On repeat evaluation, the patient was noted to be unresponsive to painful stimuli and was intubated. The patient's condition further deteriorated and he was declared brain-dead 48 hours later. His family consented to organ donation.

Further reading

Chyatte D, Tindall G, Cooper P. Diagnosis and management of aneurismal SAH. In *The Practice of Neurosurgery*. Philadelphia, PA: Williams and Wilkins, 1996.

Inagawa T. What are the actual incidence and mortality rates of subarachnoid hemorrhage? *Surg Neurol* 1997;**47**(1):47–52.

Jayaraman MV, Mayo-Smith WW, Tung GA. Detection of intracranial aneurysms: multi-detector row CT angiography compared with DSA. *Radiology* 2004;**230**(2):510–18.

Case #4

History

A 72-year-old right-handed man presents to the ED brought in by ambulance with a complaint of headache, which is new over the past 2 months. He describes the headache as being dull or "achy" in character, mild to moderate in severity, and located bifrontally. It is intermittent in nature, with maximal severity on awakening, and aggravation with coughing. There is mild associated nausea. Today, his headache is different, in that it is more persistent, has taken on a "throbbing" quality, and has become localized to the right temporal region. The patient denies any history of headaches prior to the past 2 months. He denies vision or speech changes associated with this headache, though his wife describes some "slurring" of his words today. Per EMS, the patient was hypertensive en route to the ED and received metoprolol 10 mg and enalapril 2.5 mg intravenously. EMS also reports that the patient had subtle left-sided weakness, though the patient subjectively denies any new weakness or sensory changes. Review of systems is otherwise unremarkable at this time.

Past medical history

The patient has a history of hypertension, remote GI bleed secondary to NSAID use, and spinal stenosis. He had a left scalp melanoma resected last year and was found to have one lymph node positive, for which he completed three cycles of radiotherapy, the most recent of which was 2 months ago. He has a remote smoking history of 30 pack-years, having quit in 1968. He denies alcohol or illicit drug use and works as a pharmacist.

Medications

The patient's medications include baby aspirin, amlodipine/benazepril, valsartan, hydrochlorothiazide, labetalol, and methyldopa.

Allergies

The patient has no known drug allergies.

Physical exam and ancillary studies

- *Vital signs:* en route with EMS, the patient's blood pressure was 195/114 and his heart rate was 62. The patient's blood pressure is currently 177/96, his heart rate is 74, his tympanic temperature is 36.3°C, his respiratory rate is 10, and his room air oxygen saturation is 99%.
- *General:* he is comfortable-appearing and non-toxic.
- *Mental status:* the patient is awake, alert and oriented times three, with no aphasia or dysarthria. He follows commands briskly, including crossed commands.

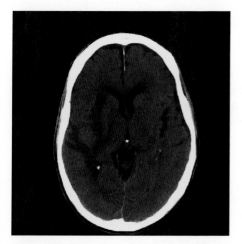

Figure 8.2. The patient's noncontrast head CT confirms a right parietal mass with surrounding edema and resulting left midline shift.

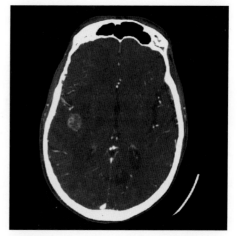

Figure 8.3. The patient's head CT angiography reveals increased vascularity surrounding the intracranial mass, a finding often seen with malignant tumors.

- *Cranial nerves:* the patient's pupils are equal, round, and reactive to light. His extraocular movements are intact and his visual fields are full. There is no nystagmus. The patient's tongue is midline on protrusion without tremor. His palatal elevation is symmetric, his trigeminal nerve branches V1–V3 are intact, and his fundoscopic exam is normal. There is slight blunting of the left nasolabial fold.
- *Neurologic:* the patient displays 5/5 power in all four extremities, proximally and distally. There is subtle downward drift of his left upper and lower extremities, with no pronator drift. His deep tendon reflexes (DTRs) are 2+/2+ and symmetric throughout. His plantar responses are downgoing bilaterally. The patient's sensation is intact to light touch, pinprick, vibratory, and proprioceptive sense throughout. He displays no extinction or neglect. The patient's cerebellar exam shows mildly dysmetric finger-nose-finger testing in the left upper extremity, proportional to the degree of weakness. His finger-nose-finger in right upper extremity and bilateral heel-to-shin testing are intact. The patient's station and gait are normal.
- *Pertinent labs:* the patient's complete blood count and basic metabolic panel are within normal limits, and cardiac markers are negative.
- *EKG:* the patient's EKG shows normal sinus rhythm at 68 bpm without ST or T wave abnormalities.
- *Imaging:* the patient's chest X-ray is normal. Representative cuts of the patient's noncontrast head CT and CT angiography are shown in Figures 8.2 and 8.3.

Questions for thought

- Based on his pattern of headache, what are your initial thoughts regarding the etiology of this patient's symptoms?

- What is your differential diagnosis for this patient, and what are his risk factors for each differential?
- Why is this patient weak?
- What other diagnostic tools can you use to make a definitive diagnosis?
- Which consultations need to be called from the emergency department?
- Which possible treatments can be offered to this patient?

Diagnosis

Intracranial metastatic malignant melanoma.

Discussion

- *Epidemiology:* new-onset insidious headaches in middle or later life, and headaches associated with focal neurologic findings or papilledema, should raise the concern for intracranial mass lesions. Roughly one-third of patients with intracranial tumors present with headache as an initial complaint.
- *Pathophysiology:* headaches associated with intracranial tumors can be directly related to the neoplasm, or attributed to increased intracranial pressure (ICP) or hydrocephalus caused by the neoplasm. Such headaches are thought to be related to traction on pain-sensitive structures within the skull, such as the meninges and dural venous sinuses. Mass lesions, therefore, may not produce headaches until they grow to such a size that they begin to compress or distort pain-sensitive structures.
- *Presentation:* headaches due to intracranial tumors tend to be nonspecific in character, described as "dull," of mild to moderate severity, and intermittent. They can occur bifrontally, then may progress to be worse and ipsilateral to the side of the tumor (in cases of supratentorial lesions) or posteriorly (in cases of posterior fossa lesions). They are usually maximal on awakening and aggravated by changes in position or maneuvers that increase intracranial pressure, such as the Valsalva maneuver that occurs with coughing, sneezing, bending, lifting, and straining with stool. If hydrocephalus and increased intracranial pressure develop, a triad of headache, nausea, and papilledema may be seen. Headaches related to intracranial masses and hydrocephalus can, less commonly, present with sudden paroxysms of pain which subside rapidly and may be associated with changes in mental status and loss of consciousness events.
- *Diagnosis:* suspicion of an intracranial mass lesion warrants prompt neuroimaging, which may help to identify the nature of the lesion and has importance for pre-operative planning. Head CT is easily performed on an urgent basis in most emergency departments and can reveal intracranial masses with surrounding edema. CT angiography may reveal increased vascularity with malignant tumors. Brain MRI with gadolinium enhancement is best for evaluating intracranial tumors, particularly of the posterior fossa. Spectroscopy (MR or CT), functional MRI, perfusion MRI, and PET scans may also be helpful in terms of diagnosis and pre-operative planning. Although intracranial tumors can have characteristic appearances on these imaging modalities, the gold standard for definitive diagnosis remains histopathology, with tissue often obtained during tumor resection or via biopsy.

- *Treatment:* the treatment for headache related to intracranial mass lesions is symptomatic. When mass lesions are small or slow-growing, they are often associated with more mild, nonspecific headaches that are adequately controlled with over-the-counter nonsteroidal anti-inflammatory agents and do not require emergency attention. As masses increase in size and begin to compress pain-sensitive structures or cause hydrocephalus, headache management consists of measures meant to decrease intracranial pressure. Cortico-steroids, osmotic diuretics, hyperventilation, and head elevation can be used early. However, persistent clinical features of elevated pressures warrant placement of intracranial pressure (ICP) monitors and may indicate a need for more aggressive management, such as therapeutic hypothermia, deep sedation, cerebrospinal fluid (CSF) drainage, and surgical decompression. These patients generally require ICU care, as close monitoring and correction of hemodynamic and electrolyte changes, and maintenance of euvolemia and normo- to hyperosmolarity are required. Prophylaxis with antiepileptic medications is often used in cases of large mass lesions or lesions adjacent to the cortex, as seizures can both complicate and contribute to elevated intracranial pressures.
- *Definitive therapy:* the definitive treatment for headache related to an intracranial mass is tumor debulking or resection. Obtaining tissue for histopathologic diagnosis is important for both prognostication and planning of adjuvant therapies. Early neurosurgical and neuro-oncologic involvement are, therefore, of critical importance, and neurologic evaluation is often sought for assistance with suspected seizure activity.

Clinical course

The keys to this patient's diagnosis are careful attention to his past medical history, pattern of headache and progression of symptoms, recognition of his focal neurologic deficits, and proper use of emergency neuroimaging.

Historical clues	Physical findings	Ancillary studies
• New-onset headache in middle-aged man	• Focal motor deficits of left face, arm, and leg	• Head CT with right hemispheric mass lesion and edema extending to posterior limb of internal capsule with relative sparing of sensory cortex and thalamus
• More mild, nonspecific headache progressing to more persistent, focal one	• No sensory deficits	• No hydrocephalus
• Headache aggravation on awakening or with Valsalva maneuvers	• No cerebellar signs	• Increased vascularity of lesion on CTA
• Associated nausea	• No cranial nerve or brainstem dysfunction	
• Recent node-positive malignant melanoma	• No papilledema	

This man was felt to have an intracranial metastasis related to malignant melanoma based on his characteristic headache pattern, past medical history, neurologic examination, and head CT. Neurologic and neurosurgical consultations were obtained, and the patient was placed on intravenous corticosteroids and prophylactic antiepileptic medications. He eventually underwent a gadolinium-enhanced MRI and tumor resection. Tissue confirmation of metastatic malignant melanoma was made. Evaluation by neuro-oncology followed tissue diagnosis and adjuvant therapy was initiated.

Further reading

Forsyth PA, Posner JB. Headaches in patients with brain tumors: a study of 111 patients. *Neurology* 1993;**43**:1678.

Ropper AH, Brown RH, eds. *Adams and Victor's Principles of Neurology*, 8th edition. New York: McGraw-Hill, 2005, pp. 158–9.

Headache Classification Subcommittee of the International Headache Society (IHS). The International Classification of Headache Disorders, 2nd edition. *Cephalalgia* 2004;**24**(Suppl 1):1–160.

Case #5

History

A 32-year-old woman comes to the ED after experiencing what she describes as an "optical illusion" and numbness to the left side of her face. The vision in her left eye was suddenly obscured by a "sunburst with a zig-zag line hanging down from it." It persisted even when she blinked or looked away from her computer. She then felt numbness and tingling to the left side of her face. The entire episode lasted about 5 minutes, then completely resolved. She became worried that she may have had a stroke and immediately called her husband. By the time he arrived at her office she was upset, anxious, and had developed a gradual-onset throbbing headache that she describes as 8/10 in intensity.

Past medical history

The patient has a history of anxiety and depression. She smokes half a pack of cigarettes daily and drinks alcohol 1–2 times per month. Her last menstrual period was 3 weeks ago. She is the mother of twins delivered by cesarean section 2 years ago.

Medications

The patient's medications include paroxetine and oral contraceptives.

Allergies

The patient has no known drug allergies.

Physical exam and ancillary studies

- *Vital signs:* the patient's tympanic temperature is 37.1°C, her blood pressure is 116/72, her heart rate is 84, her respiratory rate is 16, and her room air oxygen saturation is 99%.
- *General:* the patient is awake and alert, squinting her eyes, and occasionally holding her hand to the left side of her head.
- *Head and neck:* the patient's pupils are equally round and reactive to light, with some photophobia on examination. Her visual acuity is normal. There is no papilledema or ptosis. The patient's mucous membranes are moist. Her headache is exacerbated by swift head or neck movements, but her neck is supple and not painful. Her thyroid is normal to palpation.
- *Cardiovascular:* the patient's heart has regular rate and rhythm, her peripheral pulses are bounding, and she has normal capillary refill.
- *Lungs:* her lungs are clear to auscultation throughout all fields.
- *Extremities and skin:* there is no edema or tenderness to palpation. The patient has no rashes, petechiae, or purpura.
- *Neurologic:* the patient's GCS is 15 and her cranial nerves are intact. Her motor strength and sensation are normal and symmetric in both upper and lower extremities. Her DTRs

are 2+ bilaterally. She has normal finger-to-nose testing and performs rapid alternating movements. The patient's gait is normal. Her Romberg's test is negative.

- *Ancillary studies:* no studies were obtained.

Questions for thought

- What is the differential diagnosis for this patient?
- What risk factors (present or absent) help to make the diagnosis?
- What type of imaging is indicated?
- What are appropriate actions to treat this patient?
- Which medications should be used with caution in this patient?
- How should the patient be counseled to prevent future episodes?

Diagnosis

Migraine with aura (classic migraine).

Discussion

- *Epidemiology:* migraine is a common cause of headache and affects 5–20% of the general population. It is most prevalent in the third decade of life and over 90% of migraineurs will have experienced symptoms before age 40. Females represent 60–75% of all migraine patients. Migraine *without* aura is the most common presentation, accounting for 80% of migraines.
- *Pathophysiology:* the pathophysiology of migraine is a heavily debated topic. It is complex and certainly multifactorial. Intracranial vasoconstriction followed by rebound dilatation has long been thought to be a contributing factor. However, more recent research suggests that this is in response to a primary defect in neuronal function. Imbalance of neurotransmitters such as serotonin, dopamine, and calcitonin gene-related peptide has also been implicated. A family history of migraines is present about 60% of the time, suggesting a genetic component as well.
- *Presentation:* the presentation of our patient is classic for migraine with aura. Visual disturbances (usually involving scotomata, flashing lights, or hemianopic field defects) are the most common type of aura, followed by sensory deficits (numbness and tingling of the lower face, in the case of our patient). Patients can also have aphasic, motor, or other types of auras. A unilateral, throbbing headache is characteristic of migraine. Photophobia and nausea are common symptoms.
- *Diagnosis:* the diagnosis of migraine is a clinical one. Diagnostic testing such as CT, MRI, or lumbar puncture might be used to exclude other dangerous etiologies of headache such as bacterial meningitis, subarachnoid hemorrhage, or intracranial mass. Neuroimaging is not necessary in most patients with migraine, but should be considered when the patient has an abnormal neurologic examination or atypical symptoms.
- *Treatment:* emergency department treatment of migraine is aimed at abortive therapy. Dopamine antagonists (such as prochlorperazine or metoclopramide) are very effective in ameliorating headache, especially when nausea or vomiting is present. Patients may

also benefit from IV fluid administration. Other treatment agents include ergots, triptans, NSAIDs, steroids, and caffeine. Narcotic analgesia should be avoided if possible because it can contribute to the development of chronic rebound headaches, as well as repeat ED visits.

- *Definitive therapy:* patients should follow up with their primary care provider to identify and avoid migraine triggers and to find effective symptomatic therapy. Those patients who have frequent, long-lasting, or disabling headaches may benefit from migraine prophylaxis and follow-up with a neurologist.

Clinical course

The keys to this patient's diagnosis are careful attention to her history and exam.

Historical clues	Physical findings	Ancillary studies
• Headache onset preceded by aura	• Normal temperature	
• Unilateral location	• Normal neurologic exam	
• Patient's age	• Absence of meningeal signs	
• Patient's gender	• Photophobia	

This woman had a classic presentation for migraine with aura. She had symptoms very typical of migraine with no signs of meningitis and a normal neurologic examination, therefore no further workup was warranted. She was treated with 1 liter of normal saline IV and 10 mg of prochlorperazine IV with 25 mg of diphenhydramine IV to prevent akathisia or dystonia. After 1 hour, her headache had improved to 2/10 in intensity and she was discharged to follow up with her primary care provider.

Further reading

Bajwa ZH, et al. Acute treatment of migraine in adults. www.uptodate.com. Last updated April 15, 2008.

Bajwa ZH, et al. Pathophysiology, clinical manifestations, and diagnosis of migraine in adults. www.uptodate.com. Last updated May 19, 2008

Lipton RB, et al. Migraine prevalence, disease burden, and the need for preventative therapy. *Neurology* 2007;**68**:343.

Silberstein SD. Practice parameter: evidence-based guidelines for migraine headache (an evidence-based review): report of the quality standards subcommittee of the American Academy of Neurology. *Neurology* 2000;**55**:754

Simon, RP et al. *Clinical Neurology*, 4th edition. Norwalk, CT: Appleton & Lange, 1999. pp. 93–8.

Case #6

History

> A 60-year-old woman presents to the ED complaining of a severe headache
> which came on just before going to bed. She describes the headache as constant,
> "driving," and concentrated in her forehead and left eye. Her vision is
> intermittently blurry and cloudy. The patient is nauseated and vomited prior to
> arrival. She denies recent fevers or chills. There is no history of recent trauma.

Past medical history

The patient has a history of hypertension, non-insulin-dependent diabetes, and melanoma
removal from her left arm 4 years ago. She has a remote history of migraines, which have
decreased in frequency since her menopause 10 years ago. She currently is affected by
migraines 1–2 times per year, which she treats successfully with ibuprofen alone. She is married and works part-time as a librarian in an elementary school that is undergoing construction. She wears glasses for reading only. She does not smoke.

Medications

The patient's medications include metoprolol, altace, glyburide, metformin, flaxseed, and
calcium.

Allergies

The patient has no known drug allergies.

Physical exam and ancillary studies

- *Vital signs:* the patient's tympanic temperature is 37°C, her pulse is 91, her blood pressure
  is 145/91, her respiratory rate is 20, and her room air oxygen saturation is 97%.
- *General:* the patient is awake and alert, but in obvious pain as she occasionally holds the
  left side of her head.
- *Head and neck:* the patient's head is normocephalic and atraumatic. Her left eye is red
  and injected, but without discharge. The patient's right pupil is reactive. Her left pupil is
  slightly dilated and nonreactive. Her cornea appears hazy. The patient's tympanic membranes are clear bilaterally. Her neck is non-tender and supple, with free range of motion.
- *Cardiovascular:* the patient's heart has regular rate and rhythm without rubs. She has
  normal peripheral pulses.
- *Lungs:* her lungs are clear bilaterally.
- *Extremities and skin:* the patient has no edema. Her skin is warm and dry, with normal
  capillary refill. She has no rashes.
- *Neurologic:* the patient reports decreased, blurry vision in the left eye (20/200). Her vision
  is unchanged in right eye (20/25). The rest of the patient's cranial nerves are normal.
  She has normal motor strength and sensation, her reflexes are 2+ bilaterally, and she has

normal finger-to-nose testing with rapid alternating movements. Her gait and balance are normal.

- *Ancillary studies:* no studies were obtained.

Questions for thought

- What is the differential diagnosis for this patient?
- What physical exam findings help to make the diagnosis?
- What further tests should be performed to confirm the diagnosis?
- What risk factors are associated with this condition?
- What are appropriate actions to treat this patient?

Diagnosis

Acute angle-closure glaucoma.

Discussion

- *Epidemiology:* acute angle-closure glaucoma (AACG) is the most common form of glaucoma globally, but accounts for only about 10% of all glaucoma cases in the United States. It most frequently affects patients in their 60s and 70s. Family history of AACG and race (especially Asian or Inuit) are risk factors, as is diabetes and female gender.
- *Pathophysiology:* aqueous humor flows from the ciliary bodies in the posterior chamber (formed by the lens posteriorly and the iris anteriorly) through the pupil into the anterior chamber (bounded by the iris posteriorly and the cornea anteriorly), then through a trabecular meshwork that filters it out of the eye and into the bloodstream. In AACG, the flow is blocked when the iris comes in physical contact with the lens. This typically occurs during normal pupil dilatation, such as when ambient light is dim or when midriatics are applied. Pressure within the eye builds when the aqueous humor's drainage is impaired. The angle is further compromised when the iris bows forward from the buildup of the fluid. Increased intraocular pressure causes the cornea to become edematous and cloudy, and with time can directly damage the optic nerve. Those with anatomical variations including a thinner ciliary body or more anteriorly positioned iris or lens are more susceptible to AACG. Women are at a higher risk for AACG because of their shallower anterior chamber.
- *Presentation:* most patients who present with AACG are elderly, with no history of previous glaucoma. "Classic" presentations occur when the pupil dilates rapidly after being exposed to dimmed lights, such as in a movie theater or when the lights are turned out at bedtime. Many patients will describe eye pain or blurry vision, but can also present with complaints of headache, nausea, or even abdominal pain.
- *Diagnosis:* the diagnosis of AACG is made when the physical exam demonstrates visual loss and a mid-dilated, fixed pupil. It is confirmed with the measurement of increased intraocular pressure (IOP) by tonometry reading. Normal IOP is between 10 and 21 mmHg.

- *Treatment:* the goal of therapy is to reduce intraocular pressure and to eventually correct the angle deficit. Ophthalmic beta-blockers (such as timolol and betaxolol) will decrease aqueous production and increase outflow, and should be administered along with a topical alpha-agonist (apraclonidine). Prostaglandin analogs (travoprost) are also used to sometimes dramatically lower IOP through an increase in uveo-scleral outflow, although the exact mechanism is not clear. Carbonic anhydrase inhibitors (acetazolamide) also inhibit the production of aqueous humor and are typically administered intravenously since many patients are already nauseated. Hyperosmotic drugs (mannitol and glycerol) can be given systemically to decrease intraocular volume, by creating an osmotic gradient between the aqueous humor and the blood. Because inflammation is present, a topical steroid (prednisolone acetate) should be coadministered to reduce optic nerve damage. Finally, a topical cholinergic drug (miotic) such as pilocarpine will constrict the pupil and allow for angle widening, once the intraocular pressure has been reduced. Patients should lie supine to allow gravity to move the lens more posteriorly. Urgent ophthalmologic consultation is essential.
- *Definitive therapy:* laser peripheral iridotomy, in which tiny holes are created in the iris, is considered the definitive treatment for AACG.

Clinical course

Intraocular pressure was measured at 10 mmHg in the right eye and 42 in the left. The patient was treated with the appropriate medications while awaiting ophthalmologic consultation. Intraocular pressure was checked hourly and normalized over the next 24 hours. The patient underwent laser peripheral iridotomy 48 hours later and was discharged home with full visual recovery.

Historical clues	Physical findings	Ancillary studies
• Onset in evening (when lights are lower)	• "Red eye"	
• Age over 50	• Partially dilated, non-reactive pupil	
• Female gender	• Decreased vision	
• Diabetes	• Hazy cornea	
• Farsightedness	• Elevated intra-ocular pressure	

Further reading

Darkeh AK. Glaucoma, acute angle-closure. www.emedicine.com/topic752.htm. Last updated October 3, 2007.

Soltau JB, Thorn TJ. Changing paradigms in the medical treatment of glaucoma. Surv Ophthamol 2002;**47**(supplement 1);S2–S5.

Weizer JS, et al. Angle-closure glaucoma. www.uptodate.com. Last updated March 21, 2008.

Case #7

History

An 18-year-old male presents to the ED complaining of a headache. He states it started as a mild headache and has become worse throughout the day. He states that this is a constant headache that is worse with standing. He also admits to feeling dizzy with standing up quickly. The patient's last urine output was this morning, approximately 12 hours ago. He states that he has been outside all day in the hot weather practicing soccer for tryouts next week. The patient denies any photophobia, nausea, vomiting, neck pain, or difficulty with ambulation. He also denies any falls or head trauma. The patient denies any chest pain, palpitations, or shortness of breath. He denies taking any medication for his complaint.

Past medical history

The patient has a history of seasonal allergies.

Past surgical history

He had an appendectomy 8 years ago.

Social history

He denies any illicit drug usage. The patient also denies any sick contacts or travel outside the country.

Medications

The patient takes fexofenadine.

Allergies

The patient has no known drug allergies.

Physical exam and ancillary studies

- *Vital signs:* the patient's temperature is 36.2°C, his heart rate is 128 bpm, his blood pressure is 100/56, his respiratory rate is 16, and his room air oxygen saturation is 99%.
- *General:* the patient is awake, alert, and oriented.
- *Head and neck:* he has no signs of trauma. His pupils are equally round and reactive to light, with no photophobia. His extraocular movements are intact. The patient's mucous membranes are dry.
- *Cardiovascular:* the patient's heart has a regular tachycardia without murmurs, rubs, or gallops. He has no carotid bruits or thrills.
- *Lungs:* the patient's lungs are clear to auscultation bilaterally. He has good air movement.

- *Neurologic:* the patient's cranial nerves are intact. He has normal speech. Ambulation was not attempted secondary to the patient's lightheadedness.
- *Extremities and skin:* his skin is dry with tenting present. He has no peripheral edema or cyanosis.
- *Pertinent abnormal labs:* the patient's urine shows a specific gravity of 1.030 and it is positive for ketones. The patient's hematocrit is elevated at 54%. The remainder of the urine, hematology, and chemistry studies are normal or negative.

Questions for thought

- Why does this patient have a headache?
- What are the appropriate initial actions to take to stabilize this patient?
- Once stable, what are other diagnostic tools you can use to make a diagnosis?
- How does one ugently treat this condition in the ED?
- What is definitive treatment of this condition?

Diagnosis

Headache secondary to dehydration.

Discussion

- *Epidemiology:* dehydration is a common cause of headache. The most common causes of dehydration are gastroenteritis and inadequate fluid intake. Other frequent causes include excessive bleeding, excessive sweating, fever, and diabetes.
- *Pathophysiology:* patients with dehydration have decreased fluid intake, increased fluid loss, or both. In the early phases of dehydration, the healthy body will compensate by retaining fluid and limiting urinary output. In the setting of renal disease, this may not occur, leading to earlier signs and symptoms. Once dehydration has progressed to the point where the body is unable to compensate, the patient tends to become more symptomatic and has laboratory abnormalities. If the patient's source of dehydration is not corrected and the patient is not hydrated, this can lead to hypovolemic shock and even death.
- *Presentation:* this presentation is typical for dehydration from any cause. Severity of symptoms is based on total volume of fluid deficit. Patients typically present with thirst, dry mouth, dark urine, dizziness, muscle cramps, headache, and decreased urination. In cases of early or mild dehydration, physical exam and laboratory testing may give little or no indication of the patient's volume status. Patients will develop abnormal vital signs when dehydration is moderate to severe. In these cases, patients have an elevated heart rate, elevated respiratory rate, and decreased blood pressure. On exam, very dehydrated patients may have dry mucous membranes, delayed capillary refill time, and tenting of the skin. On laboratory evaluation, they may have evidence of concentrated urine, with a high specific gravity, or evidence of hemoconcentration, with elevated hematocrit and/or sodium levels. If the dehydration has been subacute in course, the patient may also have renal failure.

- *Treatment:* initial treatment of the patient with dehydration is fluid replacement. The ideal route would be by mouth; however, if the patient presents with vomiting or is unable to tolerate fluids by mouth, then the route of rehydration needs to be intravenous. Electrolytes also should be replaced if the patient appears to have moderate to severe dehydration. Most sports beverages as well as pediatric oral rehydration solutions are good sources of oral rehydration. If the patient needs IV rehydration, he should receive a 20 ml/kg bolus of normal saline over a 30-minute duration. Patients should be reassessed after each bolus for improving clinical appearance, vital signs, and urine output. Severely dehydrated patients may need three or even four boluses.

- *Definitive therapy:* since most of the underlying causes of dehydration are acute and short-lived in nature, the patient typically only requires treatment in the ED. Once the patient has been rehydrated, he may be safely discharged so long as he is able to take fluids by mouth. If the patient has evidence of end-organ damage from dehydration, such as renal failure, or has underlying comorbidities such as diabetes or heart disease, he may need to be admitted for closer monitoring of volume status.

Clinical course

The keys to this patient's diagnosis are careful attention to his history, physical exam, and ancillary studies.

Historical clues	Physical findings	Ancillary studies
• Thirst	• Tachycardia	• Elevated hematocrit
• Dry mouth	• Hypotension	• Elevated specific gravity on urinalysis
• Dizziness	• Dry mucous membranes	• Ketones on urinalysis
• Headache	• Skin tenting	
• Decrease urination		
• Dark urine		
• Fatigue		

This man was suspected to be dehydrated based on his history and physical exam. Dehydration is a clinical diagnosis, but in his case it was supported by his ancillary studies. The patient did not have any vomiting, so he was given oral rehydration fluids. He drank 2 liters of fluid in the ED prior to having any urine output. After the fluid, the patient's headache and dizziness resolved. His vitals signs were rechecked and it was noted that his tachycardia and hypotension had resolved. The patient was discharged and instructed on the importance of staying well hydrated while playing sports, especially in a hot environment.

Further reading

Tobleman R, Stone K. Headache. In Stone CK, Humphries RL, eds., *Current Diagnosis and Treatment Emergency Medicine*, 8th edition. New York: McGraw-Hill, 2005, pp. 158–9.

Kasper D, Braunwald E, Fauce A, et al. Headache. In *Harrison's Principles of Internal Medicine*, 16th edition. New York: McGraw-Hill, 2005, p. 399.

Counihan TJ. Headache, neck pain, and other painful disorders. In Andreoli D, Carpenter C, Griggs R, et al., eds. *Cecil Essentials of Medicine*, 5th edition. Philadelphia, PA: WB Saunders, 2001, p. 909.

Case #8

History

A 17-year-old female presents to the ED after a head injury. She had been struck in the left side of her head with a softball 3 days ago. She had a witnessed 30–60 seconds of unconsciousness immediately after the injury. Following the event, she had a headache. She has not had visual changes, nausea, vomiting, seizure activity, or gait disturbances. She rated the headache immediately after the trauma as 5/10 on a pain scale. Today, she presents with a 3 day history of intermittent mild headache which is now about 2/10 on the pain scale. She also complains of fatigue, dizziness, and nausea without vomiting. She has been treating herself with ibuprofen intermittently over the past 3 days.

Past medical history

The patient is healthy. She has a history of bladder surgery performed at the age of 9.

Medications

The patient takes only ibuprofen.

Allergies

She has no known drug allergies.

Social history

The patient is a high-school student who lives with her parents. She denies violence or abuse, and does not smoke or drink.

Physical exam and ancillary studies

- *Vitals signs:* the patient's temperature is 36.8°C, her blood pressure is 126/59 mmHg, her heart rate is 63 bpm, her respiratory rate is 16, and her oxygen saturation on room air is100%.
- *General:* the patient is awake and alert. She is not in any acute distress. She is ambulatory without any gait disturbance. She has appropriate affect. She is very interactive.
- *Head and neck:* the patient's head is normocephalic without bruising or soft tissue swelling, but she has tenderness over the left parietal-occipital area on palpation. Her pupils are equal, round, and briskly reactive to light. Her extraocular motions are intact. The patient's fundoscopic exam shows sharp disk margins. There is no tenderness on palpation of her c-spine. There is no facial asymmetry. Her tympanic membranes are normal bilaterally.
- *Cardiovascular:* the patient's heart is regular, without murmurs or rubs.
- *Respiratory:* her lungs are clear and equal, and she has no chest wall tenderness.

- *Abdominal:* the patient's abdomen is soft and non-tender. She has no organomegaly.
- *Extremities and skin:* the patient's extremities are warm and well-perfused. She has no clubbing, cyanosis, or edema.
- *Neurologic:* the patient's cranial nerves II–XII are intact. Rapid alternating hand motion, finger-to-nose and heel-to-shin are intact. The patient is able to heel-and-toe walk without difficulty and her Rhomberg is negative. Her strength is 5/5 in all four extremities. Her deep tendon reflexes are normal, equal and symmetrical in all four extremities.
- *Psychological:* the patient is alert and oriented, with appropriate memory and insight.

Questions for thought

- When should you obtain a CT scan for remote head trauma?
- Are diagnostic strategies different based on extremes of age or comorbidities?
- How valuable is a history of loss of consciousness in making a diagnosis?
- How would you handle the public expectation of obtaining a head CT when it isn't clinically indicated?
- What are the consequences and long-term complications of this diagnosis?

Diagnosis

Post-concussive syndrome.

Discussion

- *Epidemiology:* post-concussive syndrome (PCS) is a sequela of minor traumatic brain injury. It is a symptom complex that includes headaches (25–80%), dizziness (50%), neuropsychiatric symptoms (irritability, anxiety, depression), and cognitive impairment (impaired memory and concentration, as well as noise or light sensitivity). Thirty to eighty percent of patients with mild to moderate brain injury experience some symptoms of PCS. The severity of the injury does not correlate with the risk of PCS; however, increasing age and female gender increase the risk.
- *Pathophysiology:* most medical experts feel PCS is both biochemical and psychological in origin. In patients with PCS, neuroimaging (SPECT, PET, and functional MRI) have documented areas of abnormalities not seen on head CTs. However, these neuroimaging findings are not specific to head injuries and are also noted in patients with migraines and depression.
- *Presentation:* the presentation 3 days post-event is a typical timeframe for PCS. When a patient presents remotely from the injury with the symptomatology of dizziness, headache, and nausea accompanied by a completely negative neurologic exam, ominous intracranial pathology such as subdural or epidural hematoma is exceedingly unlikely. Patients usually come in at this time because they believe that symptoms referable to the head injury should have abated after a day or two; however, the PCS syndrome doesn't usually start improving until 7–10 days post-injury. It is not necessary to subject these patients to radiographic evaluation. However, the settings of impairment by mind-altering substances, extremes of age, inability to complete a good neurologic exam

or comorbities such as anticoagulation or dementia should lower the threshold for neuroimaging when someone presents in delayed fashion to the ED.

- *Treatment:* PCS is treated supportively. Mild headache management includes advocating rest, use of acetaminophen analgesia and excluding use of aspirin and ibuprofen, and a step-wise return to routine activities. This would preclude return to vigorous sports activities until resolution of all physical and cognitive symptoms to allow the concussed brain to heal and prevent re-injury. Nausea and dizziness are best managed with rest and maintaining hydration. These symptoms rarely require prescription anti-emetics. Patients should be discouraged from engaging in activities that trigger a return or worsening of their symptoms. Reassurance is the cornerstone of treatment. The disability of PCS is greatest in the first 7–10 days for the majority of patients. Most patients will be largely recovered by 3 months. An estimated 10–15% of patients will have symptoms which persist 1 year or longer. Close follow-up with a primary care provider is indicated.

Clinical course

The keys to this patient's diagnosis are careful attention to her history and physical exam.

Historical clues	Physical findings
• Head injury	• Normal neurologic exam
• Ongoing mild headache	• Normal fundoscopic exam
• Nausea	• Minimal signs of trauma

The absence of focal abnormal neurologic findings was paramount to this young patient's diagnosis. PCS diagnosis is primarily based on a normal physical exam. While her history certainly pointed to a minor traumatic brain injury with sequela of post-concussive syndrome, there was an absence of focal abnormal signs to indicate a need for CT scan. In addition, our patient had no comorbidities which would warrant consideration for delayed imaging. Often head CTs are obtained for the reassurance of the patient and family; however, newer studies indicate that this is not without danger, as the radiation exposure is significant. Therefore, CT scanning was not performed on our patient. She and her family were reassured and educated as to the natural course of this disease entity. The patient followed up with her primary care doctor 1 month after her initial injury, and had complete resolution of her symptoms.

Further reading

Bazarian JJ, Wong T, Harris M, et al. Epidemiology and the predictors of post-concussive syndrome after minor head injury in the emergency population. *Brain Inj* 1999;**13**:173.

Bazarian JJ, Atabaki S. Predicting postconcussion syndrome after minor tramatic brain injury. *Acad Emerg Med* 2001;**8**:788.

Chen SH, Kareken DA, Fastenau PS, et al. A study of the persistent post-concussion syndrome in mild head injuries using position emission tomography. *J Neurol Neurosurg Psychiatry* 2003;**74**:326.

Iverson GL. Outcome from mild traumatic brain injury. *Curr Opin Psychiatry* 2005;**18**:301.

Stein R. Too much of a good thing? The growing use of CT scans fuels medical concern about radiation exposure. *Washington Post*, January 15, 2008, p. HE01.

Case #9

History

A 54-year-old white female presents to the ED complaining of a 2-day history of headache. She describes the headache as "all over her head," and different from her usual migraine headache. She also complains of some vague left-sided chest pressure, rated approximately 6/10 on a pain scale. She denies any shortness of breath, palpitations, radiation of chest pain, or radiation of headache pain. She is on hemodialysis for end-stage renal disease, and had her last treatment yesterday. Her renal disease is secondary to hypertension. She has a history of noncompliance with medications, and has not taken her blood pressure medications.

Past medical history

The patient has end-stage renal disease as a result of uncontrolled hypertension. She also has a history of diabetes, hypercholesterolemia, anemia of chronic disease, degenerative joint disease, and gastroesophageal reflux. She has a history of a stroke 7 years ago. She is a current smoker, with a 32 pack-year history. She denies any alcohol or illicit drug use.

Medications

She is supposed to be on carvedilol, lisinopril, clonidine patch, esomeprazole, insulin, darbepoeitin, aspirin, and clopidogrel, but is noncompliant.

Allergies

Patient has no known drug allergies.

Physical exam and ancillary studies

- *Vital signs:* the patient's temperature is 36.8°C, her pulse is 107 bpm, her blood pressure is 225/131, her respiratory rate is 20, and her room air oxygen saturation is 96%.
- *General:* the patient appears non-toxic, and is in no acute distress.
- *Head and neck:* the patient's head is normocephalic and atraumatic. On eye exam, her conjunctivae are pale, her pupils are equally round and reactive to light, and her disk margins appear normal. She has moist oral mucosa, with no lesions in the oropharynx.
- *Cardiovascular:* the patient's heart sounds are regular, with no appreciable murmur.
- *Respiratory:* her lungs are clear to auscultation bilaterally.
- *Abdomen:* the patient's abdomen is soft, obese, and non-tender to palpation; no appreciable organomegaly.
- *Extremities:* her extremities are warm and well-perfused, with no clubbing, cyanosis, or edema.
- *Neurologic:* the patient's cranial nerves are intact. She has normal strength and sensation bilaterally, with intact reflexes.

- *Pertinent labs:* the patient's blood urea nitrogen is 83 with a creatinine of 9.8. Her potassium is 5.0. The remainder of her labs are normal or negative for acute disease
- *Radiographs:* the patient's head CT and chest X-ray are both negative for any acute disease.
- *EKG:* the patient's electrocardiogram shows no abnormalities.

Questions for thought

- What are the signs of end-organ damage in a patient with hypertension?
- What are the key differences between hypertensive emergency and hypertensive urgency?
- How should this patient be treated in the emergency department?
- What is a possible etiology for the patient's hypertension?

Diagnosis

Hypertensive urgency.

Discussion

- *Epidemiology:* hypertension is considered severe when the systolic blood pressure exceeds 180 mmHg and/or the diastolic blood pressure exceeds 120 mmHg. When the blood pressure reaches these levels, it may cause end-organ damage, which is termed hypertensive emergency. A patient with extremely elevated blood pressure, but without evidence of end-organ damage, fits into the hypertensive urgency category. This commonly occurs in patients who are noncompliant with their long-term antihypertensive regimen.
- *Presentation:* the hypertensive urgency patient may present with a headache, and upon review of vital signs, will be noted to be extremely hypertensive. However, physical exam and diagnostic studies will not reveal any signs of end-organ damage such as encephalopathy, retinal hemorrhages, congestive heart failure, myocardial infarction, or acute renal failure. Although this patient has an elevated blood urea nitrogen and creatinine, she is also a chronic hemodialysis patient, so this is not considered acute.
- *Treatment:* the goal of treatment is to lower the blood pressure to less than or equal to 160/100 mmHg over the span of several hours to days. The patient should be kept in a relatively quiet environment. Previous antihypertensive agents should be restarted, sometimes in higher doses. Other agents may be added on to the existing regimen. In patients who are naïve to any medications, the initiation of a thiazide diuretic or an angiotensin-converting enzyme (ACE) inhibitor may be appropriate. In choosing an antihypertensive, one must consider the appropriate antihypertensive for long-term treatment. Some choices may include beta-blockers, ACE inhibitors, thiazide diuretics, loop diuretics, alpha blockers, or calcium-channel blockers.
- *Definitive therapy:* patients with hypertensive urgency may require admission to the hospital if they have multiple comorbidities or if they are at high risk for cardiovascular events. Patients require close monitoring until their blood pressure is seen to be stable or improving. They will require close follow-up with a provider in order to evaluate for further complications of longstanding hypertension or medication-induced hypotension. Medications should be titrated or added on as necessary to achieve blood pressure goals.

Clinical course

The keys to this patient's diagnosis are careful attention to her history and physical exam, with ancillary studies which rule out hypertensive emergency.

Historical clues	Physical findings	Ancillary studies
• Headache	• No papilledema	• No evidence of acute end-organ damage on radiographic and laboratory evaluation
• Medication noncompliance	• No evidence of heart failure	
• Prior history of hypertension	• No focal neurologic findings	
• Multiple drug therapy for hypertension	• Very elevated blood pressure	

This patient had an elevated blood pressure, although she had no definitive signs of target end-organ damage on exam. This led to concern that the patient might have a hypertensive emergency, so ancillary studies were performed to seek evidence of end-organ damage. These were all negative. Although the patient complained of headache, she had no evidence of intracranial pathology or papilledema on exam. Therefore, she was given IV labetalol in the ED, with a small improvement on her blood pressure. She was admitted for further management of her hypertension given her multiple comorbidities. Her high blood pressure improved with re-initiation and titration of her oral medications.

Further reading

Cherney D, Straus S. Management of patients with hypertensive urgencies and emergencies: a systematic review of the literature. *J Gen Intern Med* 2002;**17**:937.

Chobanian AV, et al. The Seventh Report of the Joint National Committee on the Detection, Evaluation, and Treatment of High Blood Pressure: the JNC 7 report. *JAMA* 2003;**289**:2560–72.

Elliot WJ. Hypertensive emergencies. *Crit Care Clin* 2001;**17**:435.

Moser M, Setaro J. Resistant or difficult-to-control hypertension. *N Engl J Med* 2006;**355**:385–92.

Case #10

History

A 48-year-old woman is brought to the ED by her husband with complaints of progressively worsening headache. Initially, the headache was worst in the morning but now persists throughout the day. There is associated nausea, and she vomited three times earlier today. Her husband also reports that she has become increasingly lethargic over the past 24 hours. The patient denies chest pain, shortness of breath, neck stiffness, photophobia, or phonophobia.

Past medical history

The patient had an intracranial aneurysm that had ruptured 3 weeks prior, resulting in intra-ventricular hemorrhage and diffuse subarachnoid hemorrhage. The aneurysm was treated with endovascular coiling, and the patient was discharged to home after spending 10 days in the hospital. She also has a history of hypertension, hypercholesterolemia, and a 38 pack-year history of tobacco use.

Medications

The patient's medications are metoprolol, lisinopril, hydrochlorothiazide, lovastatin, and albuterol.

Allergies

The patient has an allergy to morphine.

Physical exam and ancillary studies

- *Vital signs:* the patient's temperature is 36.9°C, her heart rate is 62 bpm, her blood pressure is 156/94, her respiratory rate is 20, and her room air oxygen saturation is 96%.
- *General:* the patient is lethargic, and is in moderate distress due to her headache.
- *Head and neck:* the patient's pupils are equally round and reactive to light. Mild papilledema is seen on fundoscopic examination. Her visual fields are full and normal. Her speech reveals orientation to self and place only. The remainder of the cranial nerve exam is normal. There is no meningismus.
- *Cardiovascular:* the patient's heart is regular, with no murmurs or rubs.
- *Lungs:* her lungs are clear to auscultation bilaterally.
- *Neurologic:* the patient is able to follow simple commands but slowly drifts off to sleep during prolonged questioning. Her extremity exam reveals symmetric movements with no focal deficits.
- *Pertinent laboratory values:* the patient's complete blood count, urinalysis, and comprehensive metabolic profile are all normal.
- *Radiographs:* the patient's chest X-ray is normal. Two representative cuts from her head CT are shown in Figures 8.4 and 8.5.

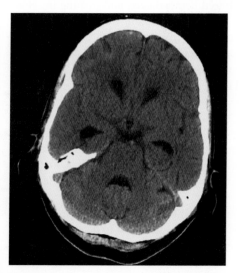

Figure 8.4. The patient has no evidence of bleeding on noncontrast cranial CT. She has enlarged ventricles.

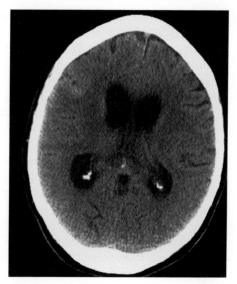

Figure 8.5. CT angiogram of the head and neck reveals intracranial aneurysm to be fully coiled. No other vascular abnormalities are seen.

Questions for thought

- What are the appropriate initial actions to stabilize this patient?
- What are possible ugent treatments for this condition in the ED?
- What is the definitive treatment for this condition?
- Why does the patient have a headache? Nausea and vomiting? Papilledema?

Diagnosis

Communicating hydrocephalus due to previous subarachnoid hemorrhage and intraventricular hemorrhage.

Discussion

- *Epidemiology:* hydrocephalus is a condition that has many causes: tumor, infection, trauma, hemorrhage, and complications of prematurity are just some examples. It has been estimated that approximately 69 000 hospital admissions per year in the United States are related to hydrocephalus.
- *Pathophysiology:* hydrocephalus results from an excessive accumulation of cerebrospinal fluid (CSF) within the ventricular system of the brain. With the rare exception of a tumor arising from the choroid plexus overproducing CSF, hydrocephalus is always due to an obstruction of flow. It can be divided into two categories: communicating and noncommunicating. Communicating hydrocephalus occurs when there is obstruction to CSF reabsorption into the large intracranial venous sinuses around the cerebral convexities.

This is more common after trauma, subarachnoid hemorrhages, and meningitis. Non-communicating hydrocephalus occurs when there is obstruction within the ventricular system, preventing flow of CSF out of the ventricles. This occurs with intraventricular tumors or hemorrhages and anatomical abnormalities such as aqueductal stenosis.

- *Presentation:* this patient's presentation is typical for the development of hydrocephalus in an adult. Symptoms are those of increased intracranial pressure and include headache, nausea, vomiting, diplopia, lethargy, ataxia, and seizures. Signs of increased intracranial pressure include an upward gaze palsy ("setting sun sign," or Parinaud's syndrome), abducens nerve palsy, visual field cuts, and papilledema. In young children in whom the skull's sutures are not fully fused, additional presenting signs and symptoms may be present, such as rapid increase in head growth, irritability, poor head control, fontanelle fullness or bulging, enlargement of scalp veins, irregular respirations with apneic spells, and splaying of cranial sutures.
- *Diagnosis:* hydrocephalus is diagnosed through a combination of clinical presentation and cranial imaging. Noncontrast head CT is a rapid, adequate test to detect ventricular enlargement. There are specialized MRI sequences that can determine CSF flow, but these are unnecessary in the acute setting.
- *Treatment:* the goal of acute treatment of hydrocephalus is aimed at decreasing intracranial pressure, as this can be a potentially fatal illness, and to protect the brain from subsequent deterioration in neurologic function. CSF diversion is required to achieve these goals. In the setting of communicating hydrocephalus, a determination can be made by a neurosurgeon to perform a lumbar puncture and remove a high volume of CSF (~40 mL). In non-communicating hydrocephalus, this would not be prudent as the obstruction is proximal to the lumbar CSF cistern. Instead, a ventriculostomy may be required.
- *Definitive therapy:* although some cases of hydrocephalus resulting in increased intracranial pressure may be transient and resolve after a brief trial of CSF diversion, many cases will require a longer-lasting treatment. This often involves placement of a catheter, shunting CSF from the ventricular system to another fluid cavity, usually the peritoneum.

Clinical course

The keys to this patient's diagnosis are careful attention to her history, physical exam, and noncontrast head CT.

Historical clues	Physical findings	Ancillary studies
• Recent aneurysm rupture with intraventricular and subarachnoid blood	• Lethargy	• CT with enlargement of the ventricular system without obstruction
• Progressive headache	• Papilledema	
• Nausea and vomiting	• Confusion	

The patient was quickly determined to have communicating hydrocephalus based on her history, clinical presentation, and noncontrast cranial CT. Fluid resuscitation was provided with a liter of normal saline. A prompt neurosurgical consultation was obtained. As the cranial CT revealed no cranial mass lesion or ventricular obstruction, an urgent lumbar puncture was performed by the neurosurgeon, removing 40 mL of xanthrochromic cerebrospinal fluid. The following morning, the patient had a ventriculoperitoneal shunt placed in the operating room. She subsequently had a full recovery and was discharged home on the first post-operative day.

Further reading

Van Gijn J, Kerr RS, Rinkel GJ. Subarachnoid hemorrhage. *Lancet* 2007;**369**:306–18.

Bergsneider M. Management of hydrocephalus with programmable valves after traumatic brain injury and subarachnoid hemorrhage. *Curr Opin Neurol* 2000;**13**:661–4.

Tsakanikas D, Relkin N. Normal pressure hydrocephalus. *Semin Neurol* 2007;**27**:58–65.

Rekate HL. Treatment of hydrocephalus. In Albright AL, ed., *Principles and Practice of Pediatric Neurosurgery*. New York: Thieme Medical, 2008, pp. 95–107.

Jones JS, Nevai J, Freeman MP, et al. Emergency department presentation of idiopathic intracranial hypertension. *Am J Emerg Med* 1999;**17**:517–21.

Shemie S, Jay V, Rutka J, et al. Acute obstructive hydrocephalus and sudden death in children. *Ann Emerg Med* 1997;**29**:524–8.

Cohen BH. Headaches as a symptom of neurological disease. *Semin Pediatr Neurol* 1995;**2**:144–50.

Detsky ME, McDonald DR, Baerlocher MO, et al. Does this patient with headache have a migraine or need neuroimaging? *JAMA* 2006;**296**:1274–83.

James HE. Hydrocephalus in infancy and childhood. *Am Fam Physician* 1992;**45**:733–42.

Case #11

History

A 65-year-old man presents to the emergency department complaining of dizziness since arising. He is somewhat vague and confused, and his wife states that he arose at 5:00 a.m. visibly unsteady, and that he seemed disoriented as well. The patient states that the dizziness has continued, and he has been intermittently disoriented throughout the day. In addition, the patient states that he had a 20 minute episode of transient blindness, during which he describes his vision going "completely white." His vision gradually returned, although the patient complains that things "seem blurry." He also complains of "floaters" in his visual fields. He feels dyspneic, but denies chest pain or pressure, and denies nausea or vomiting. Despite his illness, the patient admits to drinking alcohol today.

Past medical history

The patient has a history of nasopharyngeal cancer, for which he underwent lymph node dissection as well as radiation and chemotherapy.

Social history

The patient smokes a pack of cigarettes daily. He does not work, and admits to drinking at least four alcoholic beverages daily.

Medications

The patient takes no regular medication.

Allergies

The patient has no known drug allergies.

Physical exam and ancillary studies

- *Vital signs:* the patient's vital signs include a temperature of 36.4°C, a heart rate of 74 bpm, blood pressure of 162/100 mmHg, a respiratory rate of 18, and a room air saturation of 99%.
- *General:* the patient is ill-appearing and confused, but is oriented to time and place.
- *Head and neck:* his pupils are somewhat dilated, and are equally round and reactive to light. There is no scleral injection or icterus. On exam, his optic disk is hyperemic. His oral mucosa is moist, and there is no JVD.
- *Cardiovascular:* the patient's heart has a regular rate and rhythm, without murmurs, rubs, or gallops.
- *Lungs:* his lungs are clear bilaterally.
- *Abdomen:* his abdominal exam is benign.

- *Neurologic:* the patient's Glasgow coma scale is 15, and cranial nerves II–XII are intact. The patient's speech is somewhat slurred. He has no other abnormalities on neurologic exam.
- *Extremities and skin:* the patient's extremities and skin show no clubbing, cyanosis, edema, or lesions.
- *Pertinent labs:* the patient's labs show the following: sodium 136, potassium 4.8, chloride 105, bicarbonate 7, BUN 9, creatinine 1.0, glucose 95, blood pH 7.08. His comprehensive blood count is unremarkable, and his cardiac enzymes are negative.
- *EKG:* his electrocardiogram shows no arrhythmia or ischemia.

Questions for thought

- Why does this patient have a marked metabolic acidosis?
- What caused the patient's transient episode of blindness?
- What organ systems are in jeopardy in this patient?
- How does one urgently treat this condition in the emergency department?
- What is the definitive treatment of this condition?

Diagnosis

Acute methanol toxicity.

Discussion

- *Epidemiology:* methanol poisoning is relatively rare, with a bit over 2000 cases a year reported. Poisonings can occur when methanol-containing substances are ingested accidentally, either when residual methanol is left in a container re-used for other purposes, or when drunk directly. Methanol can appear in home-distilled liquors ("moonshine"), and desperate alcoholics have been known to drink methanol either accidentally or in an attempt to become intoxicated.
- *Pathophysiology:* methanol itself is a central nervous system depressant, much like ethanol. When methanol is metabolized in the liver by alcohol dehydrogenase and aldehyde dehydrogenase, formaldehyde and, subsequently, formate are produced. Formate causes retinal injury and can lead to permanent blindness. In addition, these acidic metabolites cause a profound metabolic acidosis with a large anion gap.
- *Presentation:* patients present with either frank intoxication or nonspecific mental status changes. In addition, patients with methanol poisoning often have visual complaints including visual acuity changes, central scotoma, or even blindness. Patients also present with headache.
- *Treatment:* supportive care of the patient's airway, breathing, and circulation is vital. For severe metabolic acidosis, sodium bicarbonate can be given as a temporizing measure to help with cardiac contractility problems secondary to acidosis. It is not curative, however. To prevent further degeneration of vision, alcohol dehydrogenase needs to be inhibited, blocking production of toxic metabolites and acids. This can be accomplished with ethanol infusion or with fomepizole. Fomepizole is advantageous because it does not depress mental status, but it is very expensive.

- *Definitive therapy:* patients with methanol toxicity often require urgent hemodialysis to aid in the elimination of the toxic metabolites of the parent alcohol. This should be initiated in anyone who has ingested more than 30 mL of methanol, anyone with visual dysfunction, and in patients with severe acidosis.

Clinical course

The keys to this patient's diagnosis are careful attention to his history, especially his social history. Prompt ordering of laboratory studies proved vital in this case, whereas physical exam findings were helpful, but nonspecific.

Historical clues	Physical findings	Ancillary studies
• Dizziness and disorientation	• Slurred speech	• Marked metabolic acidosis
• Transient blindness	• Confusion	• Normal serum glucose
• History of alcohol abuse	• Decreased visual acuity	
	• Mydriasis	
	• Disk hyperemia	

The patient was felt to have a possible toxic ingestion based on his confusion, his history of regular alcohol use, and the physical finding of mydriasis. Many people with methanol toxicity will have findings on eye exam, including retinal edema, mydriasis, or optic disk hyperemia, which was present in this case.

This man was noted to have a metabolic acidosis with large anion gap, which is often the first clue to this diagnosis. Some patients will also have elevated BUN and creatinine. The provider should be suspicious of methanol poisoning in any intoxicated patient with visual acuity changes and a metabolic acidosis, especially if the patient is euglycemic.

Once the metabolic acidosis was noted, a serum alcohol screen was ordered and the patient was found to have a methanol level of 108. A dialysis catheter was placed urgently in the ED, and treatment with IV sodium bicarbonate and fomepizole was initiated. The hospital renal service was consulted, and the patient had urgent dialysis performed. During the course of his stay, the patient was seen by the ophthalmology service, and gradually made a full recovery.

Further reading

Garibotto G, Sofia A, Robaudo C. Kidney protein dynamics and ammoniagenesis in humans with chronic metabolic acidosis. *J Am Soc Nephrol* 2004;**15**:1606.

Gabow PA, Kaehny WD, Fennessey PV, et al. Diagnostic importance of an increased anion gap. *N Engl J Med* 1980;**303**:854.

Rose BD, Post TW. *Clinical Physiology of Acid-Base and Electrolyte Disorders*, 5th edition. New York: McGraw-Hill, 2001, pp. 628–33.

Barceloux DG, Bond GR, Krenzelok EP, et al. American Academy of Clinical Toxicology practice guidelines on the treatment of methanol poisoning. *J Toxicol Clin Toxicol* 2002;**40**:415.

Hojer J. Severe metabolic acidosis in the alcoholic: differential diagnosis and management. *Hum Exp Toxicol* 1996;**15**:482.

Jacobsen D, McMartin KE. Antidotes for methanol and ethylene glycol poisoning. *J Toxicol Clin Toxicol* 1997;**35**:127.

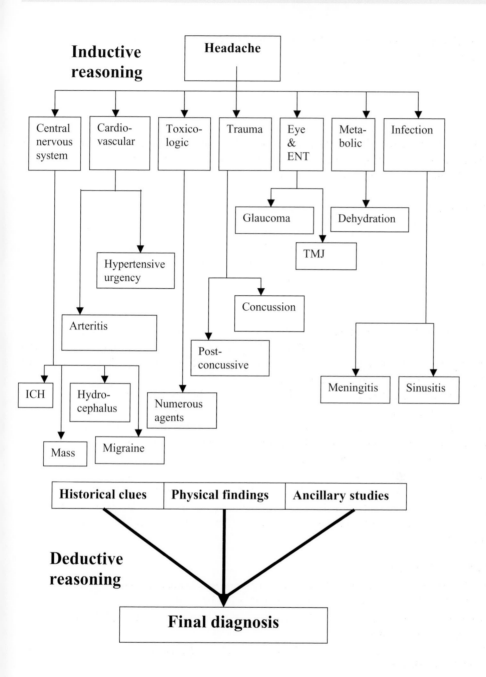

Chapter

9

Chief complaint: back pain

Donald Jeanmonod, Anna Margaritz Hernandez–Silen, Damian R. Compa,
Devin Minior, Wendy Wooley, Pamela Y. Young, Lorraine Thibodeau

Case #1

History

An 82-year-old male patient presents to the emergency department with a chief
complaint of back pain and dizziness. The patient states that he has been having
several days of "achy" poorly localized back pain which radiates into his
abdomen. Approximately an hour prior to presentation, the patient had a
worsening of the abdominal pain in the supraumbilical region associated with
lightheadedness. The patient's wife stated that she noted that the patient looked
"a little gray" and was clammy before coming in. The patient denies fever, reports
that he feels a little nauseous, but has not vomited. The patient states that his last
bowel movement was the preceding day. The patient notes difficulty initiating a
urinary stream, but this is not new for him.

Past medical history

History of hypertension and hypercholesterolemia. He quit smoking 17 years ago and has a
60 pack-year history.

Medications

Atenolol, potassium, furosemide, aspirin, and lovastatin.

Allergies

No known drug allergies.

Physical exam and ancillary studies

- *Vital signs:* temperature 37.7°C, heart rate 65 bpm, blood pressure 82/62, respiratory rate
  24, room air saturation 96%.
- *General:* awake and alert, ashen and diaphoretic.

Case Studies in Emergency Medicine, ed. R. Jeanmonod, M. Tomassi and D. Mayer.
Published by Cambridge University Press © Cambridge University Press 2010.

- *Head and neck:* pupils are equally round and reactive to light, cranial nerves intact. The patient's mucous membranes are dry. His neck is supple with a midline trachea and no JVD.
- *Cardiovascular:* regular rate and rhythm, peripheral pulses are thready. No murmurs or gallops.
- *Lungs:* clear to auscultation bilaterally. No wheezes, rales, or rhonchi.
- *Abdomen:* decreased bowel sounds throughout, obese, generalized tenderness. Fullness is noted in the right lower quadrant radiating into the right flank. Rectal examination reveals brown stool which is guaiac-positive.
- *Extremities and skin:* trace bilateral edema, no clubbing, no calf tenderness, poor capillary refill throughout with pale skin.
- *Back:* no midline or paraspinal tenderness is elicited. No stepoffs are appreciated. Slight right-sided CVA discomfort with percussion.
- *Pertinent abnormal labs:* WBC 9.4, HGB 11.4, HCT 33.2%. Na 136, K 3.6, Cl 103, CO_2 18, BUN 26, Cr 1.6, GLU 133. Alk phos, ALT, AST, and lipase are normal. CPK is normal, troponin 0.21.
- *EKG:* nonspecific ST-T wave changes.
- *Chest X-ray:* negative.

Questions for thought

- What are the appropriate initial actions to take to stabilize this patient?
- What is the differential diagnosis for this presentation?
- What bedside tests can be used to assist with the diagnosis?
- Once stable, what other diagnostic tools can be used to make a diagnosis?
- What is definitive treatment of this condition?

Diagnosis

Ruptured abdominal aortic aneurysm.

Discussion

- *Epidemiology:* abdominal aortic aneurysm (AAA) is a relatively common, potentially fatal condition. The incidence of abdominal aortic aneurysm is about 2% in the adult population, with greater than 75% of patients with AAA over the age of 65. AAA is more common in Caucasians and males. Risk factors include a history of hypertension, smoking, male sex, advanced age, and history of peripheral vascular disease.
- *Pathophysiology:* abdominal aortic aneurysms occur as a result of vessel wall weakness secondary to degeneration of the vascular media, most frequently associated with atherosclerosis but can be the result of infection or connective tissue disorders. The majority of aneurysms are fusiform and occur in the infrarenal portion of the abdominal aorta proximal to the iliac takeoff. Any portion of the infrarenal aorta larger than 3 cm in diameter or with dilatation of greater than 50% of the diameter of the normal aorta is considered aneurysmal. Laplace's law for wall tension states that wall tension is directly

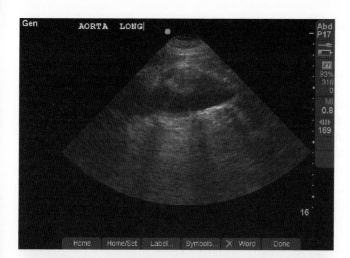

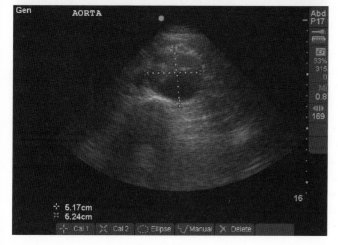

Figure 9.1 Bedside abdominal aortic ultrasound longitudinal and transverse views.

proportional to the radius and the pressure and inversely proportional to wall thickness. Therefore as the vessel radius increases, the wall becomes thinner and is under greater tension, eventually overcoming vessel integrity, resulting in rupture. The risk of rupture has been demonstrated to increase as vessel diameter increases above 5.5 cm.

- *Presentation:* the majority of patients with AAA are asymptomatic and the aneurysm is either detected on screening exam or as an incidental finding on radiologic imaging studies. Patients may be found to have a pulsatile mass or abdominal bruit on exam. If the aneurysm is dissecting, rapidly expanding, or ruptures, patients might present with abdominal or back pain. Other findings can include syncope, groin pain, and paralysis from involvement of lumbar arterial branches or acute aortic thrombosis. The classic presentation of tachycardia, hypotension, and palpable pulsatile mass is present in only 30–50% of cases.

- *Diagnosis:* if a stable patient is suspected to have an abdominal aortic aneurysm, the test of choice is a CT scan of the abdomen and pelvis with IV contrast. The sensitivity is nearly 100% and it will identify suprarenal involvement, the presence of rupture, and involvement of abdominal and retroperitoneal arterial branches and other pathology. The CT is not limited by obesity or bowel gas, but does carry risks of radiation exposure and IV contrast load to the kidneys. Ultrasound is a rapid, inexpensive screening test that can be used as a bedside tool to permit the emergency physician to quickly assess for the presence of AAA in the undifferentiated patient presenting with shock or severe abdominal pain. The downside to ultrasound is that it can be nondiagnostic in 15–20% of patients because of inability to fully visualize the aorta or accurately measure the aneurysm if a clot is present, and it cannot assess for the presence of retroperitoneal hemorrhage. A common pitfall in emergency management of AAA is to place a patient with a dissecting or leaking AAA into the CT scan without arranging for definitive care as a back-up.

- *Treatment:* emergency department management of a patient suspected of having a ruptured AAA includes ensuring adequate IV access with two large-bore peripheral IVs, reversing coagulopathy if present, and obtaining blood products for volume resuscitation. In patients who present with hypertension, beta-blockers such as IV labetalol or esmolol should be administered to decrease the pulse pressure, decreasing the wall tension. A vascular surgeon should be consulted early in all cases of rupture or high suspicion of rupture or if a known aneurysm has increased more than 0.5 cm in 6 months.

- *Definitive therapy:* unruptured AAA is often followed with serial evaluations if they are small or if the patient is a poor operative candidate. Ultimately surgical management with either an open repair with graft or endovascular placement of an endograft is required to form a new lumen and decrease the pressure on the inner vascular wall.

Clinical course

Maintaining a high index of suspicion in the appropriate clinical scenario and aggressively managing the patient's volume status and blood pressure are paramount. Although the differential diagnosis would include other life-threatening etiologies such as acute MI, severe pancreatitis, abdominal viscus perforation with septic shock, and mesenteric ischemia with septic shock, early use of bedside ultrasound was instrumental in leading to a timely diagnosis.

Historical clues	Physical findings	Ancillary studies
• Presence of risk factors, hypertension and tobacco use	• Hypotension	• Low hematocrit
• Abdominal pain	• Pallor	• Presence of renal insufficiency
• Back pain	• Poor peripheral perfusion	• Presence of anion gap acidosis
• Near syncope		• Presence of AAA on bedside ultrasound

This patient was recognized to have an AAA on bedside ultrasound, which was presumed to have ruptured given the worsening abdominal and back pain associated with his hypotension. The patient was prepared for the operating room and the vascular surgery department was consulted. The patient was permitted to remain hypotensive to minimize further bleeding and underwent a rapid CT scan on his way to the operating room to assist with staging for surgery. His AAA was leaking into his retroperitoneum and was repaired using an endograft.

Further reading

Zankl AR, Schumacher H, Krumsdorf U, et al. Pathology, natural history and treatment of abdominal aortic aneurysms. *Clin Res Cardiol* 2007;**96**:140–51.

Bentz S, Jones J. Towards evidence-based emergency medicine: best BETs from the Manchester Royal Infirmary. Accuracy of emergency department ultrasound scanning in detecting abdominal aortic aneurysm. *Emerg Med J* 2006;**23**:803–4.

Roberts K, Revell M, Youssef H, et al. Hypotensive resuscitation in patients with ruptured abdominal aortic aneurysm. *Eur J Vasc Endovasc Surg* 2006;**31**:339–44.

Isselbacher EM. Thoracic and abdominal aortic aneurysms. *Circulation* 2005;**111**:816–28.

Case #2

History

A 43-year-old male presents as a walk-in to the emergency department with a chief complaint of low back pain. The patient reports that the pain was noted on waking 3 days ago, has been continuous, and is made worse with certain movements, bending, and standing for too long. The patient reports that he has missed work for the past 2 days because he is unable to perform his duties, which include lifting boxes. The patient denies direct trauma and on questioning denies incontinence of bowels and bladder or any numbness or weakness in his lower extremities. He denies fever. The patient states that he has taken ibuprofen without experiencing relief of his symptoms.

Past medical history

The patient denies significant medical history. He states that he had an appendectomy at age 15. The patient has smoked two packs of cigarettes per day for the past 27 years. The patient admits that he drinks about six beers per day. The patient reports recreational marijuana usage. He denies other drug use including IV drug use, but states that he has used cocaine in the past.

Medications

The patient reports taking ibuprofen only.

Allergies

The patient has no known drug allergies.

Physical exam and ancillary studies

- *Vital signs:* temperature 36.4°C, heart rate 92 bpm, blood pressure 152/82, respiratory rate 24, room air saturation 95%.
- *General:* awake and alert, lying recumbent on a stretcher with his legs bent.
- *Head and neck:* conjunctivae are pink and the sclerae are anicteric. The patient has full, painless range of motion of his neck.
- *Cardiovascular:* regular rate and rhythm without murmurs, rubs, or gallops.
- *Lungs:* mild end expiratory wheezing throughout.
- *Abdomen:* right lower quadrant scar. Non-distended and non-tender throughout. No midline pulsatile masses.
- *Back:* tender to palpation in the midline lower lumbar spine with bilateral lumbar paraspinal musculature tenderness. The patient has a tender 3 cm nodular area in the right lumbar paraspinal muscle.

- *Extremities and skin:* no edema or calf tenderness. Palpable bilateral dorsalis pedis and posterior tibial pulses. Negative straight leg raise bilaterally.
- *Neurologic:* ambulatory with a slow gait, walking slightly bent over at the waist. Motor 5/5 bilateral lower extremities. Intact patellar and ankle reflexes. Sensation grossly intact.

Questions for thought

- What further diagnostic studies are necessary to evaluate this patient?
- What are some historical elements or physical findings that would trigger a more thorough evaluation?
- What are the possible treatment choices for this patient?

Diagnosis

Acute low back strain.

Discussion

- *Epidemiology:* acute low back pain is a very common problem, effecting up to 90% of adults in their lifetime. At any point in time, approximately 15–20% of the population will report having low back pain, 1% will be temporarily disabled from their low back pain, and 1% will be chronically disabled. The direct costs associated with treating low back pain are estimated to exceed $24 billion and over $50 billion in costs are estimated when indirect disability costs are included. The majority of cases are of benign etiology and approximately 90% of cases will resolve spontaneously within 6 weeks of onset. In primary care practice, the prevalence of potentially severe causes of acute low back pain have been reported as 4% for compression fractures, 1–3% for herniated disks, 0.7% for neoplasm, 0.04% for cauda equina syndrome, and 0.01% for paraspinal infection.
- *Pathophysiology:* mechanical musculo-ligamentous injury accounts for the majority of low back pain. There are multiple structures including paravertebral muscles, ligaments, facet joints, vertebral body periosteum, annulus fibrosis, and nerve roots that can be responsible for a patient's pain. However, approximately 85% of patients with low back pain will not have a precise neuroanatomical diagnosis and studies that have investigated all patients with MRI, regardless of the presence of pain, have found that only the minority with identified abnormalities report having associated pain.
- *Presentation:* patients will complain of low back pain. A herniated lumbar disk is unlikely in the absence of radicular symptoms or sciatica. Other neurologic symptoms could include neurogenic claudication, which mimics vascular claudication in the presence of leg pain on standing or after walking, but differs in its persistence after rest until the patient assumes a position of flexion at the hips. "Red flag" indicators that might prompt more extensive investigation for malignancy include history of cancer, advanced age, prolonged duration, or unexplained weight loss. Presence of unexplained fever, history of IV drug use, or immunosuppression might prompt investigation for infection. Cauda equina syndrome is suggested by the presence of low back pain with loss of bowel or bladder control, saddle anesthesia, or symmetric distal lower extremity numbness or weakness.

- *Diagnosis:* the diagnosis of acute low back strain is made clinically after excluding more serious etiologies with history and physical studies including aortic abnormalities, cancer, cauda equina syndrome, perivertebral infections, and occult fractures. No further diagnostic studies need to be performed in the absence of "red flag" indicators. Should a "red flag" be present, radiographic modalities might include X-ray or CT for fracture or MRI to evaluate for infection or cord involvement.
- *Treatment:* the mainstay of treatment for acute low back strain is nonsteroidal anti-inflammatory drugs (NSAIDs). Randomized, controlled trials have demonstrated the superiority of NSAIDs over placebo, but have not demonstrated superiority of one NSAID over another. NSAIDs tend to be well tolerated for short-term treatment, with the principal side effects reported to be gastrointestinal. Skeletal muscle relaxants have been shown to be as effective as NSAIDs for the treatment of acute low back strain, but are not as effective for chronic low back strain. Studies of NSAIDs plus muscle relaxants versus NSAIDs plus placebo have yielded conflicting results. The primary limitation to the use of muscle relaxants are the central nervous system and GI side effects. For patients with severe pain or pain failing NSAID treatment opiates can be prescribed. Other modalities demonstrating some promise for the treatment of acute low back strain include heat therapy and physical therapy. Conventional teaching of several days of bed rest has been proven to be deleterious, so patients should be encouraged to return to their previous level of activity and reassured that they will not further damage their backs with exercise.

Clinical course

This patient's presentation is fairly straightforward and is a frequent presentation to the emergency department. Because this presentation is so common, the emergency physician must stay vigilant and receptive to the possibility of underlying pathology.

Historical clues	Physical findings	Ancillary studies
• Non-traumatic mechanism of pain	• Afebrile	
• Absence of "red flag" symptoms (numbness or tingling, weakness, or incontinence of urine or stool)	• Back tenderness in lumbar paraspinal muscles	
	• Intact pulses	
	• Lack of palpable aortic aneurysm	
	• Intact distal neurological examination	

This patient was diagnosed as having acute lumbar back strain. He was prescribed an anti-inflammatory dose of ibuprofen to be taken with a muscle relaxant. The patient was given a prescription for a limited number of narcotic pain medications to be taken for breakthrough pain. The patient was encouraged to return to work and was instructed to follow up with his primary care physician for re-evaluation.

Further reading

Gilligan P, Kitching G, Taylor A, et al. SOCRATES 7 (synopsis of Cochrane Reviews applicable to emergency services). *Emerg Med J* 2005;**22**(5):368–9.

Hansen GR. Management of chronic pain in the acute care setting. *Emerg Med Clin North Am* 2005;**23**(2):307–38.

McCarberg BH, Adler JA. Updates on managing acute and chronic pain in primary care practice–optimizing pain reduction, minimizing adverse events. *J Am Acad Physician Assist Suppl Pain* 2008;1–13.

Malanga GA, Dennis RL. Use of medications in the treatment of acute low back pain. *Clin Occup Environ Med* 2006;5(3):643–53.

Della-Giustina DA. Emergency department evaluation and treatment of back pain *Emerg Med Clin North Am* 1999;17(4):877–93.

Case #3

History

An 18-year-old female G_4P_{0120} at 22 weeks and zero days of pregnancy with dichorionic-diamniotic twins presents to the ED complaining of lower back pain that started 2 days ago. The pain is on and off and is now severe and radiates into her abdomen. She had some light vaginal spotting earlier today, but denies any leakage of fluid per vagina. She denies dysuria, frequency, fever/chills, nausea, and vomiting. She has felt fetal movements twice.

Past medical history

This is an undesired pregnancy. She had one previous delivery at 23 weeks and two surgical elective terminations of pregnancy. Menstrual history: menarche at age 10, monthly and regular lasting 4 days. She is unsure of her LMP. *Chlamydia* and *Trichomonas* infections were successfully treated. She had an abnormal Pap smear 1 year ago, but follow-up smears were normal. She has chronic anemia presumed to be due to poor diet. She smokes a half pack per day and denies alcohol or drug use.

Medications

Prenatal vitamins, folic acid, iron.

Allergies

No known drug allergies.

Physical exam and ancillary studies

- *Vital signs:* temperature 37.6°C, heart rate 84 bpm, blood pressure 124/74, respiratory rate 18, room air saturation 99%.
- *General:* awake and alert, no acute distress.
- *Head and neck:* pupils are equally round and reactive to light, cranial nerves intact. The patient's mucous membranes are dry. Her neck is supple.
- *Cardiovascular:* regular tachycardia without rubs.
- *Lungs:* clear to auscultation bilaterally.
- *Abdomen:* bowel sounds are present in the four quadrants. Gravid uterus non-tender to palpation with fundal height 6 cm above the umbilicus.
- *Sterile speculum exam:* grossly normal female external genitalia. No vaginal bleeding or discharge. Cervix is visually closed with no grossly apparent lesions. It is soft, not dilated, 50% effaced, and the presentation is high.
- *Extremities and skin:* +1 bilateral pedal edema, no calf tenderness, and good capillary refill. Normal motor and sensation bilaterally.

- *External tocometer:* irregular contractions moderately strong with normal fetal heart rate variability.
- *Pertinent abnormal labs:* CBC: WBC 14.0, Hb 7.4, Hct 28.2, platelets 170. Urinalysis negative.
- *Transvaginal ultrasound:* baby A vertex presentation, placenta is anterior, amniotic fluid index is within normal limits, estimated fetal weight 48%. Baby B transverse lie, posterior placenta, amniotic fluid index within normal limits, estimated fetal weight 25%. Cervical length 1.5 cm, no funneling.

Questions for thought

- What are the appropriate initial actions to take?
- What are the diagnostic tools you can use to make a diagnosis?
- How does one urgently treat this condition in the emergency department?
- What is definitive treatment of this condition?

Diagnosis

Preterm labor (PTL)/preterm birth (PTB).

Discussion

- *Definition:* PTB is a birth that occurs before 37 completed weeks of gestation. Due to its sequelae, it is the leading cause of infant mortality in the United States.
- *Epidemiology:* the incidence of PTB in 2005 in the United States was 12.7% of all pregnancies that progressed past the second trimester.
- *Pathophysiology:* 70–80% of PTBs occur spontaneously. PTL is the most common cause of PTB, leading to approximately 40% of PTBs. The next most common cause of PTB is preterm rupture of membranes (20–30%), and the third is intervention due to maternal and/or fetal problems (20–30%). The four primary processes involved in PTB are: infection, decidual hemorrhage, pathologic uterine distension, and activation of the maternal/fetal hypothalamic-pituitary-adrenal axis.
- *Presentation:* the clinical presentation is nonspecific. Patients usually present with lower abdominal or back pain, cramping, or vaginal bleeding.
- *Diagnosis:* the clinical diagnosis should be considered in all pregnant patients with lower back pain and cramping. The transvaginal ultrasound is helpful for measuring the cervix and looking for funneling, a characteristic sign of preterm labor.
- *Treatment:* there is no evidence that any type of treatment will affect the course of PTL or PTB. Tocolysis has not been shown to be effective when there is true labor. Some tocolytic agents are: magnesium sulfate, terbutaline, nifedipine, and indomethacin. The goal is to prevent PTB from happening, with a minimum goal of being able to give two doses of betamethasone in order to reduce the morbidity and mortality associated with prematurity. When PTL is due to dehydration, the contractions usually stop after adequate IV hydration. If the patient is not about to deliver, the decision to deliver should be made

with the input of a high-risk maternal fetal medicine consultant. There are many complex ethical and medical issues in the decision to deliver a preterm infant.

Clinical course

The keys to this patient's diagnosis are careful attention to her history and physical exam.

Historical clues	Physical findings	Ancillary studies
• Previous PTB	• Cervix not dilated	• Cervical length 1.5 cm
• Multiple gestation	• Occasional contractions on the monitor	• Anemia
• Age < 18		• U/A negative
• Low socioeconomic status		
• Single		
• Sexually transmitted diseases		
• Abnormal Pap smears		
• Smoker		
• Vaginal bleeding		

This woman was recognized as probably having PTL due to the risk factors and clinical presentation. The patient was sent to the labor and delivery area for further evaluation, monitoring, and initiation of tocolysis and betamethasone therapy.

Further reading

Seibel-Seamon J, Berghella V, Baxter J, et al. Tocolytics for preterm premature rupture of membranes. *Cochrane Database Syst Rev* 2008;**2**:CD007062.

Reddy UM. Prediction and prevention of recurrent stillbirth. *Obstet Gynecol* 2007;**110**(5):1151–64.

Cunningham G, Leveno K, Bloom S, eds. Chapter 36. Preterm birth. In *Williams Obstetrics*, 22nd edition. New York: McGraw-Hill, 2005.

Lockwood CJ. Preterm labor. In DS Basow, ed., *UpToDate*. Waltham, MA: UpToDate, 2008.

ACOG Practice Bulletin: management of Preterm Labor Number 43, May 2003. *Int J Gynecol Obstet* 2003;**82**:127–35.

Case #4

History

A 63-year-old Hispanic female with HIV/AIDS presents to the emergency department complaining of midepigastric abdominal pain, nausea, and vomiting, which has progressively worsened over the past 2 days. She describes the pain as sharp and radiating through to her mid-back. It is worsened when she is in the supine position and relieved when leaning forward. She has no history of recurrent abdominal discomfort and denies chest, neck, or arm pain. She has not noted yellowing of her eyes or skin, nor melena or bright red blood per rectum. There has been no recent trauma to her chest, back, or abdomen. She does complain of chills and mild loose stools without pus. She notes breathing more quickly over the past day without an associated cough. Acetaminophen every 6 hours has not provided relief. She denies alcohol or illicit drug use and has no known history of gallbladder disease or hyperlipidemia. She reports full compliance with her home medicines with no history of intolerance or adverse effects.

Past medical and surgical history

HIV/AIDS was acquired when she used intravenous drugs in the remote past. Her most recent CD4 count was 230 cells/mm^3 and the most recent viral load was <50 copies/mL. She had a hysterectomy at age 35 for bleeding fibroids and tonsillectomy as a child. She also has a history of hypertension.

Medication

Didanosine 400 mg per day, tenofovir DF 300 mg per day, efavirenz 600 mg per day, amlodipine 5 mg per day.

Allergies

No known drug allergies.

Physical exam and ancillary studies

- *Vital signs:* temperature 38.4°C, heart rate is regular at 130 bpm, blood pressure 145/81, respiratory rate 26, room air saturation 96%, pain 8/10.
- *General:* awake, alert, anxious, in significant discomfort with shallow respirations.
- *Head and neck:* pupils are equally round and reactive to light, cranial nerves intact. There is no scleral icterus. The patient's mucous membranes are dry. Her neck is supple with a midline trachea. There is no jugular venous distension or adenopathy.
- *Abdominal:* scaphoid, tympanitic to percussion. Scant bowel sounds. Tender diffusely with moderate palpation, particularly in the left upper quadrant. There is guarding without rebound. There is no ecchymotic discoloration around the umbilicus (Cullen's sign) or at the flanks (Grey-Turner's sign). There is no hepatosplenomegaly and no masses.

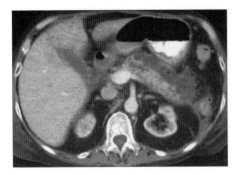

Figure 9.2 CT abdomen. This demonstrates inflammation involving the pancreas diffusely.

- *Back:* no bony deformity or step-offs. No tenderness.
- *Cardiovascular:* regular tachycardia with a systolic flow murmur. There is no rub or gallop.
- *Lungs:* resonant to percussion, without wheezes, rales, or rhonchi. No change in tactile fremitus.
- *Extremities and skin:* no edema or clubbing, no calf tenderness. Skin without jaundice, ecchymosis, petechiae or other lesions.
- *Pertinent studies:* WBC 14.0 with 12 % band forms, HCT 45% (38% 8 weeks earlier). Corrected calcium 7.8, bicarbonate 21, amylase 2100, lipase 3468, triglycerides 188. Abdominal film and ultrasound were normal. A CT scan is shown in Figure 9.2.

Questions for thought

- Does antiretroviral therapy commonly cause pancreatitis?
- Are there specific antiretroviral medications that are more commonly associated with pancreatitis?
- Should more common causes of pancreatitis be ruled out?
- Do patients who are re-challenged with didanosine often experience recurrence?

Diagnosis

Acute pancreatitis secondary to antiretroviral therapy medications.

Discussion

- *Epidemiology:* the incidence of acute pancreatitis ranges from 4 to 30 per 100 000 depending on the diagnostic criteria and the population studied. The most common etiologies include gallstones and alcohol abuse, but a broad differential including infection, trauma, and medications, amongst others, must be entertained. Pancreatitis is more common in patients with HIV when compared to the general population, perhaps secondary to the HIV itself or co-infection with opportunistic organisms. The incidence and severity of pancreatitis show a predictable inverse relationship with the CD4 lymphocyte count. Nucleoside reverse transcriptase inhibitors (NRTI) didanosine (ddI) and stavudine (d4T) appear to increase the baseline risk of acute pancreatitis, which should be suspected in the right clinical context.

- *Pathophysiology:* the pathophysiology of pancreatitis depends upon the etiology, but the final common pathway involves pancreatic destruction by inactivated digestive enzymes called zymogens. The zymogens are secreted by the pancreas into the intestine in a bicarbonate-rich fluid, where they are activated. Activation of zymogens within the pancreatic bed is destructive. The specific pathogenesis of NRTIs is not fully understood, but is most probably due to mitochondrial dysfunction. Other clinical manifestations of impaired mitochondrial function may include myopathy, neuropathy, or lactic acidosis.
- *Presentation:* this patient's presentation is typical for pancreatitis. The clinical syndrome caused by antiretroviral therapy can be more insidious and result in delayed diagnosis and therapy. Midepigastric abdominal pain is the most common symptom, often accompanied by nausea and vomiting. Radiation to the back in a band-like manner is often described. Abdominal signs range from mild tenderness to peritonitis with rebound and guarding. Blue-gray discoloration of the flanks (Grey-Turner sign) or around the umbilicus (Cullen's sign) represents exudation of hemorrhagic fluid into the subcutaneous tissue and is a clinical sign of a worse prognosis.
- *Diagnosis:* typical clinical features of pancreatitis are based on an elevated serum concentration of amylase or lipase. Serum amylase is more sensitive but less specific than lipase as a diagnostic tool. Therapy varies greatly from emergency endoscopic retrograde cholangiopancreatography (ERCP) to simply discontinuing the offending medication. Other diagnostic studies in the ED may include an abdominal plain film, ultrasound, or a CT scan. An abdominal film may suggest an alternative diagnosis such as obstruction or bowel perforation. X-ray findings in acute pancreatitis may include a localized ileus referred to as a "sentinal loop." An abdominal ultrasound may reveal an enlarged pancreas, gallstones in the gallbladder, or an enlarged bile duct. CT scan may be necessary to make the diagnosis when other clinical indicators are equivocal and may show hemorrhage, necrosis, or pseudocyst formation.
- *Treatment:* the treatment in our case was discontinuation of the antiretroviral therapy with supportive care. Some patients will experience recurrence of pancreatitis when re-challenged with didanosine, while others will not. It is impossible to predict who will fail a re-challenge and concurrent use with tenofovir or hydroxyurea may increase the risk. In general, the initial management of acute pancreatitis is aggressive fluid administration to replace the existing volume deficit and keep up with ongoing losses. Pain control, bowel rest, and attention to electrolyte imbalances are the priorities. In severe cases, intensive care unit monitoring is appropriate and a central venous catheter, bladder catheter, and arterial line are commonly employed.

Historical clues	Physical findings	Ancillary studies
• Severe abdominal pain radiating to the back	• Diffuse abdominal tenderness in the epigastrium	• Lipase is very specific and amylase very sensitive for pancreatitis.
• Vomiting		• Abdominal CT scan shows the extent of damage
• History of antiretroviral drugs		

Clinical course

The patient was admitted to the intensive care unit for monitoring. Her symptoms resolved with aggressive fluid administration, bowel rest, and judicious pain control. Antiretroviral therapy was discontinued and she recovered without complication. She was eventually re-challenged with didanosine and experienced a recurrence of acute pancreatitis within 2 weeks.

Further reading

Dutta SK, Ting CD, Lai LL. Study of prevalence, severity, and etiological factors associated with acute pancreatitis in patients infected with human immunodeficiency virus. *Am J Gastroenterol* 1997;**92**(11):2044–8.

Reisler RB, Murphy RL, Redfield RR, et al. Incidence of pancreatitis in HIV-1-infected individuals enrolled in 20 adult AIDS clinical trials group studies lessons learned. *J Acquir Immune Defic Syndr* 2005;**39**(2):159–66.

Vissers Robert J, Abu-Laban Riyad B. Chapter 87. Acute and chronic pancreatitis. In Tintinalli JE, Kelen GD, Stapczynski JS, Ma OJ, Cline DM, eds., *Tintinalli's Emergency Medicine: A Comprehensive Study Guide*, 6th edition. New York: McGraw-Hill, 2004.

Case #5

History

A 63-year-old woman presents to the ED at 2:00 a.m. complaining of back pain that began 1 hour ago. The patient states she was gardening earlier in the day and when the pain woke her from sleep, she thought it might have been related to overexertion. The pain is intrascapular, without radiation. She has no nausea, vomiting, or diarrhea and denies diaphoresis and palpitations. She has never had symptoms like this in the past. She is unable to find a position of comfort. Antacids have not helped.

Past medical history

The patient has a 10-year history of hypertension. In addition, she has a history of hyperlipidemia and elevated cholesterol. She quit smoking 5 years ago and drinks alcohol occasionally.

Medications

The patient's medications are lisinopril and atorvastatin.

Allergies

The patient has no known drug allergies.

Physical exam and ancillary studies

- *Vital signs:* temperature 36.2°C, heart rate 115 bpm, blood pressure 185/116, respiratory rate 24, room air saturation 98%.
- *General:* awake and alert, clearly uncomfortable.
- *Head and neck:* pupils are equally round and reactive to light, cranial nerves intact. The patient's mucous membranes are moist. Her neck is supple with a midline trachea.
- *Cardiovascular:* regular tachycardia with a diastolic murmur heard best over the aortic region. There are no rubs, no third or fourth heart sounds, peripheral pulses present throughout.
- *Lungs:* clear.
- *Back:* no areas of reproducible tenderness.
- *Extremities and skin:* no bilateral edema, no clubbing, no calf tenderness.
- *EKG:* left ventricular hypertrophy with strain and sinus tachycardia.
- CXR: shows a widened mediastinum.
- CT of chest: see Figure 9.3.

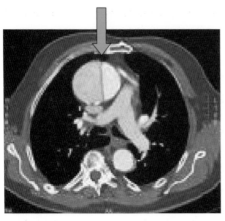

Figure 9.3. Chest CT showing the dissection flap with blood flow on one side (gray) and intimal bleeding on the other (white).

Questions for thought

- What are the appropriate initial actions to take to stabilize this patient?
- What other diagnostic modalities are appropriate in the emergency department?
- What therapeutic interventions are appropriate?
- How does ED treatment differ based on the abilities of the institution?
- What are indications for transfer?
- What is optimal EMS care?

Diagnosis

Type A aortic dissection.

Discussion

- *Epidemiology:* aortic dissection is a potentially fatal condition. Although the true incidence is not known, thoracic aortic dissection is twice as common as rupture of an abdominal aortic aneurysm. Without treatment, mortality rates approach 50% within the first 48 hours. Aortic dissection is more common in white than in black Americans and in men than in women. Most occur between the ages of 40 and 70.
- *Pathophysiology:* degenerative changes within the muscular wall of the aorta result in breakdown of collagen and elastin. This normal aging process is accelerated by hypertension, diabetes, hyperlipidemia, and inherited disorders of collagen formation, such as Marfan's syndrome or Ehler Danlos syndrome. A small tear in the intima of the aorta allows blood to dissect along the tissue planes of the vessel wall, causing pain. Additional symptoms are due to vascular occlusion of branch vessels, retrograde dissection into the pericardial sac, causing cardiac tamponade, or free rupture with resulting blood

loss. Aortic dissections are Type A if they involve any portion of the ascending aorta or the aortic arch and Type B if they involve the descending aorta alone.

- *Presentation:* classic symptoms include a sudden onset of intrascapular back pain in a patient at risk based on age and comorbidities. Additional symptoms will depend on the exact location of the dissection, but may include acute myocardial ischemia, lateralizing neurologic symptoms, limb ischemia, bowel ischemia, acute renal dysfunction, spinal cord ischemia, or shock from cardiac tamponade or blood loss. Painless dissection occurs in up to 10% of patients. In these, the diagnosis is suspected on the basis of ischemic symptoms.
- *Diagnosis:* diagnosis begins with a clinical suspicion. Chest radiographs should be obtained but may be normal. EKG should be done to rule out other causes of chest pain and to ensure there is no sign of compromise to the coronary arteries from dissection. Definitive diagnosis can be made with CT angiography, which will show the dissection and entry point as well as suggest areas of ischemia. Alternatively, transesophageal echocardiography will demonstrate the presence and location of dissection. Multiple studies have confirmed the diagnostic accuracy of both study modalities and the modality chosen depends on the ready availability of each at your institution.
- *Treatment:* initial treatment should be aimed at lowering the blood pressure and the shear force of the blood as it enters the aorta. This is best done with beta-blockers to control heart rate, blood pressure and heart contractility. Short-acting beta-blockers are preferred so that dose can be closely titrated to response. This can be done as a temporizing modality while the patient is transferred to a tertiary care center for definitive treatment.
- *Definitive therapy:* additional therapy will depend on the location of the dissection and the consequences of resulting ischemia. Type A dissections require urgent surgical repair and urgent transfer to a tertiary center is usually required. Type B dissections are treated with medical therapy alone unless there is evidence of rupture or impending rupture.

Clinical course

The keys to this patient's diagnosis are careful attention to her history, physical exam, and ancillary studies.

Historical clues	Physical findings	Ancillary studies
• Acute-onset intrascapular pain	• Lack of reproducible findings to support a musculoskeletal etiology	• CXR
• Patient with risk factors	• Hypertension	• CT angiogram of the chest

This patient's diagnosis was suspected based on her age, presentation and presence of risk factors. Her hypertension and tachycardia responded well to intravenous beta-blockade. The CT angiogram confirmed the diagnosis of an ascending aortic dissection. She was transferred to a tertiary care center and taken urgently to the operating suites for repair. She recovered uneventfully and was discharged to home on the sixth post-operative day.

Further reading

Hagan PG, Nienaber CA, Isselbacher EM, et al. The International Registry of Acute Aortic Dissection (IRAD): new insights into an old disease. *JAMA* 2000;**283**(7):897–903.

Knaut AL, Cleveland JC. Aortic emergencies. *Emerg Med Clin North Am* 2003;**21**(4):817–45.

Rogers RL, McCormack R. Aortic disasters. *Emerg Med Clin North Am* 2004;**22**(4):887–908.

Case #6

History

A 17-year-old female presents to the ED with a complaint of 10/10 back pain. Patient states the pain starts on the left side of her back and radiates around her flank to involve her entire abdomen. She states she has had these symptoms for about a week and they have been getting progressively worse. She was seen in the ED 2 days ago for similar pain that was associated with a fever. She was diagnosed with a urinary tract infection (UTI) and discharged home on a 3 day course of oral antibiotics. She is returning to the ED today because the pain is worse and she now has associated nausea and vomiting. She states that she has been unable to keep anything down today. She noticed that her fever has disappeared since being on the antibiotics. She does report some urinary frequency and dysuria. She denies any diarrhea or constipation. She does report some light-headedness upon standing.

Past medical history

She denies any significant medical history except an elective termination of a pregnancy last year. She is G_1P_{0010} and states her periods have been regular since her termination.

Medications

She is on an antibiotic that was prescribed 2 days ago. She doesn't remember the name and states that she vomited today's dose.

Allergies

No known drug allergies.

Physical exam and ancillary studies

- *Vital signs:* temp 36.8°C, heart rate 106 bpm, blood pressure 102/66, respiratory rate 22, room air saturation 100%.
- *General:* awake and alert, non-toxic-appearing and in no acute respiratory distress but appears markedly uncomfortable.
- *Cardiovascular:* regular rhythm with tachycardia. No murmurs appreciated. 2+ palpable peripheral pulses throughout.
- *Respiratory:* lungs are clear to auscultation with adequate air entry in all fields. No rales, rhonchi, or wheeze.
- *Musculoskeletal:* no deformities noted. Positive costovertebral angle (CVA) tenderness present on the left.
- *Abdomen:* voluntary guarding. She is diffusely tender to palpation without rebound, greater on the left side. She has a negative Murphy's sign.
- *Skin:* warm and dry without rashes or lesions.

- *Pertinent abnormal labs:* urine dip: 1+ protein, 1+ leukocyte esterase, 1+ bilirubin, urobilinogen > 8, urine pregnancy test is negative. Microscopic urinalysis: 50–100 WBCs, 5–10 RBCs, + casts. CBC: Hgb 9.5, Hct 27, WBC 8.5 and CMP is normal except for a potassium of 3.0 and BUN of 5.

Questions for thought

- What are the most appropriate initial actions?
- What other diagnostic tests/modalities should be considered?
- What is the differential diagnosis for this patient presentation?
- How should this patient be treated in the emergency department?
- What is the most appropriate disposition for this patient?
- What are the complications of this condition?

Diagnosis

Acute pyelonephritis.

Discussion

- *Epidemiology:* pyelonephritis is a common infection of the kidneys. Most cases are due to ascending infections from bowel organisms that enter the lower urinary tract. It typically starts as a cystitis or prostatitis that ascends to involve the renal tissue. It is more common in females than males and there is some suspicion that many women presenting with lower tract symptoms have pyelonephritis.
- *Pathophysiology:* acute pyelonephritis is caused by bacterial invasion of the renal parenchyma. It can be an ascending infection from the lower urinary tract or by direct hematogenous spread to the kidney. The factors that increase the risk for pyelonephritis include pregnancy, frequent lower urinary tract infections, structural abnormalities or instrumentation of the urinary tract, immunocompromised state and comorbidities, including diabetes mellitus.
- *Presentation:* the presentation of pyelonephritis can vary from dramatic with shaking chills, fevers, and flank pain associated with dysuria and frequency, to a more subtle presentation that may be very difficult to diagnose. In infants and the elderly, the symptoms may be very nonspecific so the clinician needs to maintain a high index of suspicion. Typically, pyelonephritis will present with dysuria and frequency associated with systemic symptoms and flank pain. The urine will often show the presence of white blood cell casts in addition to the typical findings of bacteria, leukocyte esterase, and nitrites.
- *Diagnosis:* the diagnosis of pyelonephritis is made based on clinical suspicion from symptoms and urinalysis. The microscopic urinalysis typically will present with pyuria (WBC > 2 to 5/hpf), white blood cell casts, and bacteria. Urine cultures should be obtained to isolate the bacteria responsible and to help guide antibiotic therapy. Imaging is only needed to evaluate for other causes of the symptoms or to look for complications from the infection.

- *Treatment:* antibiotics are the mainstay of therapy as pyelonephritis is a bacterial infection. Most regimens will include nitrofurantoin, trimethoprim/sulfamethoxazole or a flouroquinolone. A third-generation cephalosporin given intravenously can be used to initiate therapy in the hospital and the patient can be discharged on cephalexin. However, it is important to be aware of local resistance patterns and treat accordingly. When urine culture and sensitivity results are available they can be used to guide the choice of antibiotic therapy. Therapy should be continued for 10–14 days in the presence of upper tract disease. The patient with acute pyelonephritis who is vomiting will usually require admission for intravenous hydration and symptomatic management of pain and nausea.
- *Disposition:* young, healthy females with uncomplicated pyelonephritis can be managed as outpatients provided they are able to tolerate oral antibiotics. Patients who cannot tolerate oral antibiotics or who are pregnant, immunocompromised, or diabetic require admission for parenteral antibiotics.
- *Complications:* acute pyelonephritis can have many complications, including scarring of the renal tissue, papillary necrosis, acute renal failure or obstruction, perinephric abscess formation, sepsis, and even death. Host factors contribute to the prognosis, with young, healthy patients experiencing the fewest complications.

Clinical course

The patient's diagnosis was made based on careful attention to the history, physical exam, and ancillary studies. She had a prior diagnosis of UTI with urinary frequency and dysuria. She was now presenting with worsening back and flank pain as well as vomiting. The patient had CVA tenderness present on examination. Her urine dip was significant for urobilinogen and leukocyte esterase. The formal urinalysis showed the presence of white blood cells and casts.

Historical clues	Physical findings	Ancillary studies
• Flank pain	• Tachycardia	• Urinalysis positive for white blood cells and bacteria
• Fever and chills	• CVA tenderness	
• Nausea and vomiting		
• Dysuria or frequency of urination		

The diagnosis of acute pyelonephritis was accurately recognized and, due to the fact that it was complicated by vomiting and inability to tolerate oral medications, the patient was appropriately admitted to the hospital. She was admitted for IV antibiotics and made a rapid recovery and 2 days later was discharged on oral antibiotics.

Further reading

Bogner MP, Howes DS. Chapter 94. Urinary tract infections. In Tintinalli JE, Kelen GD, Stapczynski JS, Ma OJ, Cline DM, eds., *Tintinalli's Emergency Medicine: A Comprehensive Study Guide*, 6th edition. New York: McGraw-Hill, 2004.

Jaffe J, Morris J. Chapter 40. Upper urinary tract infection (pyelonephritis). In Stone CK, Humphries RL, eds., *Current Diagnosis and Treatment: Emergency Medicine*, 6th edition. New York: McGraw-Hill, 2008.

Shoff WH, et al. Pyelonephritis, acute. *Emedicine*, Topic 2843. February 2007.

Case #7

History

An 84-year-old Caucasian female presents to the emergency room after a fall at home. She is accompanied by her daughter, who reports that she witnessed the patient slip on ice-covered stairs and land on her back. The patient denies striking her head but complains of a moderate amount of pain in her mid-back. She was able to stand and ambulate on her own after the fall, but with some difficulty secondary to the pain. She denies radiation of the pain, extremity weakness, paraesthesia, or hypoesthesia.

Past medical history

Chronic low back pain, hypertension, hypercholesterolemia, hypothyroidism, and osteoporosis.

Medications

Lisinopril, hydrochlorothiazide, atorvastatin, levothyroxine, alendronate, calcium, vitamin D.

Allergies

No known drug allergies.

Physical exam and ancillary studies

- *Vital signs:* temperature 37.1°C, heart rate 85 bpm, blood pressure 148/91, respiratory rate 14, room air saturation 96%, height 5′5″, weight 115 lb.
- *General:* awake and alert, moderate distress due to back pain. Oriented times three.
- *Head and neck:* head was normocephalic and non-traumatic. Pupils are equal, round, and reactive to light. Cranial nerves intact. No Battle's or Raccoon's sign. Tympanic membranes are normal with no hemotympanum. Her neck is supple with a midline trachea and without spinal process tenderness.
- *Cardiovascular:* regular rate. Peripheral pulses palpable and symmetric.
- *Lungs:* clear bilaterally without rales, rhonchi, or wheezes.
- *Extremities and skin:* no edema or clubbing. Normal capillary refill.
- *Musculoskeletal:* minimal tenderness to midline palpation posteriorly at the level of the thoracolumbar junction. Motor, sensory, and reflex examination is normal and symmetric throughout.
- *Radiograph and MRI:* see Figure 9.4.

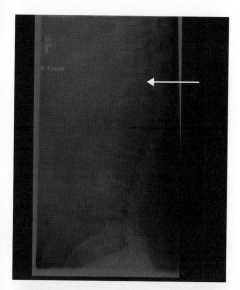

Figure 9.4 Lateral lumbar radiograph and spinal T2-weighted sagittal magnetic resonance imaging showing compression fractures.

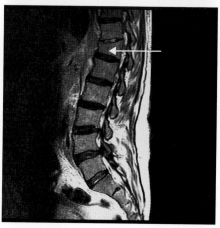

Questions for thought

- What is the underlying disease process responsible for this patient's current problem?
- What factors must be considered in acutely and chronically managing this patient?
- When does this condition require the consultation of a specialist?
- What is the definitive treatment of this condition?

Diagnosis

Acute on chronic back pain secondary to osteoporotic vertebral compression fractures (OVCF).

Discussion

- *Epidemiology:* approximately 700 000 vertebral compression fractures (VCFs) occur annually in the United States. There are twice as many of these as hip fractures. The most common metabolic disorder of bone, osteoporosis, is responsible for a significant portion of these fractures. At least 25% of American women reaching menopause will suffer at least one OVCF in their lifetime. In addition, osteoporosis affects one-third of men over the age of 75. After experiencing one VCF, an individual is five times more likely to develop subsequent fractures.

- *Pathophysiology:* osteoporotic bone has decreased mineralization and increased porosity and elastic resistance. Loss of bone integrity occurs due to an imbalance between bone resorption and formation. A high turnover state is due to excessive osteoclastic activity, the mechanism believed to be responsible for postmenopausal osteoporosis. In osteoporosis of the elderly, inefficient osteoblasts are thought to be the cause. In both cases, there exists diminished structural support of the osseous spinal column, predisposing individuals to fractures with even relatively minor traumatic events.

- *Presentation:* roughly two-thirds of OVCFs are asymptomatic and found incidentally on radiographs. With relatively atraumatic activities, such as standing or forceful sneezing, or with minor trauma, such as low-impact falls, patients may experience sudden or acute pain. Often the paraspinal musculature is suspected as the etiology rather than a spinal fracture when the symptoms are mild. The pain may not be localized to the exact site of the vertebral fracture. Significant and intense pain is due to irritation of the periosteum and joint capsule. This should be suspected when there is radiation of the pain or direct tenderness over the site.

- *Diagnosis:* spinal radiographs are the diagnostic study of choice and usually reveal the classic "wedge" fracture. This consists of loss of anterior vertebral body height with minimal to no posterior vertebral body involvement. The thoracolumbar junction is the most commonly involved area of the spine, followed by the mid-thoracic region. Computed tomography should be utilized to better define the fracture and ensure that it doesn't extend beyond the spine's anterior column, creating a potentially unstable injury. Since many OVCFs are asymptomatic and only identified incidentally it may be difficult to distinguish an acute from a chronic fracture. The latter may show some sclerosis or osteophyte formation along the fracture line. Magnetic resonance imaging, bone scintigraphy, or positron emission tomography may be helpful to determine the timing of the injury and to detect other pathologies, such as neoplasm or infection.

- *Treatment:* those patients with vertebral compression fractures that are symptomatic usually follow a relatively benign course. Pain generally improves over a 6–8 week course. Initially, for some patients, the pain may be intense, necessitating inpatient admission for pain control. Bed rest should be limited to a few days, after which the patient should be mobilized. If necessary, bracing with a spinal orthosis may help ameliorate pain associated with ambulation. Analgesia should be provided as appropriate. There are now some promising therapeutic devices for restoration of vertebral height and referral to a spine surgeon should be strongly considered.

- *Definitive therapy:* some OVCFs may progress, and regular surveillance is required to treat symptoms and prevent long-term complications. Acutely, transient ileus, urinary retention, and rarely spinal cord compression from fracture progression may occur and constitute a neurosurgical emergency. With multiple, significant fractures, chronic problems, such as kyphosis-induced breathing difficulties, extreme back pain, and ambulation limitations, may result. Every patient should be evaluated for osteoporosis and bone mineral density and treated with the proper medical management (e.g., bisphosphonates, hormone-replacement drugs, parathormone analogs, calcitonin, calcium, and vitamin D supplementation). Patients with chronic pain after vertebral compression fracture can be treated surgically with vertebral body augmentation techniques. These include kyphoplasty and vertebroplasty, minimally invasive options with relatively low risk and high clinical success rates.

Clinical course

The keys to this patient's diagnosis are careful attention to her history, physical exam, and ancillary studies.

Historical clues	Physical findings	Ancillary studies
• Chronic back pain	• Tenderness to posterior midline palpation	• Lateral lumbar radiograph demonstrating compression fractures and poor bone density
• Osteoporosis	• Normal motor, sensory, and reflex examination	• MRI showing compression fracture
• Caucasian	• No signs of spinal cord compression or radiculopathy	

The patient detailed above was recognized to have a compression fracture of the T12 vertebra. There was no radiographic evidence of compression of the neural elements nor any clinical signs of neurologic deficit. An attempt was made to mobilize the patient in the emergency department after the administration of oral analgesia. She was somewhat limited by her pain. After the application of a spinal orthosis, her pain with ambulation improved. The patient was instructed to wear the brace only when upright or ambulatory and cautioned against the potential skin breakdown that might occur. Discharged with oral opiate analgesia, she was told to follow up with her primary physician for any necessary modifications of her osteoporosis medications. She was informed of the option of surgical intervention if her pain persisted chronically and that the decision to pursue such treatments should be made with her primary physician.

Further reading

Kim DH, Vaccaro AR. Osteoporotic compression fractures of the spine; current opinions and considerations for treatment. *Spine J* 2006;**6**:479–87.

Wu SS, Lachmann E, Nagler W. Current medical, rehabilitation, and surgical management of vertebral compression fractures. *J Women's Health* 2003;**12**:17–26.

Prather H, Watson JO, Gilul LA. Nonoperative management of osteoporotic vertebral compression fractures. *Injury* 2007;**38**(Suppl 3):S40–8.

Barrocas AM, Eskey CJ, Hirsch JA. Vertebral augmentation in osteoporotic fractures. 2007; *Injury* **38**(Suppl 3):S88–96.

Case #8

History

A 46-year-old male presents to the ED complaining of severe low back pain which has become progressively worse over the past several days. He states that he works unloading trucks for a living, and does a great deal of heavy lifting every day. He was fine until 8 weeks ago, when he developed lower back pain after work. He had no weakness, incontinence, numbness, or tingling in his lower extremities. He saw his primary doctor, who gave him muscle relaxants and anti-inflammatories and narcotics. He improved a bit but still had significant pain. His primary care provider referred him to a pain management physician who did an epidural injection 2 weeks ago. Afterwards he felt significant relief for 5 days, but then his pain returned, getting progressively worse since then. He has been feeling feverish for the past day but he did not take his temperature. He could not get an appointment with his primary care physician until next month and so he came to the emergency department for help.

Past medical history

He has had back strains several times in the past. He smokes one pack a day, and denies any alcohol or recreational drug use.

Medications

Ibuprofen, hydrocodone, and orphenadrine.

Allergies

No known drug allergies.

Physical exam

- *Vital signs:* temperature 38.0°C, heart rate 110 bpm, blood pressure 148/84, respiratory rate 18, room air saturation 98%.
- *General:* awake and alert, in obvious pain.
- *Head and neck:* pupils are equally round and reactive to light, cranial nerves intact. The patient's mucous membranes are dry. His neck is supple with a midline trachea. He has no jugular venous distension.
- *Cardiovascular:* regular rate and rhythm with a normal S1 and S2. No murmurs or rubs.
- *Lungs:* clear and equal breath sounds with a few scattered wheezes. No rales or rhonchi.
- *Abdomen:* soft, non-tender, no palpable aneurysm, no guarding or rebound.
- *Back:* tender to palpation of entire lumbosacral region with obvious spasm. No erythema, no scoliosis. No point tenderness. No swelling.

- *Neurologic:* awake, alert, and oriented times three. Cranial nerves II–XII are intact. Sensation is intact to light touch and two point discrimination and motor functions are 5/5 throughout. Reflexes are two plus throughout. Gait is slow secondary to pain, but there are no gross abnormalities.
- *Extremities:* no edema, swelling or tenderness.
- *Skin:* no rash or lesions. No track marks.
- *Laboratory results:* WBC 11.8. The remainder of labs are normal or negative. A blood culture was obtained and is pending.

Questions for thought

- Does this patient require acute intervention in the emergency department?
- Is there anything in this patient's history that makes him different from the typical patient with back pain?
- Is radiographic testing warranted, and if so what type?
- What are the "red flags" of back pain?

Diagnosis

Spinal epidural abscess as a complication of epidural injection.

Discussion

- *Epidemiology:* back pain is a frequent complaint of ED patients. Epidural abscess is very rare, often very subtle in presentation, and can be a neurologically devastating cause of back pain. Most patients have predisposing conditions: underlying disease processes, recent instrumentation, or IV drug use. These are some of the 'red flags' for this diagnosis. Many of these predisposing conditions allow bacteria to enter the bloodstream via the skin, thus accounting for the high percentage of *Staphylococcus aureus* seen in epidural abscesses.
- *Pathophysiology:* patients with a spinal epidural abscess have an infection in their epidural space. Half of the cases arise from hematogenous spread, one-third from contiguous spread, and the remainder will have no identifiable source. Most patients will have at least one predisposing factor, including immunocompromise from HIV, diabetes, transplant, alcoholism or other causes, or a potential site allowing bacteria to enter the blood such as skin infection, concurrent infections such as osteomyelitis, IV drug use, indwelling vascular devices, tattoos, or injections such as epidural nerve blocks. As the infection progresses, the spinal cord can be damaged because of direct compression by the abscess or vascular occlusion secondary to septic thrombophlebitis. The most common bacteria involved is *S. aureus*, but a variety of others can cause infection as well depending on the source.
- *Presentation:* this presentation is typical for spinal epidural abscess from any cause. Patients with this condition can be differentiated from the multitude of patients who present with routine back pain by the presence of distinguishing features such as the predisposing factors listed above. Three-quarters of spinal epidural abscess patients present

with back pain, half with fever, and one-third with neurological deficit. The classic triad of fever, back pain, and neurological compromise is the exception rather than the norm and patients presenting early in the disease are usually indistinguishable from those with muscular back pain. Spinal epidural abscess goes through a predictable progression of illness from back pain at the level of infection without any other signs or symptoms, to nerve root symptoms with radiating pain, to frank neurological compromise with motor weakness and/or sensory deficits, and finally complete paralysis.

- *Diagnosis:* if the diagnosis of spinal epidural abscess is in question, an MRI with IV gadolinium is the test of choice to perform. Although CT may reveal the presence of diskitis and osteomyelitis it is not as specific or sensitive as MRI. Laboratory studies may reveal elevated white counts, although these are neither sensitive nor specific.
- *Treatment:* treatment of the patient with spinal epidural abscess is rapid administration of IV antibiotics and emergency consultation with the spine surgery service. Many patients will be candidates for a decompressive laminectomy and debridement of infected tissue. While cultures are pending, empirical antibiotic therapy should cover staphylococci and include vancomycin to cover MRSA in addition to a second agent such as third- or fourth-generation cephalosporin to cover Gram-negative bacilli.

Clinical course

The keys to this patient's diagnosis are careful attention to his history with his predisposing factors, as well as his physical exam and ancillary studies.

Historical clues	Physical findings	Ancillary studies
• Recent epidural injection	• Fever	• Mild leukocytosis
• Back pain	• Back tenderness	
• Fever		
• Worsening symptoms over time		

This man was correctly recognized to have a probable spinal epidural abscess based on his history of predisposing factors. Therefore, after IV placement and laboratory studies, broad-spectrum IV antibiotics were administered and the patient was sent for emergency MRI. The neurosurgical team was notified and reviewed the MRI upon its completion. The patient was taken urgently to the operating room for drainage of the abscess and completed a successful recovery without any neurological sequelae.

Further reading

Pradilla G, Ardila GP, Hsu W, et al. Epidural abscesses of the CNS. *Lancet Neurol* 2009;**8**(3):292–300.

Ziai WC, Lewin III JJ. Update in the diagnosis and management of central nervous system infections. *Neurol Clin* 2008;**26**(2):427–68.

Sendi P, Bregenzer T, Zimmerli W. Spinal epidural abscess in clinical practice. *QJM* 2008;**101**(1):1–12.

Fischer B. Complications of regional anaesthesia. *Anaesthesia Intensive Care Med* 2007;**8**(4):151–4.

Case #9

History

A 66-year-old female presents to the emergency department complaining of low back pain for a month. She denies any trauma but states it started when she turned suddenly to speak with her grandchild. The pain is now 10+/10. She had been evaluated by her primary doctor, and given oxycodone without relief. She had been seen at a neighboring hospital ED the prior evening, complaining of increased pain. They performed an abdominal workup, including a CT scan. She was discharged on Lortab and Flexeril without relief. The pain radiated around to bilateral hips and to the front of her thighs. She described the pain as a burning sensation. She denied GI complaints and urinary or bowel changes. She also denied extremity weakness and incontinence, fever, chills, lightheadedness, dizziness, chest pain, and shortness of breath.

Past medical history

Swelling in left arm 5 years ago, diagnosed as rheumatoid arthritis. MRI of upper spine was negative. Hypercholesterolemia.

Social history

Patient quit smoking approximately 25 years ago after a 20 pack-year history. She is retired. She has an occasional alcoholic drink.

Family history

Father deceased of lung cancer. Mother deceased of breast cancer.

Medications

Oxycodone, rosuvastatin, cyclobenzaprine, alendronate, calcium supplements.

Drug allergies

None.

Physical exam and ancillary studies

- *Vital signs*: temperature 36.7°C orally, pulse 95 bpm, respiratory rate 16, blood pressure 143/87, oxygen saturation 97% on room air.
- *General*: alert and oriented times three, pleasant, ambulatory with stiffened gait, non-toxic.
- *HEENT*: normocephalic, atraumatic. Pupils equally round and reactive, oral mucosa moist with dentures in place, neck non-tender to palpation, no JVD, no carotid bruits.

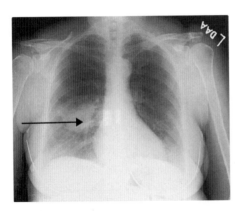

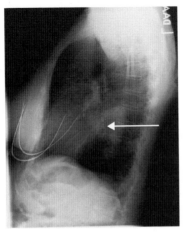

Figure 9.5 Chest X-ray demonstrating a lung mass.

- *Cardiovascular:* normal rate and rhythm, no murmurs, rubs, or gallops.
- *Respiratory:* lungs clear to auscultation bilaterally. No wheezes, rales, rhonchi.
- *Musculoskeletal:* full range of motion in all extremities. Strength 5/5 × 4. DTRs 2+ throughout.
- *Back:* no tenderness to palpation of lumbar or thoracic spine. Tenderness to palpation of bilateral paraspinal muscles in upper lumbar and lumbosacral area. Negative straight leg raise and crossed straight leg raise. No pain with hip palpation or movement.
- *Pertinent labs:* WBC 3.3, Hgb 11, Hct 32.1, alk phos normal, calcium normal.
- *Chest X-ray:* see Figure 9.5.

Questions for thought

- What was the likely source of the patient's pain?
- Why didn't the patient feel short of breath?

Diagnosis

New lung mass, metastatic bone lesions to L4 and rib.

Discussion

- *Epidemiology:* lung cancer is the most common cause of cancer morbidity and mortality worldwide for both men and women. Smoking is the most important risk factor but others include radiation therapy, environment toxins, pulmonary fibrosis, HIV infection, genetics, and diet.
- *Pathology:* there are five major histological cell types of lung cancer. These are; adenocarcinoma, squamous cell carcinoma, large-cell carcinoma, small-cell carcinoma and other non-small-cell carcinomas or undefined types.
- *Clinical presentation:* because cancer is usually asymptomatic at onset, most patients present with symptoms of advanced disease. Intrathoracic effects may cause cough, hemoptysis, chest pain, and dyspnea. Persistent hoarseness in a smoker may be indicative of either laryngeal cancer or lung cancer. Malignant effusion secondary to pleural involvement is considered a sign of an incurable cancer. Extrathoracic metastases usually present later in the course of the disease, with the most frequent sites of metastasis in the liver, adrenal glands, bones, and brain. Bone lesions frequently present with pain and may be associated with markedly elevated levels of serum alkaline phosphatase or calcium. Bone metastases most commonly involve the ribs, pelvis, and vertebrae, with 70% found in the thoracic spine. Pain from pathological fracture is the most common symptom. This may develop over weeks, with increased severity at night. If there are associated neurological symptoms, evaluation for spinal cord compression must be done.
- *Diagnosis:* plain X-rays of the spine are the initial diagnostic modality but may only detect osteolytic lesions. Osteoblastic lesions are best detected via radionuclide bone scanning. MRI is the most sensitive method of detecting bone metastases of either type.
- *Treatment:* treatment depends on the underlying malignancy. Local radiation therapy is one option for treatment. Hormonally responsive tumors may respond to hormone blockade therapy. Bisphosphonates are an adjunctive therapy used both for pain and to maintain bone density. Steroid therapy may also help with pain and immediate therapy is high-dose dexamethasone. Surgery is an effective treatment for spinal metastasis stabilization and depends on location of the tumor within the vertebral body and the extent of the lesion.
- *Prognosis:* early detection and treatment is an important prognostic factor, as is the general health of the patient at time of diagnosis. Adenocarcinoma has the greatest survival rate, followed by squamous carcinoma. The prognosis for patients with metastatic disease to the spine is poor. Those classified as stage I, tumor less than 3 cm without metastasis have a 5 year survival rate of 60–80%, while those with bony metastasis have a 5 year survival rate of less than 5%.

Hospital course

The patient was treated for pain with a combination of ketorlac 30 mg IV, morphine 4 mg IV and diazepam 5 mg IV. Approximately 10 minutes after receiving medication, the patient became confused and extremely somnolent. Vital signs were reassessed and oxygen saturation was 89–90% on room air. She was placed on 2 liters of oxygen via nasal cannula, which raised her saturation.

Historical clues	Physical findings	Ancillary studies
• Increasing low back pain	• Back tenderness	• Low hematocrit
• Shortness of breath		• Mass on chest X-ray

She returned to normal mentation but saturation remained in the high 80s, dropping to low 80s with ambulation. Patient denied ever feeling short of breath. Her lung mass was diagnosed, and she went on to have a metastatic evaluation, revealing her metastases. She was referred to oncology for further palliative treatment. She was eventually sent for chest X-ray, at which time she noted significant decrease in back pain.

Further reading

Bilsky MH, Lis E, Raizer J, Lee H, Boland P. The diagnosis and treatment of metastatic spinal tumor. *Oncologist* 1999;**4**(6):459–69.

Schuster JM, Grady MS. Medical management and adjuvant therapies in spinal metastatic disease. *Neurosurg Focus* 2001;**11**(6):article 3.

White AP, Kwon BK, Lindskog DM, Friedlaender GE, Grauer JN. Metastatic disease of the spine. *J Am Acad Orthop Surg* 2006;**14**(11):587–98.

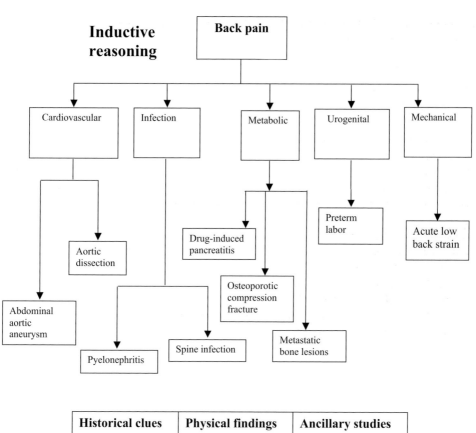

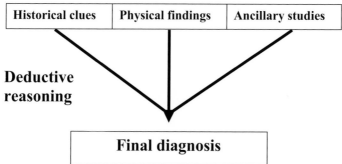

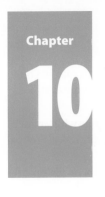
Chief complaint: altered mental status

Shellie Asher, Timothy Barcomb, Luke Day, Antoinette Eng, Ravi Ghandi, Edward Lisenby, Jeremy Lux, Amee Mapara-Shah, Shankar Perumal, Sheetal Sharma

Case #1

History

A 63-year-old woman presents to the ED with her husband, who reports that approximately 2 hours prior to presentation she complained of a severe headache which came on suddenly. It was not associated with exertion. She vomited several times, and subsequently became confused and lethargic. She is unable to give any history. Her husband denies any recent illnesses.

Past medical history

She has a history of coronary artery disease with a stent placed 1 year ago. She also has type II diabetes mellitus, hypertension, and chronic obstructive pulmonary disease.

Medications

The patient's medications include metoprolol, quinapril, metformin, theophylline, and insulin. Her husband believes she has been taking her medications.

Allergies

The patient is allergic to penicillins.

Family history

Both parents deceased due to hypertension and heart disease.

Social history

The patient smokes a half pack of cigarettes per day. Per her husband, she does not use alcohol or illicit drugs.

Case Studies in Emergency Medicine, ed. R. Jeanmonod, M. Tomassi and D. Mayer.
Published by Cambridge University Press © Cambridge University Press 2010.

Physical exam and ancillary studies

- *Vital signs:* the patient's vital signs are as follows: temperature 36.7°C, heart rate 103 bpm, blood pressure 222/143 mmHg, respiratory rate 14, room air oxygen saturation 98%.
- *General:* the patient is lethargic, but responds to verbal stimuli.
- *Head and neck:* the patient's mucous membranes are dry. Her neck is supple without jugular venous distension or bruit. Sclerae are non-icteric. Fundoscopic exam reveals retinal hemorrhages and mild papilledema.
- *Cardiovascular:* her heart is regularly tachycardic without murmur, rub, or gallop. Her distal pulses are normal in all four extremities.
- *Lungs:* the chest wall has equal expansion without retractions. Breath sounds are equal and clear without rales, wheezes, or rhonchi.
- *Abdomen:* the patient's abdomen is soft without apparent tenderness. There are no masses or organomegaly.
- *Extremities and skin:* her skin is dry without rashes. There is no peripheral edema. Her legs are of equal size with no palpable cords.
- *Neurologic:* the patient's pupils are equal and react normally to light. Her tongue is midline. She does not follow commands, but moves all four extremities equally. She withdraws equally to pain. Her gait was not tested. Her reflexes are 2+ throughout.
- *Psychiatric:* the patient is lethargic but responds to verbal stimuli. She is oriented to self but not place or time. Her speech is confused.
- *Pertinent labs:* her complete blood count is normal. Her chemistries are significant for a blood glucose of 517. They are otherwise normal, and her anion gap is 9. Her cardiac enzymes are normal. Her ammonia and liver enzymes are normal. Her cerebrospinal fluid studies are normal.
- EKG: see Figure 10.1.
- *Radiographs:* the patient's chest X-ray is unremarkable. Her head CT shows no abnormalities.

Questions for thought

- What are the appropriate initial actions to take to stabilize this patient?
- What medications should be avoided in this patient?
- How does one urgently treat this condition in the emergency department?
- What is definitive treatment of this condition?
- What is causing this patient's altered mental status?

Diagnosis

Hypertensive encephalopathy.

Discussion

- *Epidemiology:* of the 60 million or more persons in the United States with hypertension, fewer than 1% will develop a hypertensive emergency, defined as acute organ dysfunction

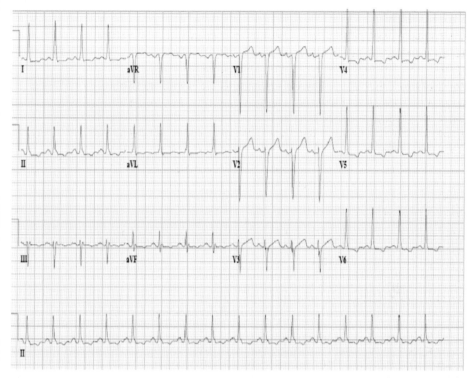

Figure 10.1. This EKG demonstrates a normal sinus rhythm with evidence of left ventricular hypertrophy (QRS complex in lead aVL greater than 11 mm). There are flipped T waves laterally, which is commonly seen with left ventricular hypertrophy. This is consistent with longstanding hypertension.

related to hypertension. The central nervous, cardiac, respiratory, and renal systems may be affected.

- *Pathophysiology:* elevated blood pressure outside the limits of cerebral autoregulation results in leakage of fluid across the blood–brain barrier, causing cerebral edema. While the most common cause is acute elevation of blood pressure in the chronic hypertensive, other secondary causes must be considered.
- *Presentation:* most patients have underlying diagnosed hypertension. They may or may not be compliant with their antihypertensive medications. Symptoms may be vague, and include headache, confusion, visual changes, new-onset seizures, nausea, and vomiting. Progression of symptoms to altered mental status occurs over 24–48 hours.
- *Treatment:* antihypertensives are the mainstay of treatment. Because these patients are usually hypertensive at baseline, normal blood pressure is not the goal. The mean arterial pressure should be lowered by about 25%. Commonly used medications include short-acting beta-blockers, calcium-channel blockers, and nitroprusside. Patients should be admitted to an intensive care setting for monitoring of hemodynamics and end-organ function.
- *Definitive therapy:* patients should be maintained on outpatient antihypertensive medications of the class which were effective in treating their acute hypertensive emergency, with frequent reassessments. Lifestyle modifications also may improve outpatient blood pressure control.

Clinical course

The keys to this patient's diagnosis are careful attention to history, physical exam, and the use of ancillary studies to rule out other pathology.

Historical clues	Physical findings	Ancillary studies
• History of hypertension	• Severely elevated blood pressure	• EKG with left ventricular hypertrophy and repolarization abnormalities consistent with hypertension
• Sudden-onset headache	• Presence of papilledema	• Otherwise negative lab and radiographic workup, excluding other pathology
• Vomiting and altered mental status suggesting elevated intracranial pressure		

The patient's clinical picture suggested hypertensive encephalopathy, or central nervous system end-organ dysfunction secondary to acute hypertensive emergency. She had papilledema and retinal hemorrhaging on fundoscopic exam, which is not uncommon with hypertensive emergencies. Typical of people with hypertensive encephalopathy, her neurologic exam revealed deficits in a non-anatomic pattern, with some elements of confusion and alteration in level of consciousness. Although not present in this patient, some patients have lab evidence of cardiac, respiratory, or renal involvement. This patient's EKG showed changes associated with longstanding severe hypertension, but the remainder of her findings showed isolated neurologic involvement.

Since the patient's chest X-ray showed no evidence of pulmonary edema or lung disease and her head CT showed no evidence of hemorrhage or stroke, these were excluded as possible sources of her altered mental status. Likewise, she did not have evidence of ischemia on her EKG. Hypertensive encephalopathy is a diagnosis of exclusion once other causes of alteration in mental status have been ruled out, and this patient had no other likely cause.

Our patient was treated in the emergency department with a labetalol drip. Her blood pressure decreased and her mental status improved. She was admitted to the cardiac ICU, where she was switched to a new oral antihypertensive regimen, and discharged a few days after admission with a complete resolution of symptoms.

Further reading

Chang R. Encephalopathy, hypertensive. Retrieved April 1, 2008, from eMedicine.com.

Case #2

History

An 81-year-old man presents to the emergency department after being found by his neighbor on the floor in his home in an altered state. He was brought in by EMS, and noted to be confused and mildly lethargic. He had been complaining of frequent urination and excessive thirst for the last several days. He also had complained of generalized weakness and fatigue, mild dizziness, and had "turned against food." He had had a recent bout of community-acquired pneumonia and was still being treated with a quinolone. Over the last 2 days, he had tried to decrease his fluid intake, as he was "peeing too much." He denies fever or chills, but admits to mild nausea without vomiting, and several episodes of loose bowel movements. He denies any other complaints.

Past medical history

The patient has been treated for community-acquired pneumonia for the last 7 days. He also has a history of psoriasis, significant hypertension, and hemorrhoids. His surgical history is remarkable for a tonsillectomy.

Medications

The patient's medications include lisinopril, metoprolol, omeprazole, hydrochlorothiazide, and verapamil. He is on day 7 of 10 of gatifloxacin treatment for pneumonia, and had completed several days of guiafenesin.

Allergies

The patient has no known drug allergies.

Social history

He was a 120 pack-year smoker, who quit 10 years prior. He also has a history of prior alcohol abuse, but denies current alcohol use. He lives at home alone.

Physical exam and ancillary studies

- *Vital signs:* the patient's temperature is 35.6°C, his heart rate is 73 bpm, his blood pressure is 144/62 mmHg, his respiratory rate is 14, and his room air oxygen saturation is 96%. His orthostatic blood pressures are significant for a drop of 22 mmHg in his systolic blood pressure upon standing.
- *General:* the patient is arousable, but is somewhat lethargic. He speaks slowly. He is not oriented to time.

- *Head and neck:* his pupils are equally round and reactive to light, without icterus or conjunctival pallor. The patient's mucous membranes are notably dry. His neck is supple without jugular venous distension.
- *Cardiovascular:* the patient's heart is regular without murmurs. His peripheral pulses are normal.
- *Lungs:* his lungs are clear throughout, without wheezes or crackles.
- *Extremities and skin:* the patient has no evidence of edema, cyanosis, or clubbing on extremity exam. His skin is noted to have poor turgor.
- *Neurological:* his cranial nerves are intact. He moves all extremities equally, and has normal tone and reflexes. His power is mildly reduced globally.
- *Pertinent labs:* the patient's complete blood count shows a white cell count of 9.2 and a hematocrit of 40.1%. His electrolytes are remarkable for a sodium of 122, potassium of 6.1, chloride of 86, and bicarbonate of 27. His creatinine is 3.0. The patient's glucose is 1024. His serum osmolarity is 323. His urine shows a glucose greater than 1000, no ketones, and specific gravity of 1.023. His arterial blood gas is notable for a pH of 7.36.
- Electrocardiogram: his EKG is normal.
- *Radiographs:* the patient's chest X-ray is read as normal.

Questions for thought

- What are the appropriate initial actions to take to stabilize this patient?
- Once stable, what are other diagnostic tools you can use to make a diagnosis?
- How does one urgently treat this condition in the emergency department?
- What is the definitive treatment of this condition?
- Why is this patient lethargic?
- Why are there electrolyte abnormalities?

Diagnosis

Hyperosmolar hyperglycemic nonketotic syndrome.

Discussion

- *Epidemiology:* hyperosmolar hyperglycemic nonketotic syndrome (HHNS) is a relatively common condition seen in the ED. It is most commonly seen in older individuals with previously undiagnosed diabetes, although it can occur in all age groups. The mean age of onset is in the seventh decade of life, with a slightly female predominance. The prevalence of this condition will probably rise with the ever-aging demographic, as well as with the increasing rise in obesity and diabetes in the general population.
- *Pathophysiology:* in HHNS, the patient has a relative lack of insulin as well as some degree of insulin resistance. This leads to glucosuria diuresis, and inhibits the kidney from concentrating urine. This results in dehydration and prerenal azotemia, ultimately decreasing glomerular filtration and further increasing glucose in the serum (since less is then filtered out). The blood level of insulin in these patients is enough to inhibit ketoacid production, but is not sufficient to prevent hyperglycemia. This is what distinguishes these

patients from those with diabetic ketoacidosis, although some overlap is present in many situations.

- *Presentation:* patients with HHNS typically present with polyuria, polydipsia, and a degree of neurological dysfunction ranging from mild changes to coma. The symptoms typically develop over days, as initially patients are able to replenish fluids to counteract their osmotic diuresis. Once they are no longer able to effectively replenish fluids, symptoms worsen rapidly. Many patients have inciting factors, including infections (most commonly pneumonia or urinary tract infections) or noncompliance with prescribed diabetic medications. Other causes include medications, such as beta-blockers, diuretics, antihistamines, steroids, and antibiotics (gatifloxacin). Substance abuse (alcohol), underlying Cushing's syndrome, or pancreatitis may also precipitate HHNS. Patients typically have signs of hypovolemia, including poor skin turgor, dry mucous membranes, orthostatic hypotension, tachycardia, sunken eyes, and altered mental status. As serum osmolarity rises, altered mental status worsens. Coma is more common at values beyond 350 mOsm. As hyperglycemia worsens and hypovolemia continues, acute renal failure, pseudo-hyponatremia, and hyperkalemia can develop.

- *Treatment:* initial treatment of the patient with HHNS is aggressive fluid resuscitation with normal saline. Insulin therapy is commonly initiated with 10 units IV, and then IV infusion of 0.1 units/kg. Many patients will have rapid correction of hyperglycemia with fluids and, since rebound hypoglycemia can occur with insulin administration, frequent blood sugar measurements should be taken. Dangers of rapid overcorrection of hyperglycemia include cerebral edema or clinically significant hypoglycemia. Undercorrection of severe hypovolemia can result in myocardial and bowel ischemia. Close monitoring of electrolyte abnormalities is warranted to prevent arrhythmias or worsening of mental status. These patients often require electrolyte replacement. Patients with HHNS typically have 9 liters fluid total body deficit, so early therapy with fluid resuscitation is essential.

- *Definitive therapy:* therapy includes managing any precipitants, such as infections or medications. In addition, therapy typically includes eventual discharge from the hospital with oral hypoglycemic agents or insulin therapy. Long-term management of diabetes and its potential complications is also necessary.

Clinical course

This patient's diagnosis hinges on careful attention to his recent medical history, physical findings, and laboratory values.

Historical clues	Physical findings	Ancillary studies
• Recent URI and antibiotics	• Orthostatic hypotension	• Hyperglycemia without urinary ketones
• Polyuria	• Dry mucous membranes	• Elevated serum osmolarity
• Polydipsia	• Poor skin turgor	• Renal failure
• Altered mental status	• Lethargy	• Pseudohyponatremia
• Sub-acute symptom development		• Normal range ABG pH of 7.36
		• No anion gap

This patient was recognized to have HHNS based on his presentation and symptoms in the days prior to admission. Therefore, after IV placement, aggressive fluid resuscitation was begun in the ED, with 4 liters of normal saline as a bolus. The patient was placed on a cardiac monitor. The patient's labs revealed the typical findings of HHNS, including a glucose of greater than 600 mg/dL and a serum osmolarity of greater than 320 mOsm. The patient's pH was greater than 7.3 and he had little to no urine ketones, which ruled out diabetic ketoacidosis (DKA) as a diagnosis. He had acute renal failure, which is also common in these patients.

The patient's gatifloxacin was stopped on admission to the hospital. His orthostatic hypotension improved with fluid resuscitation, as did his renal function. Over the next several days, he returned to normal serum glucose values, without further medications or insulin. The patient made a full and uneventful recovery, and was followed for future development of insulin resistance and diabetes by his primary care physician. At most recent follow-up, his blood sugars remain normal, and his antibiotic appears to have been the culprit.

Further reading

Blommel AL. Severe hyperglycemia during renally adjusted gatifloxacin therapy. *Ann Pharmacol* 2005;**39**:1349–52.

Happe MR, et al. Gatifloxacin induced hyperglycemia. *Ann Intern Med* 2004;**141**(12):968–9.

Matz R. Management of hyperosmolar hyperglycemia syndrome. *Am Fam Physician* 1999;**60**:1468–76.

Stoner GD. Hyperosmolar hyperglycemic State. *Am Fam Physician*, 2005;**71**:1723–30.

Parke-Wyllie LY, et al. Outpatient gatifloxacin therapy and dysglycemia in older adults. *N Engl J Med* 2006;**354**:1352–61.

Orlander JD. Gatifloxacin-induced hyperglycemia. *Infect Dis Clin Pract* 2004;**12**;230–2.

Yip TJ, Lee AJ. Gatifloxacin-induced hyperglycemia: a case report and summary of the current literature. *Clin Ther* 2006;**28**;1857–66.

Haerian H, et al. Gatifloxacin produces both hypoglycemia and hyperglycemia: a retrospective study. *Am J Med Sci* 2008;**335**(2):95–8.

Case #3

History

A male who appears to be in his thirties is brought in by ambulance after being found unconscious in a hotel room. It was unknown how long he had been down. There were no apparent signs of foul play or trauma, no empty pill bottles, no drug paraphernalia, and no suicide note. The room was littered with trash, emesis, and feces. Naloxone 2 mg IV yielded no response. A nasal trumpet and non-rebreather mask with 100% oxygen at 10 L/min were placed and he was transported to the emergency department.

Past medical and social history

Upon contact with family it was learned that he had a history of ethanol and tobacco abuse, with no other known medical problems. He is an armed-forces veteran and currently works as an automobile mechanic. He had recently been depressed after the suicide of his girlfriend 2 months ago.

Medications

None.

Allergies

None known.

Physical exam and ancillary studies

- *Vital signs:* the patient's vital signs reveal a temperature of 37.2°C, a heart rate of 175 bpm, a respiratory rate of 32, a blood pressure of 192/90 mmHg, and an oxygen saturation of 96% on 100% oxygen by non-rebreather.
- *General:* the patient is obtunded and unresponsive.
- *Head and neck:* there is no evidence of trauma. His pupils are 2 mm in diameter and sluggishly responsive, and he has no gag reflex.
- *Cardiovascular:* his heart is tachycardic and regular, with no rubs or murmurs.
- *Lungs:* the patient is tachypneic, with scattered rhonchi.
- *Abdomen:* his abdomen is soft and non-tender.
- *Extremities and skin:* the patient's skin is flushed and diaphoretic, with no outward signs of trauma.
- *Neurological:* his Glasgow coma scale level is 3.
- *Pertinent labs:* chemistries: Na 144, K 7.8, Cl 108, bicarbonate 10, BUN 15, Cr 2.2, glucose 148. Arterial blood gas: pH 6.90, CO_2 17, HCO_3 3. Serum osmolality: 337 mOsm/kg. CBC: WBC 38.4, hematocrit 55.4%, platelet count 348 000. Serum ethanol, salicylate, and

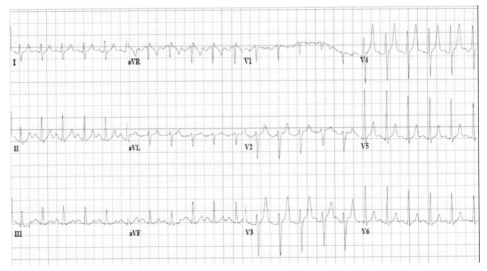

Figure 10.2. EKG showing sinus tachycardia with peaked T waves in the precordial leads, which is a common finding with hyperkalemia.

acetaminophen levels: negative. Urine cocaine, benzodiazepine, amphetamine, tricyclics: negative. Urine: no calcium oxalate crystals, no fluorescence under Woods lamp. CSF: unremarkable. Special alcohols panel: ethylene glycol 16 mg/dL.
- *EKG:* see Figure 10.2.
- *Radiographs:* the patient's chest X-ray was unremarkable. His head CT was negative.

Questions for thought

- What are the appropriate initial actions to take to stabilize this patient?
- Once stable, what other diagnostic tools can you use to make a diagnosis?
- How does one urgently treat this condition in the emergency department?
- What is definitive treatment of this condition?

Diagnosis
Ethylene glycol poisoning.

Discussion
- *Epidemiology:* ethylene glycol causes dozens of deaths per year. The most common sources of ethylene glycol are automotive antifreeze, engine coolants, and hydraulic-brake fluids. Most ingestions are accidental. Non-accidental ingestions are generally suicidal, homicidal, or attempts at self-harm; or attempts to substitute for ethanol. Pets are common unwitting victims, due to the substance's innate sweet taste.

- *Pathophysiology:* ethylene glycol itself is relatively harmless; its metabolites kill. It is metabolized by alcohol dehydrogenase to glycolic, glyoxylic, and oxalic acid. Glycolic acid contributes most to metabolic acidosis. Metabolic acidosis causes encephalopathy and cardiotoxicity. Oxalic acid chelates serum calcium. The resulting calcium oxalate crystals precipitate in renal tubules causing acute tubular necrosis and reversible renal failure. Glycolic acid itself is also toxic to the renal tubules. Ethylene glycol is absorbed rapidly after ingestion and peak serum levels occur in 1–4 hours. Serum half-life is between 3 and 9 hours. Metabolism is slowed by co-ingestion of ethanol. The lethal dose is stated to be 1 g/kg, although deaths have occurred with lower doses.
- *Presentation:* the common presentation of ethylene glycol poisoning is a person who appears intoxicated without an odor of ethanol. Three clinical stages of ethylene glycol poisoning have been described. The first is neurological, which occurs 30 minutes to 12 hours post-ingestion. This is when metabolites are at maximal serum concentration. Signs are similar to ethanol intoxication, such as slurred speech and ataxia. The patient may even be comatose. The second stage is cardiopulmonary, and occurs 12–24 hours hours post-ingestion. As the parent compound is metabolized, the patient develops metabolic acidosis with cardiopulmonary symptoms of tachypnea, tachycardia, and hypertension. Cardiopulmonary failure can occur during this time. The third clinical stage is renal, and occurs 24–72 hours post-ingestion. As calcium oxalate crystals precipitate in renal tubules, and toxic metabolites permeate the tubular tissues, acute tubular necrosis and renal failure ensue. Hypocalcemia due to calcium consumption secondary to crystal formation can result in seizures or cranial nerve palsy. In some patients, chronic cranial and sensorimotor polyneuropathies have been reported.
- *Treatment:* as always in the emergency department, treatment begins with securing airway, breathing, and circulation. Since the metabolites of ethylene glycol cause its toxicity, treatment is aimed at inhibition of alcohol dehydrogenase to prevent metabolite formation. This can be accomplished by using ethanol, either IV or by mouth, with a goal serum level of 100 mg/dL. Fomepizole is also useful for this purpose. The advantage of fomepizole is that it does not cause the central nervous system depression that ethanol can, but it is very expensive. In many patients, it is necessary to treat acidosis, as well. In less severe cases, sodium bicarbonate can be used, but with severe acidosis, renal failure, or central nervous system depression, hemodialysis is the treatment of choice. This also removes the toxic metabolites. Finally, pyridoxine and thiamine may aid in elimination of toxic metabolites, and, although there is no clear benefit, many advocate their use. Finally, many patients develop concurrent problems such as hyperkalemia that require treatment.

Clinical course

The keys to this patient's care were rapid attention to "ABCs," systematic approach to investigation of his altered mental status, and rapid recognition and treatment of his condition based on clinical patterns and lab data.

This patient was suspected to have overdosed because of the above historical clues. He appeared obtunded, but had no odor of ethanol. His labs pointed to an anion gap of 26 ($Na^+ - (Cl^- + HCO_3^-)$), which is very elevated, and is a common finding in ethylene glycol poisoning. He also had an elevated osmolar gap (($2 \times Na+$) + (BUN/2.8) + (glucose/18)).

As he became acidotic, he had a drop in serum pH to 6.9. These findings led the provider to suspect a toxic alcohol poisoning.

Historical clues	Physical findings	Ancillary studies
• History of recent depression and stressors	• Coma	• Metabolic acidosis, osmolal gap, elevated creatinine, hyperkalemia
• Potential access to toxic substance through work as mechanic	• Tachycardia	• Serum ethylene glycol
• No response to naloxone	• Hypertension	• Negative other findings
	• Tachypnea	
	• No odor of ethanol	

The patient also had elevated BUN and creatinine, probably secondary to tubule destruction from calcium oxalate crystals. Some patients will have calcium oxalate crystals on urine microscopy, but this finding is neither sensitive nor specific. Urine fluorescence under Woods lamp is helpful if it is present, since it occurs due to sodium fluorescein present in antifreeze, but this test is also not very sensitive. This patient had neither of these findings. When evaluating this patient, the medical provider tested for ethanol, methanol, and isopropanol in addition to ethylene glycol, since patients may have co-ingestants and because it can be difficult to tell these substances apart based solely on clinical presentation. The patient's toxicology showed ethylene glycol poisoning.

This patient was intubated for airway protection upon arrival. He received rapid IV fluid resuscitation with 0.9% normal saline. He was intiated on fomepizole 1.2 g IV, followed by 800 mg every 4 hours. Due to the degree of his metabolic acidosis, acute renal failure, and other evidence of end-organ damage (coma), he underwent hemodialysis. For his hyperkalemia, he was given intravenous calcium gluconate, sodium bicarbonate, insulin, and glucose. He was admitted to the medical intensive care unit, where he underwent hemodialysis until his levels of ethylene glycol were zero. He ultimately regained a normal level of consciousness and was transferred to the psychiatric inpatient unit, still undergoing hemodialysis three times per week.

Further reading

Barceloux DG, Krenzelok EP, Olson K, Watson W. American Academy of Clinical Toxicology practice guidelines on the treatment of ethylene glycol poisoning. Ad hoc committee. *J Toxicol Clin Toxicol* 1999;**37**:537.

Sivilotti MLA, Winchester JF. Methanol and ethylene glycol intoxication. *UpToDate 2007*. Retrieved November 25, 2007.

Wiener SW. Chapter 103. Toxic alcohols. In *Goldfrank's Toxicologic Emergencies*, 8th edition. New York: McGraw-Hill, 2006.

Case #4

History

A 21-year-old male active-duty soldier is brought into the emergency department by ambulance. He and one of his barracks-mates had been noted to be "acting funny" that evening, making strange noises and remarking that everyone around them "looked like midgets." When confronted by the military police, it was discovered that the two had been drinking an over-the-counter cough and cold medication in an attempt to get drunk. The ingestion occurred approximately 6 hours ago. The patient is unable to give further history and does not answer questions.

Past medical history

According to the soldier's command he is in good health, with no significant past medical or social history which is clinically relevant.

Medications

The patient takes no medications.

Allergies

The patient has no known drug allergies.

Physical exam and ancillary studies

- *Vital Signs:* his temperature is 37.8°C, his heart rate is 160 bpm, his respiratory rate is 22, his blood pressure is 176/100 mmHG, and his room air oxygen saturation is 98%.
- *General:* the patient is awake and alert but non-responsive to direct questioning. He is making noises but not speaking in sentences. He is agitated, but not combative.
- *HEENT:* the patient has no signs of trauma. His pupils are 8 mm and non-reactive.
- *Cardiovascular:* the patient's heart is tachycardic and regular. His pulses are intact.
- *Lungs:* his lungs are clear to auscultation bilaterally.
- *Abdomen:* the patient has absent bowel sounds. His agitation increases with palpation of his lower abdomen.
- *Extremities and skin:* the patient's skin is red, flushed, dry.
- *Neurological:* He is rocking back and forth on the stretcher. He responds appropriately to pain, but does not follow commands or answer questions appropriately. His motor exam is symmetric. His reflexes are intact and normal.
- *Pertinent labs:* the patient's labs are all normal or negative, including glucose, toxicology screens, chemistries, and serum creatinine kinase, with the exception of an acetaminophen level of 20 μg/mL.
- *EKG:* the EKG demonstrates sinus tachycardia with normal intervals and no other abnormalities.

Questions for thought

- What is the initial approach to the patient with delirium?
- To what condition does this constellation of symptoms point?
- How would one treat this condition in the emergency department?
- Does this patient require admission?

Diagnosis

Anticholinergic toxicity.

Discussion

- *Epidemiology:* anticholinergic toxicity is a common condition resulting from ingestion of a broad array of regularly available substances. This can occur intentionally, either as a suicide attempt or in an effort to "catch a buzz," or it can be accidental. There are over 600 prescription and over-the-counter medications with anticholinergic properties, including antihistamines (e.g. diphenhydramine), cough suppressants, tricyclic antidepressants (TCAs), anti-nausea/motion-sickness preparations (e.g. scopalomine), and anti-diarrheals. Several plants also have these properties, including Jimson weed and belladonna.
- *Pathophysiology:* anticholinergic toxicity occurs after ingestion of anticholinergic drugs, of which atropine is the prototypical agent. These substances compete with the neurotransmitter acetylcholine at post-synaptic muscarinic receptors, which are present in the central nervous system and at post-synaptic peripheral nerve junctions. They have no effect on nicotinic acetylcholine receptors, and this is indeed a good thing, as nicotinic receptors control skeletal muscles, including the diaphragm, and can compromise breathing and volitional movement.
- *Presentation:* the presentation of anticholinergic toxicity fits a classic pattern of signs and symptoms, known as a toxidrome. In this case the toxidromal symptoms have a well known and oft-repeated mnemonic associated with them: "hot as a hare, dry as a bone, red as a beet, blind as a bat, full as a flask and mad as a hatter." "Hot as a hare" refers to hyperthermia as a result of central temperature control dysregulation, "dry as a bone" describes the lack of sweat (anhidrosis) which compounds this, while "red as beet" refers to the cutaneous vasodilatation which results as a means to dissipate this excess heat. "Blind as a bat" refers to the dysfunction of mydriasis and accommodation, resulting in large, non-reactive pupils and blurred vision. "Full as a flask" refers to the lack of urination secondary to inability to relax the detrusor and urinary sphincters. "Mad as a hatter" describes the agitation, delirium, hallucinations and sometimes seizures which result with CNS muscarinic blockade. The report that people "look like midgets" is a common complaint, and is known a Lilliputianism. Other symptoms include tachycardia and decreased bowel sounds secondary to a paralytic ileus of the GI tract. The psychomotor agitation can, in severe cases, lead to widespread muscle breakdown and ultimately rhabdomyolysis.

- *Treatment:* in treating the patient with anticholinergic toxicity, supportive care is generally sufficient. If the ingestion is within about an hour of presentation, GI decontamination with activated charcoal (dosage 1 g/kg to a maximum dose of 50 g) should be undertaken. Whole bowel lavage is not used in this situation. If seizures occur they can be treated with benzodiazepines. Physostigmine, an acetylcholinesterase inhibitor, may be used judiciously in patients with severe altered mental status and profound psychomotor agitation. This reverses anticholinergic toxicity, but has some risk of cholinergic toxicity of its own, and should only be used in severe cases. Note that physostigmine is contraindicated in known or suspected TCA overdose, as this can cause the patient to become bradycardic, and eventually asystolic. If hyperthermia is severe, evaporative cooling techniques can be used. If the patient cannot urinate, you should place a Foley catheter to drain the bladder. As in all overdose patients, assessment of the patient's level of suicidality and homicidality is a necessary part of evaluation, including holding the patient for a formal psychiatric consultation if needed.

Clinical course

The keys to this patient's diagnosis and eventual treatment were careful attention to his history and physical exam, with ancillary laboratory studies to rule out other toxicologic pathology.

Historical clues	Physical findings	Ancillary studies
• History of overdose	• Toxidromal behavior	• EKG with sinus tachycardia
• Use of cold medication with anticholinergic properties	• Tachycardia	• Serum toxicology with positive acetaminophen level
	• Hyperthermia	• EKG with sinus tachycardia
	• Altered mental status	
	• Cutaneous vasodilatation	
	• Anhydrosis	
	• Pupillary dilation	
	• Urinary retention	

This patient was suspected of having anticholinergic poisoning based on his history of drinking cough syrup. When the diagnosis of anticholinergic poisoning is considered, there are few laboratory or other tests which are helpful. However, the toxidromal symptoms present in this patient are pathognomonic of antiocholinergic toxicity. Because of the very high frequency of co-ingestions, acetaminophen and aspirin levels were also checked. In this patient, the acetaminophen level came back positive, probably because of the presence of that substance in most cold medications.

In an anticholinergic patient, an EKG also may supply supporting diagnostic information. In this patient, sinus tachycardia was present, but anticholinergic toxicity can also cause QRS morphology changes, dysrhythmias, and interval prolongation.

This patient was protecting his own airway when he arrived in the emergency department. As the ingestion had occurred some hours previously, and he was already showing signs of anticholinergic toxicity, he was not given activated charcoal. There was a debate about whether to administer physostigmine or not, as this patient met some but not all criteria for this antidote. He was eventually treated with 1.6 mg of physostigmine, which produced an immediate relief of his delirium. His agitation further decreased when his bladder was drained via Foley catheter. The patient's acetaminophen levels remained below threshold at 4 hours, without creatine kinase or creatinine elevation. He was not found to be suicidal, and was admitted to the telemetry floor for overnight cardiac monitoring and serial acetaminophen levels. He was discharged into the care of the military police, and his ultimate disposition was a return to baseline health, to face the disciplinary fallout of his actions.

Further reading

Wax P. Anticholinergic toxicity. In *Tintanelli's Emergency Medicine*, 6th edition. New York: McGraw-Hill, 2004.

Su M, Goldman M. Anticholinergic poisoning. *UpToDate*, updated June 11th, 2007. Retrieved December 15, 2007, from www.uptodate.com.

Tomassoni A, Weisman R. Antihistamines and decongestants. In *Goldfrank's Toxicologic Emergencies*, 8th edition. New York: McGraw-Hill, 2006.

Case #5

History

A 79-year-old man is brought to the emergency department (ED) by ambulance after being found in his automobile in a ditch on the side of the road. Emergency medical service (EMS) personnel state the patient was found wearing his seatbelt in the driver side of the vehicle, which had only minimal front end damage. The patient was noted to be confused, oriented to person only. EMS personnel state the patient was stable in transit and that he became increasingly tachycardic a few minutes prior to arrival at the hospital. Upon arrival, the patient is awake and appears to be in no respiratory distress. He follows commands but continues to show signs of disorientation. He remembers being found in his vehicle by EMS but is unable to recall his intended destination. His only complaint is that he feels "a little tired." Given his confusion, a thorough and accurate history is unattainable but the patient specifically denies headache, shortness of breath, chest pain, abdominal pain, or recent nausea, vomiting, or diarrhea. Within a few minutes of his arrival, the patient's son is reached via telephone and reports that his father has no baseline disorientation and that he was completely lucid when he visited him for dinner yesterday evening. The son is unable to elaborate on his father's medical history any further.

Past medical history

The patient is unable to give his past medical history.

Medications

The patient had some prescription medications with him in the car and these include atorvastatin, amlodipine, metoprolol, and tamsulosin HCl.

Social history

The patient reports smoking one pack of cigarettes daily for "years and years."

Allergies

He has no known allergies.

Physical exam and ancillary studies

- *Vital signs:* the patient's temperature is 36.2°C, his heart rate is 156 bpm, his blood pressure is 137/76 mmHg, his respiratory rate is 20, and his room air saturation is 96%.
- *General:* the patient is a well-nourished, well-dressed, elderly white male who is awake and comfortable. He appears fatigued.

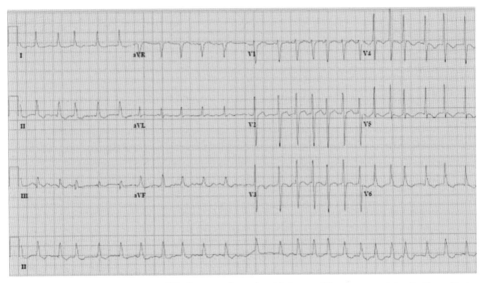

Figure 10.3. Initial EKG showing atrial fibrillation and questionably inverted T waves anterolaterally. The patient was subsequently given metoprolol 5 mg IV ×1 and he converted to sinus rhythm (see Figure 10.4 below).

- *Head and neck:* there are no signs of trauma. Pupils are equally round and reactive to light, cranial nerves intact. The patient's mucous membranes are dry. His neck is supple with a midline trachea. He has no carotid bruits.
- *Cardiovascular:* his heart has a tachycardic rate and irregular rhythm without murmurs, rubs, or gallops. Peripheral pulses are normal in all four extremities.
- *Lungs:* there is normal chest excursion. Lungs are clear to auscultation bilaterally without wheezes, rales, or rhonchi.
- *Abdomen:* his abdomen is non-tender, with no masses or abnormalities.
- *Extremities and skin:* his extremities are warm and well perfused. There is no edema, clubbing, or calf tenderness, nor is there skin breakdown.
- *Neurologic:* the patient is alert and oriented to person only. He answers simple questions pertaining to his health with "yes" and "no" answers and follows commands appropriately. His memory is impaired, with greater short-term than long-term memory deficit. His sensation is normal globally. His strength is 5/5 in all four extremities.
- *EKG:* see Figure 10.3.
- *Pertinent labs:* the patient's comprehensive blood count is within normal limits. His electrolytes, liver and thyroid function tests and urinalysis are unremarkable. The patient's cardiac enzymes are remarkable for a troponin of 1.8 ng/mL.
- *Radiographs:* the patient's chest X-ray is read as having no acute disease.

Questions for thought

- What are the appropriate initial actions to take to stabilize this patient?
- What are the emergency causes of altered mental status in the elderly?

- What is the appropriate workup in an elderly patient with altered mental status in the emergency department?
- What are the common presenting signs and symptoms of ischemic heart disease in the elderly?

Diagnoses

Altered mental status secondary to cardiac arrhythmia and non-ST-elevation myocardial infarction.

Discussion

- *Epidemiology:* acute coronary syndrome (ACS) is a fairly common cause of altered mental status among ED patients, particularly the elderly. The incidence of altered mental status in the emergency department is unclear, but recent literature has suggested that approximately 26% of patients 70 years of age and over had mental status impairment. The percentage of elderly patients presenting to the ED with altered mental status who turn out to have a significant arrhythmia or ACS is unknown.
- *Pathophysiology:* altered mental status induced by pathology of the cardiovascular system is usually a result of decreased brain perfusion by a diseased cardiovascular system. In atrial fibrillation, the underlying arrhythmia in this patient, the disorganized atrial contractions lead to a decrease in the left ventricular end diastolic volume. Similarly, large infarcts can result in a significant and even life-threatening reduction in cardiac contractility, also decreasing cardiac output. In turn, cerebral perfusion becomes compromised and altered mental status may result.
- *Presentation:* this patient's presentation of arrhythmia-induced altered mental status is actually quite common. Causes of atrial fibrillation include idiopathic hypertension, valvular disease, alcohol use ("holiday heart"), cardiac ischemia, pulmonary embolus, sick sinus syndrome, thyrotoxicosis, and chronic obstructive pulmonary disease. While this patient's atrial fibrillation may have been from any cause, it is most probably secondary to his cardiac ischemia. It is common for elderly patients to have atypical symptoms during arrhythmias or during a myocardial infarction. While chest pain has historically been thought of as the primary "typical" symptom, multiple studies have shown that between 33 and 52% of patients who are found to have ACS do not present with typical chest pain. The elderly frequently present with complaints of dyspnea, nausea, diaphoresis, weakness, or pain in the neck or limbs.
- *Treatment:* initial treatment of atrial fibrillation depends on the stability of the patient and the duration of the arrhythmia. If the patient is unstable, treatment should be with 100–200 J using synchronized cardioversion regardless of the duration. Stable patients with atrial fibrillation longer than 48 hours should be anticoagulated with heparin and will need direct visualization of the heart using a transesophageal echocardiogram to identify whether an atrial thrombus is present prior to cardioversion. Atrial fibrillation that is less than 48 hours old can be safely cardioverted either electrically or chemically (amiodarone, procainamide, or propafenone), though it is typical for the emergency physician to first control the heart rate and consult with a cardiologist to determine whether cardioversion in the ED is warranted. Rate control can be accomplished using diltiazem. Metoprolol

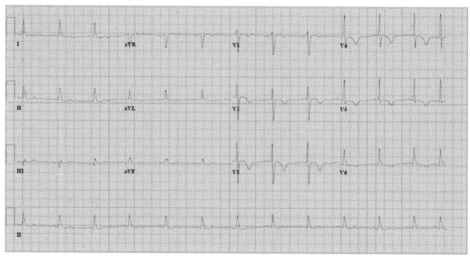

Figure 10.4. Repeat EKG performed after the patient had converted to a normal sinus rhythm revealed cardiac ischemia.

and less often digoxin can also be used. As in the patient described in this case, it is fairly common for people with new-onset atrial fibrillation to convert to a normal sinus rhythm spontaneously or following rate control in the first 24 hours.

While the treatment of ACS in the elderly is very similar to that in younger adults, it should be tailored individually based on many factors. In an elderly patient with altered mental status, the living will or healthcare proxy should be consulted to ascertain the patient's wishes regarding their desired management. Aggressive management in the elderly is sometimes not performed due to significant comorbidities where the risks may outweigh the benefits.

Clinical course

The keys to this patient's diagnosis are a thorough physical examination and comprehensive ancillary testing given the extensive differential of an elderly patient with altered mental status.

Historical clues	Physical findings	Ancillary studies
• Altered mental status	• Disorientation	• Head CT showing no acute pathology
• Patient feels "tired"	• Fatigue	• EKG #1: atrial fibrillation at 140 bpm
• Prescription drugs including antihypertensives	• Irregular tachycardia	• Following rate control, EKG #2: T-wave inversions anterolaterally
		• Elevated cardiac enzymes

In the ED, an IV was started and the patient was immediately placed on oxygen. The physician recognized the patient's altered mental status as having a possible cardiovascular origin and quickly obtained an EKG. Rapid atrial fibrillation was noted and the patient's heart rate was successfully lowered using just one dose of metoprolol 5 mg IV.

Repeat EKG performed after the patient had converted to a normal sinus rhythm revealed cardiac ischemia (Figure 10.4). The patient had ST depressions in his lateral leads. Therefore, the physician administered aspirin and heparin to the patient in the emergency department. He was admitted to the cardiology service, where he remained in normal sinus rhythm and his baseline mental status returned. He was managed medically for the non-ST-elevation myocardial infarction and was discharged home 3 days later.

Further reading

Tintinalli J, Kelen G, Stapczynski S. *Emergency Medicine: a Comprehensive Study Guide*. 6th edition. New York: McGraw-Hill, 2004.

Hustey FM, Meldon SW. The prevalence and documentation of impaired mental status in elderly emergency department patients. *Ann Emerg Med* 2002;**39**:248.

Canto JG, et al. Atypical presentations among medicare beneficiaries with unstable angina pectoris. *Am J Cardiology* 2002;**90**:248–53.

Canto JG, et al. Prevalence, clinical characteristics, and mortality among patients with myocardial infarction presenting without chest pain. *JAMA* 2000;**283**:3223–9.

Gupta M, Tabas JA, Kohn MA. Presenting complaint among patients with myocardial infarction who present to an urban, public hospital emergency department. *Ann Emerg Med* 2002;**40**:180–6.

Case #6

History

A 70-year-old right-handed man presents to the ED after being found on the floor by his wife. He was confused and had been incontinent of urine. His wife reports that he was vomiting, as well. He was sleepy when she found him, but responded to her voice. Initially he was not oriented to time or place, but was able to answer some simple yes-or-no questions. He was unable to get up off the ground. He now is agitated and combative, and unable to answer any questions. He is not moving his left arm as briskly as his right arm. Because he is not able to protect his airway, he is being intubated.

Past medical history

He has a history of hypertension. He quit smoking 30 years ago. The patient has a 9 month history of short-term memory loss according to his family, which has progressed to the point that he can't remember daily activities.

Medications

The patient's only medication is lisinopril.

Allergies

The patient has no known drug allergies.

Physical exam and ancillary studies

- *Vital signs:* the patient's temperature is 37.5°C, his heart rate is 82 bpm, he has a blood pressure of 123/83, a respiratory rate of 24, and his oxygen saturation is 100% on 40% oxygen through the ventilator.
- *General:* the patient is intubated, not responsive to verbal commands, and spontaneously moving his right arm and both legs.
- *Head and neck:* there is a minor bruise on the his forehead. His neck is supple.
- *Cardiovascular:* the patient's heart has a regular rate and rhythm, with no murmurs, rubs, or gallops.
- *Lungs:* his lungs have decreased air movement throughout, and bibasilar rales.
- *Abdomen:* his abdomen is non-distended, with no appreciable tenderness.
- *Extremities and skin:* the patient has trace bilateral lower extremity edema, with no clubbing or cyanosis.
- *Neurologic:*
  - Speech: the patient had no spontaneous speech prior to intubation.
  - Cranial nerves: the patient's pupils are 3 mm bilaterally and sluggishly reactive. He appears to be looking to the right. His corneal reflexes are intact bilaterally.

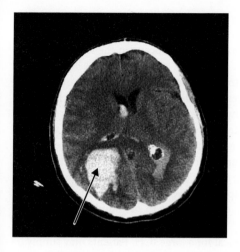

Figure 10.5. Head CT showing large intracranial hemorrhage with extension into the ventricles and mild hydrocephalus.

- Strength: the patient withdraws both legs and his right arm to noxious stimuli. On noxious stimulation of his left hand, the patient's left arm extends and turns inward.
- Sensation: the patient grimaces to noxious stimuli in all his extremities except his left upper extremity.
- Reflexes: the patient's deep tendon reflexes are 2+ in his right arm and leg, 3+ in his left arm and leg, and both his toes are upgoing on Babinski testing.

- *Pertinent labs:* the patient has a normal coagulation profile, normal complete blood count, and normal chemistries.
- *Radiographs:* see Figure 10.5.

Questions for thought

- What are the appropriate initial actions to take to stabilize this patient?
- How would you urgently treat deterioration in this patient's condition?
- What are other diagnostic studies you can use to help determine the underlying reason for this patient's problem?
- What clues are there in the history that help lead to a diagnosis?
- What is the prognosis of a patient with this condition?

Diagnosis

Intracranial lobar hemorrhage secondary to amyloid angiopathy.

Discussion

- *Epidemiology:* approximately 10% of strokes are caused by intracranial hemorrhage (ICH). Populations with higher incidence of hypertension such as African-Americans have a higher incidence of ICH, as do people of Chinese, Japanese, and Thai ancestry. ICH accounts for a higher percentage of strokes in patients younger than age 40 and those of advanced age, as in this case.

- *Pathophysiology:* ICH are formed from an extravasation of blood into the parenchymal tissue with distortion of the surrounding tissue. The hematoma will expand until it clots. The hemorrhages of cerebral amyloid angiopathy tend to occur in the lobar regions as opposed to hypertensive hemorrhages which occur most commonly in the basal ganglia, thalamus, pons, and cerebellum. Patients with amyloid angiopathy have deposits of beta-amyloid in the walls of small intracranial vessels. This leads to a fragility of the vessels and a predisposition to hemorrhage. This amyloid deposition is recognized as one of the hallmark features of Alzheimer's disease. Extension of the hemorrhage into the ventricular system, or intraventricular hemorrhage, is an important aspect to recognize because this can lead to obstruction of the ventricular system resulting in hydrocephalus. Blood in the brain parenchyma is also extremely irritating to the surrounding tissue, and will cause edema. If there is obstructive hydrocephalus or severe edema, there may be pressure on other parts of the brain and this can cause damage to surrounding brain tissues and ultimately herniation.
- *Presentation:* the patient's presentation is typical for a large ICH. Patients may simply be confused or unresponsive, but will probably have focal neurologic deficits as well if a careful exam is done. Patients may also present with convulsive or non-convulsive seizures, since the blood may be irritating the cerebral cortex. Blood in the third and fourth ventricles, as in this patient, may also cause obstructive hydrocephalus which may also cause obtundation and papilledema. If the hemorrhage involved the frontal region, the patient's eyes may be deviated towards the side of the hemorrhage.
- *Treatment:* the initial treatment is supportive. As always, the ABCs should be considered. In addition, the patient's blood pressure should be controlled using IV medications if needed. If there is a suspicion of seizure activity, the patient should receive IV antiepileptics, such as phenytoin or benzodiazepines. If the patient is on anticoagulation, it is important to reverse this urgently with vitamin K and fresh frozen plasma (FFP). Neurosurgery should be involved early to evaluate the efficacy of evacuating the hematoma. This may be indicated if there is clinical deterioration refractory to medical treatment or if the hematoma is superficial. If there is blood in the ventricular system, as in this patient, it may be necessary to perform a venticulostomy and monitor intracranial pressures in order to prevent hydrocephalus. If there is a suspicion of impending herniation, it may be necessary to acutely lower intracranial pressure with mannitol 1 g/kg IV, 3% saline IV, or possibly go to the OR urgently.
- *Definitive therapy:* ultimately, there is no definitive therapy for ICH except for supportive care, and measures to prevent edema and hydrocephalus. If there is an underlying cause for the hemorrhage such as hypertension or the use of anticoagulants, it is important to reverse these processes. If the patient's condition is refractory to medical treatment and if the hemorrhage is superficial, surgery may be indicated. Unfortunately, the prognosis is poor for a hemorrhage of this size. Approximately 30–35% of patients with medium to large-sized hematomas will die in 1–30 days. In those who survive, the chance of regaining independent function is poor.

Clinical course

The keys to this patient's diagnosis are careful attention to his history, physical exam, and ancillary studies.

Historical clues	Physical findings	Ancillary studies
• Found on the floor with urinary incontinence	• Spontaneously moving right side only	• Head CT with ICH with extension into the lateral ventricles and mild hydrocephalus
• History of dementia	• Right gaze deviation	
• Patient is not only confused, but weak as well	• Left arm posturing with noxious stimuli	
	• No sensation in left arm with noxious stimuli	

The patient was suspected of having an intracranial process based on his severely depressed mental status and focal neurologic exam. A CT was done, which is the test of choice for the diagnosis of ICH. If available, a CT angiogram can be done as well, which could rule out an underlying cause such as an arteriovenous malformation or aneurysm rupture. If an underlying anatomic cause is still suspected, MRI with gadolinium may be performed, but may have to be delayed for a few weeks because of the artifact from the intracranial blood. In this patient, this was not indicated.

The neurosurgery department was consulted and it was determined that surgical evacuation was not indicated. He was given mannitol IV and started on 3% saline to try and reduce his intracranial pressure. He was loaded with IV fosphenytoin for the possibility of a seizure. The patient was maintained on full ventilator support for the duration of his hospital stay; however, the family decided to withdraw support after a long discussion on the patient's prognosis. He passed away soon after.

Further reading

Caplan LR. *Caplan's Stroke: a Clinical Approach*. Boston: Butterworth Heinemann, 2000, pp. 383–413.

Ropper A, Brown R. *Adams and Victor's Principles of Neurology*. New York: McGraw-Hill, 2005, pp. **708**, 711–16.

Wijdicks, EFM. *The Clinical Practice of Critical Care Neurology*. New York: Oxford University Press, 2003, pp. 221–37.

Bradley WG, et al. *Neurology in Clinical Practice*. Philadelphia: Butterworth Heinemann, 2004, pp. 1251–67.

Rowland LP. *Merritt's Neurology*. Philadelphia: Lippincott, Williams and Wilkins, 2005, pp. 303–7.

Case #7

History

A 76-year-old female presents after intervention by police and a mobile psychiatric crisis unit. A neighbor had called the police because the patient was running up and down the halls yelling. Apparently she believes that Rachael Ray, Oprah, and the governor of New York are coming to visit her. She recalls that 2 months ago she read an article in the paper about some local children in the area who were not getting enough food because their parents were poor. She states she developed a successful program to feed the children, and Rachael Ray and Oprah are coming to give her an award for her efforts. She does admit to some depressive thoughts and decreased sleep. In addition, she has had no sleep in the last 3 days because she has been worried about making a speech at the upcoming award ceremony. She states that she has had decreased food intake because of her increased depression and anxiety for the last several days. She missed a scheduled cardiology appointment today and is out of her verapamil. She denies any recent falls or head trauma. She denies any suicidal or homicidal ideations. She denies any auditory or visual hallucinations. She is not in any pain at this time. Her review of symptoms is otherwise negative.

Past medical history

The patient has a history of diabetes, osteoporosis, sciatica, and atrial fibrillation. She has a recent history of shingles that resolved about a week ago, and for which she was using lidocaine patches.

Medications

The patient takes salmeterol, warfarin, esomeprazole, venlafaxine, aspirin, vitamins, verapamil, digoxin, atorvastatin, and pioglitazone.

Allergies

This patient has no known drug allergies.

Physical exam and ancillary studies

- *Vital signs:* the patient's temperature is 36.9°C, her heart rate is 98 bpm, her respiratory rate is 18, her blood pressure is 135/65 mmHg, and her room air oxygen saturation is 100%.
- *General:* she is awake and alert, and non-toxic in appearance.
- *Head and neck:* her head is normocephalic, with no evidence of trauma. Her lids and lashes are normal. Her pupils are equal, round, and reactive to light. She has moist oral mucosa.
- *Cardiovascular:* her heart is regular, with no murmurs, rubs, or gallops.

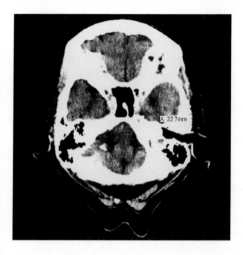

Figure 10.6. This head CT shows a left temporal mass which appears to be infiltrative, possibly a glioblastoma. There is some mass effect on the left occipital horn but no hydrocephalus.

- *Lungs:* her lungs are clear to auscultation bilaterally.
- *Abdomen:* her abdomen is soft, non-tender, and non-distended. She has normal bowel sounds.
- *Extremities and skin:* the patient has full range of motion in all four extremities. She has no petechiae or lesions. Her skin is warm and dry throughout. No lidocaine patches were found.
- *Neurologic:* the patient's GCS is 15. Her speech and strength are normal. Her gait was not assessed initially, but later determined to be unsteady per nursing.
- *Psychiatric:* she is alert with intact memory. She has normal insight with the exception of the fixed delusion about Oprah and Rachael Ray. She denies suicidal or homicidal ideation.
- *Pertinent labs:* the patient's complete blood count is notable for a white cell count of 13.8 and a hematocrit of 35%. Her chemistries are remarkable for a blood urea nitrogen of 30, a creatinine of 1.4, and a creatine kinase of 347. Her INR is 1.8. All of her other labs were normal.
- *EKG:* her EKG shows atrial fibrillation with a heart rate of 78 and no evidence of ischemia.
- *Radiographs:* the patient's chest X-ray showed no acute disease. A representative slice from her head CT is shown in Figure 10.6.

Questions for thought

- What is the differential diagnosis for altered mental status in the elderly?
- What is the difference between confusion, delirium, and dementia?
- What is the appropriate workup for a patient presenting like this?
- Does the patient need to be admitted?
- What is the definitive treatment of this condition?

Diagnosis

Altered mental status secondary to a brain mass.

Discussion

- *Epidemiology:* altered mental status is present in 10% of elderly ED patients, but only 20–30% of those cases are recognized in the ED. The 6 month mortality in patients with recognized altered mental status is 12%, compared to a mortality of 30% in the altered patients who are not recognized.
- *Pathophysiology:* the basis of altered mental status must be thoroughly investigated. Organic causation can be classified into four categories: infections or systemic disease, intracranial or neurologic processes, cardiovascular or metabolic causes, and medications or toxins. Infections and systemic diseases account for 30–40% of cases and include pneumonia, urinary tract infections, meningitis, and sepsis. Stroke, subdural hematoma, seizures, and dementia are the main neurologic and intracranial causes and account for 20–30% of cases. Cardiovascular and metabolic diseases, such as myocardial infarction, electrolyte imbalance, and endocrine disease, cause 20–30% of cases. The final 5–10% of patients have metabolic and toxic reasons for their altered mental status. Alcohol, narcotic, and anticholinergic use and withdrawal from other drugs are the most common culprits.

  It is important to recognize and treat reversible causes of altered mental status. A helpful acronym is: **D**rugs/delirium, **E**motional illness (depression), **M**etabolic/endocrine disorders (thyroid dysfunction), **E**ye/ear/environment (sensory impairment), **N**utritional (vitamin B deficits), **T**umors/trauma, **I**nfection (HIV, meningitis), **A**lcholism/anemia/atherosclerosis.
- *Presentation:* patients may present with confusion, delirium, or dementia. Confusion is often noted by someone else close to the patient and is seen as acting outside society's norm. The patient usually lacks insight into their abnormal behavior. Two percent of emergency department patients have confusion. Delirium is an acute condition with alteration in wake–sleep patterns, disorganized thinking, inattention, distractibility, and fluctuating confusion. Delirium is present in 10–15% of older patients at the time of hospital admission. Dementia is a chronic confusional state that has been slowly progressing over time. Patients often have difficulty carrying out activities of daily living due to their cognitive impairments. These conditions can also co-exist.
- *Treatment:* treatment is aimed at the underlying cause. Infectious etiologies such as urinary tract infections, pneumonia, meningitis, and sepsis will require antibiotics. Neurology or neurosurgery consultations may be needed if stroke, intracranial hemorrhage, seizure, or dementia is responsible for the altered mental status. Pharmaceutical intervention may assist in overdoses.
- *Definitive therapy:* definitive therapy depends on the cause of altered mental status. If no cause is found then psychiatric evaluation must be obtained. In the elderly, however, psychiatric illness is a diagnosis of exclusion, and should never be presumed to be present.

Clinical course

The key to diagnosis in this case is a thorough history from the patient and from neighbors, a careful physical exam, and appropriate use of ancillary studies to rule out other pathology.

Historical clues	Physical findings	Ancillary studies
• Acute change in mental status	• Unsteady gait	• Negative tox screen
	• No findings of infection or trauma	• Negative cardiac panel
		• CT scan with brain mass

Because it is uncommon for an elderly person to have an acute psychotic break without a precipitant, this patient had a very complete workup. Careful examination of medications including when the drugs were initiated may provide insight into drug reactions or unintentional overdoses. In this case, no pain patches were found on the patient. Physical examination in the acutely altered patient may point to a new neurologic deficit or source of infection. This patient had evidence of an unsteady gait, but no other evidence of systemic process. Finally, a complete investigation including EKG, CBC, electrolytes, CXR, and urinalysis revealed no other reason for altered mental status. A head CT was needed because the patient had been on Coumadin and there was a lack of other substantial findings to account for her altered mental status, so it was pertinent to rule out an intracranial hemorrhage. The CT then led to the discovery of her brain mass.

The patient was admitted to the medicine service for further management. She went on to have an MRI which showed an extra-axial mass, most likely a meningioma with accompanying edema in the left temporal lobe. She underwent steroid therapy for the edema, and is still considering surgical management.

Case #8

History

A 41-year-old man presents to the ED complaining of four or five episodes of transient confusion over the past 36 hours. He states that he has had word-finding difficulties, and is confused by simple numerical calculations. He says "I just don't feel like myself." These episodes last approximately 30–45 seconds and are associated with red and blue flashes of light that he sees mostly in his right eye. His most recent episode reportedly occurred 2 hours prior to presentation at his primary care provider's office, who instructed him to come to the ED. He denies a history of similar events prior to the past 2 days. He also denies any aggravating or alleviating factors. He denies any numbness, weakness, or tingling of the extremities, and he denies recent head trauma. He denies blurry vision. His review of systems is otherwise negative.

Past medical history

The patient reports that he was started on penicillin 6 days ago for strep throat and that he had taken two doses of valacyclovir 3 days ago for perioral "cold sores." Today, his physician discontinued the penicillin. The patient is otherwise healthy.

Medications

The patient takes no medications except as described above.

Allergies

The patient has no known drug allergies.

Physical exam

- *Vital signs:* the patient's temperature is 36.5°C, his heart rate is 94 bpm, his blood pressure is 126/95 mmHg, his respiratory rate is 16, and his room air oxygen saturation is 97%.
- *General:* the patient is awake and alert. He appears comfortable. He answers questions appropriately.
- *Head and neck:* his pupils are equally round and reactive to light, and his cranial nerves are intact. His visual acuity is 20/25 in each eye. The patient's mucous membranes are dry. His neck is supple with a midline trachea.
- *Cardiovascular:* the patient's heart has a regular rate and rhythm without murmurs, rubs, or gallops. His peripheral pulses are normal.
- *Lungs:* his lungs are clear to auscultation bilaterally without wheezes, rales, or rhonchi.
- *Extremities and skin:* his extremities are warm and well perfused. He has no edema, clubbing, or calf tenderness.

- *Neurologic:* the patient is initially alert and oriented. He answers questions without confusion and has good long- and short-term memory. His sensation is normal globally, and his strength is 5/5 in all four extremities. Near the end of the physical exam the patient suddenly begins having difficulty answering simple questions. When asked whether he is experiencing one of the "episodes" he begins to perseverate the word "no." He sniffs repeatedly and appears to be experiencing a peculiar smell lasting for approximately 30–45 seconds. He subsequently has a tonic-clonic seizure that lasts approximately 90 seconds.

Questions for thought

- What are the appropriate initial actions to take to stabilize this patient?
- How does one urgently treat this condition in the emergency department?
- Once stable, what other diagnostic tools can you use to establish an etiology for the seizure activity?
- What lab values would you expect to find immediately following the seizure?
- What is the appropriate workup in a patient with a first-time seizure?

Diagnosis

New-onset tonic-clonic seizure.

Discussion

- *Epidemiology:* approximately 100 000 new cases of seizure are diagnosed each year and an estimated 6–10% of individuals will have at least one seizure in their lifetimes. The incidence rates of seizures are highest for individuals under 20 years of age with a second increase in incidence for those over 60 years old.
- *Pathophysiology:* patients with seizures have abnormal electrical discharge of the neurons in the brain, resulting in neurological abnormalities. It is important to determine the etiology of a seizure as this can help to guide appropriate medical management. Primary seizures are those without a known cause. Secondary seizures are those that have an alternate identifiable cause, which includes but is not limited to intracranial mass or hemorrhage, toxins, metabolic abnormalities, or medication effects.
- *Presentation:* seizures are classified into two major groups, generalized and partial (focal). Generalized seizures involve a loss of consciousness and include tonic-clonic, absence (petit mal), atonic, and myoclonic seizures. Partial seizures range from no alteration in consciousness, as in simple partial seizures which are focal, to complex partial seizures which involve an alteration in consciousness. Status epilepticus is defined as seizure activity lasting greater than 30 minutes or when a patient has two or more seizures that occur without an interval return to baseline. Some physicians have proposed shortening the criteria for the diagnosis of status epilepticus to 5 minutes. Most primary seizures will not be witnessed by the ED physician. If the event is not witnessed by the ED physician or a reliable historian, it is imperative to determine whether a true seizure occurred or whether the event was more probably syncope, pseudoseizures, or another etiology.

Table 10.1. ACEP guidelines for hospital admission of patients with new-onset seizure

- Status epilepticus
- Acute head trauma
- Eclampsia
- Focal neurological deficit
- New intracranial lesion
- Central nervous system (CNS) infection
- Persistent altered mental status
- Correctable medical problem (e.g. electrolyte abnormality, hypoxia, EtOH withdrawal, etc.)

- *Treatment:* as with most emergencies in the ED, the physician should start with the ABCs in the actively seizing patient. Although it is quite difficult and typically not necessary to ventilate the seizing patient during the acute episode, one should be prepared to establish a definitive airway if the condition persists. Upon cessation of the episode, the physician should have oral suction ready and apply both an oxygen face mask and a pulse oximeter. The goal should be to ensure the patient's safety by elevating the rails of the bed and placing the patient in a lateral decubitus position to decrease aspiration. As in the patient described here, expectant management is all that is necessary in most cases. However, the longer a seizure continues, the more likely it is that a permanent neurological injury will occur. If the seizure persists beyond a few minutes and pharmacologic treatment is warranted, benzodiazepines are the primary drug of choice. Either diazepam (0.1 to 0.3 mg/kg) or lorazepam (0.05–0.1 mg/kg) IV are effective initial agents, with lorazepam preferred due to its longer duration of action (4–6 hours). Diazepam rectal gel is most often used in patients who have no IV access. If the seizure persists, an additional 0.05 mg/kg of lorazepam may be given followed by phenytoin (20 mg/kg) or fosphenytoin (20 mg "phenytoin equivalents"/kg) IV. Refractory seizures may be given barbiturates (phenobarbital or pentobarbital) and then propofol as well.
- *Definitive therapy:* patients with a "first seizure" require a more thorough workup than those with recurrent seizures, and neurology should be consulted in the emergency department or on the hospital floors if the patient is admitted. The elevated risk of recurrence following a new-onset seizure can be further stratified using an electroencephalogram (EEG), where electrodes placed on the scalp are able to record a patient's intracranial electrical activity. Patients with abnormal EEGs are twice as likely to have recurrent seizures. Most emergency departments do not have EEGs readily available and thus most patients with first seizure are admitted. However, this practice varies widely and, if prompt neurologic follow-up can be ensured, it is within the standard of practice to discharge someone with a first-time seizure. ACEP guidelines for hospital admission are listed in Table 10.1. The decision of which, if any, anticonvulsant to begin should be made in conjunction with a neurologist.

Clinical course

The keys to this patient's diagnosis are careful attention to his history and the witnessed seizure activity.

Historical clues	Physical findings	Ancillary studies
• Episodic altered mental status	• Normal exam on presentation	
• Visual aura	• Post-ictal following the seizure	
• Olfactory aura	• No focal neurological deficits	

This patient was easily recognized to have a generalized tonic-clonic seizure based on the witnessed event. He did not have an underlying seizure disorder, but historically he did have the presence of an aura, both the flashing lights he described as well as an olfactory aura. He also had loss of consciousness during the event as well as a post-ictal state after. In addition, his seizure activity lasted a little over a minute, which is fairly typical for a tonic-clonic seizure. His seizure was self-limited and after IV placement, oxygen administration, and placement on a monitor the patient had no further events. As his seizure was observed, he was known to have suffered no traumatic injuries during the episode; however, this is a concern in patients with unwitnessed seizures.

Because he had never had a seizure before, the patient was evaluated for secondary metabolic causes, such as hypoglycemia, hypocalcemia, hypomagnesemia, hyponatremia, and abnormalities in potassium. He had none of these abnormalities. A toxicology screen is also prudent in the seizure patient (negative in this patient), as well as a pregnancy test in young women with new seizures. If an infectious process is suspected, a lumbar puncture must be performed. This did not seem likely in this man. Finally, central nervous system masses or bleeding may cause new seizures. Therefore this patient underwent a head CT, which was also unremarkable.

The patient was admitted to the neurology service. He had an EEG which was unremarkable and an MRI which showed a 4 mm nonspecific white matter mass in the frontal lobe which may have been responsible for his seizures. The patient was discharged home on hospital day 2 on an anticonvulsant, and is being followed up on an ongoing basis with neurology to monitor the lesion.

Further reading

Tintinalli J, Kelen G, Stapczynski S. *Emergency Medicine: a Comprehensive Study Guide*, 6th edition. New York: McGraw-Hill, 2004.

Hauser WA, Hesdorffer DC. *Epilepsy Frequency, Causes and Consequences*. New York: Demos, 1990.

Lowenstein D, Bleck T, MacDonald R. It's time to revise the definition of status epilepticus. *Epilepsia* 1999;**40**:120–2.

American College of Emergency Physicians: clinical policy for the initial approach to patients presenting with a chief complaint of seizure who are not in status epilepticus. *Ann Emerg Med* 1997;**29**:706.

Case #9

History

A 75-year-old Hispanic male with a history of hepatitis C cirrhosis and peptic ulcer disease presents to the ED with confusion. The patient's wife states he has been sleepy and not himself for a couple of days. Upon questioning, the patient complains of abdominal pain, predominantly in the right upper quadrant and epigastric regions. He has also had melena for the past 2 days. He does not recall seeing any bright red blood in his stool. He reports feeling a little light-headed. He can't give further history, as he seems confused and can't remember any other details. He has to be woken to ask him questions. His wife reports he hasn't been eating, but he has not had any vomiting.

Past medical history

The patient has a history of hepatitis C cirrhosis, peptic ulcer disease and anemia. He also has a history of a recent non-ST elevation myocardial infarction, hypertension, legal blindness, and a history of syphilis.

Medications

The patient's medications include full-dose aspirin, famotidine, metoprolol, docusate, and senna.

Allergies

The patient has no known drug allergies.

Social history

The patient lives with his wife. He smokes a half pack of cigarettes per day. He drinks alcohol socially, but binges on the weekends. He denies recreational drug use.

Physical exam and ancillary studies

- *Vital signs:* the patient is afebrile. His blood pressure is 100/65, his heart rate is 95 bpm, and his room air oxygen saturation is 98%.
- *General:* he is an elderly male who appears sleepy, but is in no apparent distress.
- *Head and neck:* the patient has no signs of trauma. His pupils are equally round and reactive to light. He has mild scleral icterus and pale conjunctivae. His neck is supple.
- *Chest:* the patient's heart is regularly tachycardic without murmurs or rubs. His chest wall has several spider angiomata. His lungs are clear to auscultation bilaterally, with no wheezes or rhonchi.

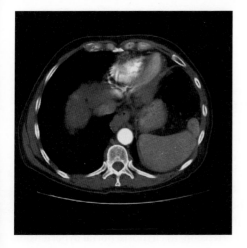

Figure 10.7. This CT of the abdomen and pelvis shows esophageal varices.

- *Abdomen:* his abdomen is soft. He has some generalized tenderness with mild distension, but no palpable masses or hepatomegaly. His bowel sounds are normal.
- *Rectal exam:* on rectal exam, the patient has black tarry stool which is guaiac-positive. There are no masses.
- *Extremities:* the patient's extremities are not tender and have normal range of motion. He has no clubbing, cyanosis, or edema.
- *Neurologic:* the patient is sleepy, but can be aroused. He is oriented to person and place, but not to time. He follows simple commands. He has some short-term memory deficits. He has no evidence of asterexis.
- *Pertinent labs:* the patient's complete blood count is remarkable for a hematocrit of 25% with a mean corpuscular volume of 98. It is otherwise normal. The patient's INR is 1.6. On chemistry evaluation, the patient has a potassium of 5.1, a blood urea nitrogen of 39, and a creatinine of 1.1. On liver testing, the patient has an albumin of 1.5, a bilirubin of 2.6, an alkaline phosphatase of 223, an AST of 421, and an ALT of 110. His ammonia level is 111.
- *Radiographs:* the patient's chest X-ray was unremarkable. Figure 10.7 shows a representative cut from the patient's CT of his abdomen and pelvis.
- *Further diagnostic studies:* the patient's emergency esophagogastroduodenoscopy (EGD) showed bleeding from the patient's esophageal varices.

Questions for thought

- What is the differential diagnosis in the patient with a gastrointestinal (GI) bleed?
- What initial resuscitative steps should be undertaken in this setting?
- What medications should be started in this patient?
- What are the next diagnostic and therapeutic steps in managing this patient?
- What is a neurologic complication of gastrointestinal bleeding in cirrhotic patients?
- What long-term treatment and follow-up is needed for this patient?

Diagnosis

Esophageal variceal bleeding in the setting of hepatitis C cirrhosis.

Discussion

- *Epidemiology:* cirrhosis affects 3.6 out of 1000 North American adults, and results in 32 000 deaths annually. A major cause of cirrhosis-related morbidity and mortality is the development of variceal hemorrhage, a direct result of portal hypertension. Variceal hemorrhage occurs in 25–40% of patients with cirrhosis. Each episode of variceal bleeding is associated with 30% mortality. The survivors of a variceal hemorrhage have a 70% chance of recurrent bleeding within 1 year. Variceal hemorrhage can result in severe neurologic compromise by causing hepatic encephalopathy, as depicted in our patient.
- *Pathophysiology:* portal hypertension can be classified as prehepatic (e.g. portal vein thrombosis), hepatic (e.g. cirrhosis) or posthepatic (e.g. Budd–Chiari syndrome). Cirrhosis is the most common cause of portal hypertension. In cirrhosis, portal hypertension results from both increased resistance to outflow through distorted hepatic parenchyma, as well as increased portal inflow due to splanchnic arteriolar vasodilation. Any form of portal hypertension can lead to the formation of portosystemic collaterals. Collateral formation through the coronary and left gastric veins to the azygos vein produces gastroesophageal varices. Varices form to decompress the hypertensive portal vein and return blood to the systemic circulation. The larger the varices, the higher the chance of bleeding. Hepatic encephalopathy is thought to be a result of an increase in ammonia concentration, which can occur in the setting of a variceal bleed, as well as from inhibitory neurotransmission through GABA receptors in the central nervous system and changes in central neurotransmitters and circulating amino acids.
- *Presentation:* esophageal varices do not produce symptoms unless they rupture and bleed. One must consider this diagnosis in the setting of cirrhosis and upper gastrointestinal bleeding. It usually presents with hemetemesis, melena or even hematochezia in the setting of massive upper GI bleeding. Patients may also have lightheadedess, fatigue, and altered mental status from hepatic encephalopathy, as in the patient described above. This is a result of digested blood in the setting of a liver unable to clear the metabolites. Signs of liver disease such as jaundice, spider angiomata, and ascites may be present. Hypotension, tachycardia, and postural drop of blood pressure suggest significant GI blood loss.
- *Treatment:* active variceal hemorrhage from varices is a medical emergency. Patients should be managed in the intensive care unit. Volume resuscitation of fluids and blood products through two large-bore IVs and optimizing the hemodynamic status are the priorities. Establish airway protection in the setting of a massive upper GI bleed, especially in the setting of altered mental status, to prevent aspiration. A continuous infusion of octreotide, which reduces splanchnic blood flow and lowers portal pressure, should immediately be initiated. Patients with esophageal varices and no prior history of hemorrhage should be treated with nonselective beta-blockers, unless a contraindication exists. The medication should be titrated to a 25% decrease in resting heart rate. Patients with cirrhosis who present with upper GI bleeding should be given prophylactic antibiotics, preferably prior to endoscopy, since this has been shown to decrease infectious complications and possible mortality. Early endoscopy should be performed, as band ligation is first-line treatment for active variceal bleeding. Sclerotherapy may be used in difficult-to-control cases. If bleeding persists despite the above measures, balloon

tamponade is a temporizing measure, but it has many complications. In refractory or recurrent variceal bleeding, a portosystemic shunt should be performed either percutaneously or surgically.

After acute bleeding has stopped, secondary prophylactic interventions lower the risk of rebleeding. This can be achieved with beta-blocker medications, or through serial endoscopic band ligation sessions to completely obliterate the varices. Once the varices are obliterated, endoscopic surveillance for recurrent varices is usually annual or biannual.

Clinical course

The keys to this patient's diagnosis are careful attention to his history, physical exam and ancillary studies.

Historical clues	Physical findings	Ancillary studies
• History of hepatitis C	• Mild hypotension	• Anemia
• Cirrhosis	• Tachycardia	• Elevated BUN
• Melena	• Scleral icterus	• Coagulopathic with INR 1.6
• Lightheadedness	• Spider angiomata	• Elevated LFTs
• Recent confusion	• Coagulopathy	• Varices on CT scan
	• Melena	• Variceal bleeding on endoscopy
	• Abdominal distention	

The patient was recognized to be at high risk for variceal bleeding based upon his underlying risk factors. This diagnosis was well supported by his physical findings and his ancillary tests. Although nasogastric lavage may be used to look for evidence of upper GI bleeding, it is not a very sensitive test. In a patient like this one who is very high risk, it is reasonable to proceed directly to endoscopy instead, which is both diagnostic and therapeutic.

The patient was hemodynamically tenuous, so two large-bore IVs were placed. He was resuscitated with crystalloid as well as 2 units of packed red blood cells. He was also given fresh frozen plasma, since he was coagulopathic.

An octreotide drip for possible variceal bleed and esomeprazole infusion for possible ulcer source were initiated. Antibiotics were also given in the setting of a GI bleed in a cirrhotic. EGD showed evidence of bleeding esophageal varices, which were successfully banded. The patient was then transferred to the medical intensive care unit (MICU).

After a few days of observation in the MICU, the patient was transferred to the floor. One night the patient was found to be unresponsive. The ammonia level was found to be 252 μmol/L. A nasogastric tube was placed for lactulose administration, and dark blood return was seen. It was deduced that the patient had developed significant hepatic encephalopathy from a recurrent variceal bleed. Despite lactulose administration, the patient never regained consciousness. He was given comfort care and subsequently expired.

Further reading

Smith JL, Graham DY. Variceal hemorrhage. A critical evaluation of survival analysis. *Gastroenterology* 1982;**82**:968.

DeDombal FT, Clarke JR, Clamp SE, et al. Prognostic factors in upper GI bleeding. *Endoscopy* 1986;**18**:6s.

Graham DY, Smith JL. The course of patients after variceal hemorrhage. *Gastroenterology* 1981;**80**:800.

Grace ND. Prevention of initial variceal hemorrhage. *Gastroenterol Clin North Am* 1992;**21**:149.

Bernard B, Grande JD, Khac EN, et al. Antibiotic prophylaxis for the prevention of bacterial infection in cirrhotic patient with gastrointestinal bleeding: a meta-analysis. *Hepatology* 1999;**29**:1655.

Yamada T, Hasler W, Inadomi J, Anderson M, Brown R. *Handbook of Gastroenterology*, 2nd edition. Philadelphia: Lippincott Williams & Wilkins, 2005.

Feldman M, Friedman L, Brandt L. *Sleisenger and Fordtran's Gastrointestinal and Liver Disease Pathophysiology, Diagnosis, Management*, 8th edition. St Louis, MO: Saunders Elsevier, 2006.

Friedman S, McQuaid K, Grendell J. *Current Diagnosis and Treatment in Gastroenterology*, 2nd edition. New York: McGraw-Hill, 2003.

Case # 10

History

A 73-year-old man presents to the ED from a local nursing home for evaluation of "not acting right." Since he is not able to give a coherent history, the nursing home is contacted. His nurse states that usually the patient is a pleasant, active elderly male who likes to flirt with the nurses. For the last couple days, he has been eating a bit less and his behavior has been withdrawn, such that he just stays in his room in bed. This morning he vomited his breakfast, and had a low-grade fever to 37.7°C. He has had no complaints of pain, no diarrhea, no new weakness, and no known falls.

Past medical history

His past medical history is remarkable for dementia, hypertension, and benign prostatic hypertrophy. He was treated for a urinary tract infection 2 months ago.

Medications

The patient takes doxazosin, aspirin, and donepezil.

Allergies

The patient has no known drug allergies.

Physical exam

- *Vital signs:* the patient's temperature is 37.8°C, his heart rate is 100 bpm, his blood pressure is 105/70 mmHg, his respiratory rate is 24, and his room air oxygen saturation is 97%.
- *General:* he is awake and frail-appearing.
- *Head and neck:* the patient has no signs of trauma. His pupils are equally round and reactive to light. His extraocular movements are intact with no nystagmus. The patient's mucous membranes are dry. His neck is supple. There is no jugular venous distension or carotid bruit.
- *Cardiovascular:* the patient's heart is regularly tachycardic with no murmur, rub, or gallop. He has full peripheral pulses throughout. His capillary refill is less than 2 seconds.
- *Lungs:* he has normal breath sounds, and his breathing is non-labored. He is slightly tachypneic.
- *Abdomen:* the patient has normal active bowel sounds. His abdomen is soft, non-tender, and non-distended, with no pulsatile mass or bruits. His stool is brown, and is guaiac-negative. His prostate is enlarged, and it is non-tender.
- *Musculoskeletal and skin:* the patient has pink, warm extremities. He has no rashes, edema, or decubiti. He has no costovertebral angle tenderness.

395

- *Neurological:* he is alert to self only. His cranial nerves are intact. He is moving all extremities symmetrically, and has intact sensation throughout. His cerebellar, reflex, and gait exams are unremarkable.
- *Pertinent labs:* the patient's complete blood count is remarkable for a white blood cell count of 14.2. His creatinine is 1.0. The patient's urinalysis shows 10–20 white blood cells per high-power field, and is positive for nitrite. Moderate bacteria are noted.

Questions for thought

- What are appropriate initial actions to take to stabilize this patient?
- What is this patient's primary problem?
- What initial differential diagnoses should be considered in this patient?
- What diagnostic tests would be helpful?

Diagnosis

Recurrent nosocomial urinary tract infection.

Discussion

- *Epidemiology:* urinary tract infection (UTI) is regarded to be the most common bacterial infection nationwide and is a common cause of altered mental status in the elderly. The annual incidence of symptomatic bacterial UTI in the elderly is high, at an estimated 10%. While uncommon in healthy young males, UTI becomes more common in elderly men due to a rise in predisposing conditions such as benign prostatic hypertrophy with bladder outlet obstruction, malignancy, neurodegenerative diseases, and diabetes. The female-to-male ratio of prevalence of bacteriuria in the young is about 30:1; by age 65 this ratio narrows to 2:1.
- *Pathophysiology:* the majority of UTIs result from bacteria that ascend the urethra to the bladder, then ascend the ureters to the kidneys. There exist hematogenous and lymphatic routes of infection, but these are much less common. Common risk factors for UTI in the elderly include ureteral strictures, bladder catheterization, benign prostatic hypertrophy, chronic bacterial prostatitis, atrophic urethritis or vaginitis, cystoscopy and prostatic cancer. Other considerations are presence of calculi or structural anomalies (vesicorectal fistula in colitis, ileal bladder diversion or urostomy, for example).

  E. coli is the most common pathogen, responsible for about 85% of outpatient and 50% of nosocomial infection. *Klebsiella* is the second most common Gram-negative aerobic species. *S. saprophyticus* is responsible for 5–15% of infections in young women. In other populations, *Enterococcus*, *Proteus*, and *Klebsiella* account for the remaining 5–15%. *Enterococcus* seems to predominate in older men with prostate abnormalities. *Proteus mirabilis* and *Morganella morganii* are more common in men (due to prevalence in preputial skin flora), those who are chronically catheterized, those with calculi (due to alkaline milieu), and those with malignancy. *Serratia*, *Enterobacter*, *Citrobacter*, *Acinetobacter*, and *Pseudomonas* species predominate in nosocomial UTI. In recurrent UTI, resistant non-*E. coli* Gram-negative and Gram-positive pathogens are typical. Specifically, think of enterococci, coagulase-negative staphylococcus and group B streptococcus. Suspect enterococcal superinfection in those who have been frequently treated for UTI with cephalosporins, quinolones, and sulfonamides.

In the setting of benign prostatic hypertrophy, as in the above patient, outlet obstruction leads to urinary retention and stasis, with subsequent bacterial overgrowth and symptomatic infection. Another proposed mechanism is that bladder muscle hypertrophies due to chronic contraction against outlet obstruction, then ultimately becomes relatively atonic with high volumes of urine retention and stasis, and then bacterial overgrowth results in infection.

- *Presentation:* the presentation of UTI encompasses a broad spectrum of signs and symptoms. Many cases of both bacteriuria and UTI are asymptomatic. Patients can have lower tract symptomatology of cystitis and upper tract symptoms of pyelonephritis, as described above. Severe infections involving bacteremia can present with septic shock and death. In the elderly, as in the above patient, symptoms are often as nonspecific as "just not acting right." The elderly can also present with confusion, and frequently will not mount a fever, or they may take longer to do so. They may also present with hypothermia instead.
- *Treatment:* it is acceptable to treat uncomplicated UTI empirically with antibiotics. Otherwise, whenever possible, treatment of UTI should be directed to the results of urine culture and sensitivities, or Gram stain. If necessary, empiric treatment of UTI will depend on local patterns of antibiotic resistance, the type of pathogen suspected based on the clinical context, the patient's own past history of infections if any, and any allergies or side effects.

Clinical course

The patient's diagnosis was not readily apparent on initial exam, but there were historical and physical exam clues that were helpful in guiding evaluation and workup.

Historical clues	Physical findings	Ancillary studies
• Recent UTI	• Low-grade temperature	• Urinalysis with evidence of infection
• History of prostate enlargement	• Tachycardia	• Elevated white blood cell count
• Vomiting	• Hypotension	
• Change in mental status		

The patient was recognized to have a UTI when his urinalysis became available. Urinalysis and urine dipstick testing are the most common way in which UTIs are diagnosed. Dipsticks detect leukocyte esterase released from white blood cells, and have a sensitivity of 77% and specificity of 54% for UTI. Nitrite is released when enterobacteriaciae metabolize urinary nitrates. The sensitivity of dipstick to pick up nitrite is 81% and specificity for UTI is 87%. The limitation to nitrite testing is that it will not be present in the absence of enterobacters. On urinalysis, greater than 5 WBC per high-power field is considered indicative of pyuria, which is strongly associated with bacterial infection. Greater than 5 RBC and 2+ bacteria are also considered indicative of UTI. The gold standard for diagnosis is culture, but the results of this are usually not available in the ED.

On reviewing the patient's previous lab work, it was noted that the pathogen from his last UTI was *Proteus mirabilis*. He was started on empiric treatment for this with intravenous levofloxacin. Parenteral treatment was chosen due to his vomiting. He improved within 48 hours and was discharged to complete his course at the nursing home. He returned to his baseline mental status within 4 days.

Further reading

Shaeffer AJ, Shaeffer EM. Infections of the urinary tract. In Wein et al., eds., *Campbell-Walsh Urology*, 9th edition, Philadelphia, PA: Saunders Elsevier, 2007, pp. 223–302.

Norris DL, Young JD. Urinary tract infections: diagnosis and management in the emergency department. *Emerg Med Clin N Am* 2008;**26**:413–30.

Stamm WE, Hooten TM. Management of urinary tract infections in adults. *N Engl J Med* 1993;**329**(18):1328–34.

Rajagopalan S. Chapter 100. Urinary tract infections. In Beers MH, et al., eds., *The Merck Manual of Geriatrics*. Whitehouse Station, NJ: Merck & Co, 2006. Retrieved October 7, 2008, from http://www.merck.com/mkgr/mmg/sec12/ch100/ch100a.jsp.

Zhanel GG, et al. Antibiotic resistance in Escherichia coli outpatient urinary isolates: final results from the North American Urinary Tract Infection Collaborative Alliance (NAUTICA). *Int J Antimicrob Agents* 2006;**27**(6):468–75.

Karlowsky JA, et al. Fluoroquinolone-resistant urinary isolates of Escherichia coli from outpatients are frequently multidrug resistant: results from the North American Urinary Tract Infection Collaborative Alliance-Quinolone Resistance study. *Antimicrob Agents Chemother* 2006;**50**(6):2251–4.

Warren JW, et al. Guidelines for antimicrobial treatment of uncomplicated acute bacterial cystitis and acute pyelonephritis in women. *Clin Infect Dis* 1999;**29**:745–58.

Gilbert DN, Sande MA, et al. Clinical approach to initial choice of antimicrobial therapy: kidney, bladder, & prostate. In *The Sanford Guide to Antimicrobial Therapy*. Sperryville. VA: Antimicrobial Therapy, 2008.

Case # 11

History

A 69-year-old right handed male is brought to the ED by his children, who state that the patient has been not acting like himself and has been complaining of a headache for the past 3 days. The patient states his headache worsens with movement and is throbbing in nature. He complains that the headaches wake him up from his sleep and are constant throughout the day. He is unable to get any relief from pain using acetaminophen and aspirin. He also admits to being increasingly unstable on his feet and feeling sleepier more often. He denies any fever, chills, night sweats, photophobia, or recent trauma.

Past medical history

The patient was recently admitted to the hospital for an ST elevation myocardial infarction, at which time he developed an arrhythmia. A pacemaker was placed at that time. He has longstanding hypertension and diabetes. Besides his pacemaker, he has had no other surgeries. He quit smoking in 1991 and denies any alcohol use. He is currently retired from being a school teacher.

Medications

The patient's medications include warfarin and aspirin, which he started taking after his recent myocardial infarction. He also takes atenolol, lisinopril, and atorvastatin.

Allergies

The patient has no known drug allergies.

Physical exam and ancillary studies

- *Vital signs:* the patient's temperature is 36.6°C, his heart rate is 90 bpm, his blood pressure is 190/100 mmHg, his respiratory rate is 20, and his room air oxygen saturation is 98%.
- *General:* the patient is well-groomed, resting on a stretcher, with no apparent distress.
- *Head and neck:* the patient has no evidence of trauma. His pupils are equally round and reactive to light, and his extraocular movements are intact. His neck is supple, with no adenopathy.
- *Cardiovascular:* the patient's heart has a regular rate and rhythm, with no murmurs, rubs, or gallops. He has good peripheral perfusion.
- *Lungs:* the patient's lungs are clear bilaterally, with no wheezes, rales, or rhonchi.
- *Abdomen:* the patient's abdomen is soft, non-tender, and non-distended. He has no organomegaly.

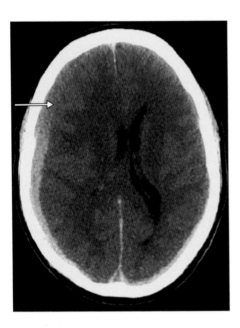

Figure 10.8. This head CT shows an acute right-sided subdural hematoma with 1–2 cm midline shift.

- *Extremities and skin:* the patient has no clubbing or cyanosis. He has no rashes.
- *Neurologic:* the patient is currently awake, alert, and oriented. He has no aphasia. He has slight dysarthria, although his repetition is intact. He follows commands briskly. On cranial nerve testing, he has slight blunting of the left nasolabial fold. Otherwise, his cranial nerves are intact. On motor exam, he has pronator drift in his left upper extremity. He has 5/5 strength in his right upper and lower extremities, and 4/5 strength in his left lower extremity. His deep tendon reflexes are symmetric bilaterally. On plantar testing, his toes are downgoing on the right and upgoing on the left. On sensory testing, the patient has a normal exam. On cerebellar testing, he has slight dysmetria of his left upper extremity. His gait is ataxic.
- *Pertinent labs:* the patient's complete blood count and chemistries are withing normal limits. His INR is 3.4.
- *EKG:* the patient's EKG shows a sinus rhythm at 68 bpm without ST or T wave abnormalities.
- *Radiographs:* the patient's chest X-ray shows cardiomegaly with no evidence of pulmonary disease. A representative cut from the patient's head CT is shown in Figure 10.8.

Questions for thought

- What are the most important initial actions to take?
- Based on this patient's pattern of symptoms, what is at the top of your differential?
- What needs to be addressed in the ED in order to expedite treatment?
- What are the treatment options?

Diagnosis

Acute subdural hematoma with midline shift.

Discussion

- *Epidemiology:* acute subdural hematomas most commonly present after traumatic events and are most common in the elderly population. They commonly present in patients with risk factors which include alcohol abuse, cerebral atrophy, seizure disorders, cerebrospinal fluid shunts, and coagulopathies, or in patients at risk for falls. Evidence of trauma is identified in less than 50% of cases.

- *Pathophysiology:* there are two suspected and commonly identified mechanisms of acute subdural hematomas found in post-trauma situations. They can be secondary to parenchymal brain injury which continues to bleed into the subdural space or secondary to tearing of bridging vessels torn from acceleration-deceleration during violent head movement. The most common non-traumatic factor is the use of anticoagulation, which has been shown to increase the risk of acute subdural hematoma in males by 7-fold and in females by 26-fold.

- *Presentation:* patients present with headaches, weakness, confusion, language difficulties, seizures, or decreased mental status. Patients may present with significant mass effect and even have cerebral herniation. Acute subdural hematomas may develop and go unnoticed, in which case patients may progress towards chronic subdural collections without recognizable symptoms. It is important when dealing with these patients to exclude spinal cord injury, adult hydrocephalus, and stroke as an etiology for symptoms. The most important features to delineate for prognosis and treatment include determining the age of the patient and evaluating for mass effect. Acute subdural hematomas (1–3 days) are hyperdense on CT, subacute (4 days to 3 weeks) are isodense on CT, and chronic (>3weeks) are hypodense but may present with mixtures of varying ages of blood.

- *Treatment:* the treatment of subdural hematomas varies largely depending on the patient's physical exam and symptoms. However, it is important to evaluate and treat risk factors. Patients on anticoagulation should have their anticoagulation reversed and stopped. Patients should be acutely optimized in the case of operative intervention including fluid balance, IV access, and hemodynamic status. Patients with a more indolent course can be observed and may avoid operative intervention altogether. Patients who present with acute neurological decline and significant subdural hematomas should be operated on within 4 hours of injury. Based on a retrospective review of 82 comatose patients, patients operated on within 4 hours had a mortality of 30% compared to 90% for those delayed beyond the 4 hours. The patient's outcome is also dictated by the patient's admission Glasgow coma score and post-operative intracranial pressure.

- *Definitive therapy:* surgery is the definitive therapy for acute subdural hematomas. Surgery can vary based on the size and location of the subdural. The goal of surgery in patients with acute neurological injury is to relieve increased pressure as rapidly as possible. Once surgical evacuation is carried out, patients often require post-operative intracranial pressure monitoring and management.

Clinical course

The keys to this patient's diagnosis are careful attention to his history, physical exam, and ancillary studies.

Historical clues	Physical findings	Ancillary studies
• Older male	• Motor weakness on left arm and left leg	• Head CT with acute right subdural hematoma
• Headache aggravated by movement	• Ataxia	• Increased INR
• Difficulty ambulating	• Decreased sensation	
• Recent anticoagulation therapy	• No cranial nerve deficit	
	• No papilledema	

This man was recognized to potentially have an intracranial process based on his history and physical exam. This prompted a CT scan, which demonstrated his subdural hematoma. This patient's pathology was most probably related to his iatrogenic anticoagulation and possibly to his increased blood pressure. The patient received vitamin K and fresh frozen plasma in order to reverse his anticoagulation. He also had strict blood pressure control as an inpatient. Cardiology was consulted in order to minimize the patient's perioperative cardiac risks. Ultimately, the patient was taken to the operating room to evacuate his subdural hematoma.

Intraoperatively, this patient underwent a craniotomy and evacuation of his acute subdural hematoma. There were no active bleeding blood vessels noted. He recovered without sequelae post-operatively and was discharged home.

Further reading

Greenberg MS. *Handbook of Neurosurgery*, 6th edition. New York: Thieme, 2005, pp. 672–6.

Kawamata T, Takeshita M, Kubo O. Management of intracranial hemorrhage associated with anticoagulation therapy. *Surg Neurol* 1995;**44**:438–43.

Seelig JM, Becker DP, Miller JD. Traumatic acute subdural hematoma: major mortality reduction in comatose patients treated within four hours. *N Engl J Med* 1981;**304**:1511–18.

Case#12

History

A 46-year-old female presents to the emergency department with gradually increasing somnolence and confusion over the last 2 days. Paramedics are bringing her in after a friend found her lethargic and confused at home. Upon questioning the family, they state she began to be "not herself" 2 days ago and has been "sleeping more." The family was not with her this morning when her friend found her in this worsened state.

Past medical history

The patient has a history of morbid obesity, and is currently being treated for chronic obstructive pulmonary disease (COPD), diabetes mellitus (non-insulin-dependent type II), depression, and hypertension.

Medications

The patient's medications include glucophage, aspirin, rosiglitazone, gabapentin, montelukast, hydrochlorothiazide, albuterol, loratidine, escitalopram, lisinopril, trazadone, buspirone, and a nicotrol inhaler as needed.

Allergies

The patient has no reported medication allergies.

Family history

The patient's family history consists of both parents having adult-onset diabetes mellitus type II and hypertension. There is no reported history of cancer or cerebrovascular accident in either parent.

Social history

The patient is quitting smoking and does not drink. She lives alone and has frequent family visitors.

Physical exam and ancillary studies

- *Vital signs:* the patient's temperature is 36.9°C, her heart rate is 103 bpm and regular, her blood pressure is 106/80 mmHg, her respiratory rate is 26 breaths per minute, and her oxygen saturation on a 100% non-rebreather mask is 100%.
- *General:* the patient is in a generally poor state of hygiene and is morbidly obese. She is arousable but very lethargic. She is very slow to answer questions, speaks very slowly, and is only oriented to person.

- *Head and neck:* her pupils are equal and slowly reactive to light, measuring 3 mm and without icterus or conjunctival pallor. Her mucus membranes are unremarkable, her neck supple, and she does not have signs of jugular venous distention.
- *Cardiovascular:* the patient's heart is without murmur and her peripheral pulses are normal throughout.
- *Lungs:* her lungs show distant but present breath sounds with minimal expiratory wheeze.
- *Abdomen:* the patient's abdomen is soft and non-tender with normal bowel sounds throughout.
- *Extremities and skin:* the patient has no evidence of edema, cyanosis, or clubbing on extremity exam.
- *Neurologic:* the patient's cranial nerves are intact. She moves all extremities equally with normal tone and reflexes. She appears to have normal strength although she is not completely cooperative with the exam. She localizes equally to pain, and her Glascow coma score is 12 (eyes 2, verbal 4, motor 6).
- *Psychiatric:* the patient is lethargic and slowly responds to verbal stimuli and follows commands with much prompting. She is oriented to self only and is verbal only with yes or no answers.
- *Pertinent labs:* her complete blood count is significant for a white blood cell count of 14.5 and hemoglobin of 10.2. Her chemistries are significant for a bicarbonate of 35. Her arterial blood gas analysis shows a pH of 7.01, pCO_2 of 152, paO_2 of 106, bicarbonate of 38, and an saO_2 of 91% on 100% 4 L nasal cannula oxygen.
- *EKG:* her EKG is grossly unremarkable, in normal sinus rhythm with a rate of 90 bpm.
- *Radiographs:* her chest X-ray is unremarkable except for chronic changes consistent with COPD, and the CT scan of her head is unremarkable.

Questions for thought

- What are the appropriate initial actions to take to stabilize this patient?
- What is the goal oxygen saturation in this patient?
- How does one urgently treat this condition in the emergency department?
- What is causing this patient's altered mental status?
- What disease processes may cause this condition?
- How can this condition be prevented?

Diagnosis

Hypercapnic encephalopathy.

Discussion

- *Pathophysiology:* hypercapnia has a profound anesthetic and depressant effect on the central nervous system. This may be attributed to cerebral vasodilatation (pH-mediated) and possible increased permeability of cerebral vasculature causing cerebral edema and increased intracerebral pressure. Common disease entities producing hypercapnia are those that cause hypoventilation, such as chronic obstructive pulmonary disease, sleep apnea, asthma, central nervous system injury, and central nervous system depression (from multiple causes such as hypoglycemia and medication/drug-induced). Overproduction of carbon dioxide is another means of causing hypercapnia, found in states of sepsis, overfeeding, lactic acidosis, or thyrotoxicosis; however, these states rarely cause clinically significant elevations in blood CO_2 levels.

- *Presentation:* acute elevations in blood carbon dioxide to 60–70 mmHg are associated with headache and mild confusion. Acute elevation of $paCO_2$ greater than 70 mmHg causes depressed levels of consciousness and coma (hypercapnic encephalopathy). Additionally, the cause of the hypercapnic state may be evident on presentation through history or physical exam, such as a history of COPD or drug use or constricted pupils in narcotic overdose.

- *Treatment:* mainstays of treatment for hypercapnia are reduction of the elevated blood CO_2 levels and resolution of the resulting acidemia. This is accomplished through treatment of the underlying hypoventilation state and the use of both invasive and non-invasive ventilatory devices. In patients with COPD, bronchodilators such as inhaled beta-agonists and inhaled anticholinergics coupled with anti-inflammatory medications such as corticosteroids (oral and IV) are used to reverse the underlying decreased alveolar ventilation or increased deadspace. Antidotes to common drug overdoses (such as naloxone with narcotics and bicarbonate with tricyclic antidepressants) improve CNS depression and therefore minute ventilation. Indications for intubation and mechanical ventilation include marked acidemia (pH < 7.20) and/or a marked depression in level of consciousness with inability to protect one's own airway. In those cooperative patients with a less severe depression in level of consciousness and who are protecting their airway, non-invasive positive-pressure ventilation (NIPPV) may be attempted to prevent endotracheal intubation. NIPPV should be avoided in patients with anticipated prolonged duration of ventilation, or who have a significant aspiration risk or facial trauma. In the patient with COPD or other conditions causing a chronic elevation of blood CO_2 levels, it is important not to over-oxygenate the non-mechanically ventilated patient. One must continue to treat life-threatening hypoxemia when it exists, but over-oxygenating may increase the patient's carbon dioxide levels. This occurs through a worsening V/Q mismatch in the lungs, the 'Haldane effect' (where oxygen displaces CO_2 molecules from RBCs), and a reduction in minute ventilation by losing the hypoxic ventilatory drive. Typical goal saO_2 in these situations is 88–90%

- *Definitive therapy:* this includes lowering the patient's blood carbon dioxide to their baseline level (usually higher than 'normal' if patient has COPD and chronic CO_2 retention) and therefore correcting the acidemia resulting from the elevated CO_2; it is also important to maintain this level via avoidance of hyper-oxygenation and maintaining adequate ventilation through reversal of hypoventilatory states by treating the underlying cause.

Clinical course

The keys to this patient's diagnosis are careful attention to history, physical exam, and ancillary studies to rule in/rule out pathology.

Historical clues	Physical exam	Ancillary studies
• History of COPD	• Change in mentation	• ABG with severely elevated CO^2 and pH abnormalities
• History of sleep apnea	• Lethargy	• Otherwise normal lab and radiographic workup (+/− chronic lung disease changes on chest X-ray), excluding other pathology
• Gradual onset of depressed cognition and mental status	• No focal deficits	
• Gradually worsening state of confusion	• Decreased air movement and wheeze on pulmonary auscultation	

The patient's clinical pictures suggested hypercapnic encephalopathy. The patient's change in mental status was a result of the direct effects of lowered pH and elevated carbon dioxide on cerebral blood flow and intracranial pressure. The overall state was probably being caused by an acute exacerbation of her chronic obstructive pulmonary disease.

Since the patient's head CT showed no evidence of hemorrhage or stroke, and her EKG was without evidence of ischemia or arrhythmia, intracranial pathology and cardiac abnormalities were excluded as possible causes for her change in mental status. Additionally, her chest X-ray showed flattening of her diaphragms and she did not have any significant chemistry abnormalities aside from a bicarbonate of 35, both consistent and common with chronic obstructive pulmonary disease and chronic carbon dioxide retention.

Our patient was treated in the emergency department initially with intravenous fluid hydration and NIPPV. When her pH of 7.01 was not affected by NIPPV, and in light of her severely depressed level of consciousness, rapid sequence endotracheal intubation was performed. She was admitted to the intensive care unit and monitored overnight on assist control mechanical ventilation. The following morning, her pH was 7.25 and her CO_2 had dropped to 80. On hospital day 2 she was fully awake and following all commands. She was successfully extubated on hospital day 3, and discharged home with steroid taper on hospital day 4.

Further reading

Brian JE. Carbon dioxide and the cerebral circulation. *Anesthesiology* 1998;**88950**:1365–86.

Celikel T, Sungur M, Ceyhan B, et al. Medical therapy in hypercapnic respiratory failure. *Chest* 1998;**114**:1636.

Hanson CW, Marshall B, Frasch HF, Marshall C. Causes of hypercarbia with oxygen therapy in patients with chronic obstructive pulmonary disease. *Crit Care Med* 1996;**24**:23.

Joosten SA, Koh MS, Bu X, et al. The effects of oxygen therapy in patients presenting to an emergency department with exacerbation of chronic obstructive pulmonary disease. *Med J Aust* 2007;**186**:235.

Matakas F, Birkle J, Cervos-Navarro J. The effect of prolonged experimental hypercapnia on the brain. *Acta Neuropathology* 1978;**41**(3):2007–10.

Robinson TD, Freiberg DB, Regnis JA, Young IH. The role of hypoventilation and ventilation-perfusion redistribution in oxygen-induced hypercapnia during acute exacerbations of chronic obstructive pulmonary disease. *Am J Respir Crit Care Med* 2000;**161**:1524.

Scala R, Naldi M, Archinucci I, et al. Noninvasive positive pressure ventilation in patients with acute exacerbations of COPD and varying levels of consciousness. *Chest* 2005;**128**:1657.

Weinberger SE, Schwartzstein RM, Weiss JW. Hypercapnia. *N Engl J Med* 1989;**321**:1223.

Case #13

History

A 58-year-old male is brought in to the ED by EMS after being found confused and combative by his wife. She states that he hasn't been feeling well since Friday. He skipped his Friday dialysis treatment. She urged him to go to the doctor but he refused. When she returned home from work this afternoon he was difficult to arouse, didn't recognize her and was not making any sense so she called 911. The patient is unable to give further history.

Past medical history

The patient's medical history is significant for diabetes, hypertension, anemia, and end-stage renal disease.

Medications

The patient's medications include metoprolol, lantus insulin, regular insulin, phos-lo, and epopoeitin injections.

Allergies

The patient has no known drug allergies.

Family history

Both parents are still living with hypertension.

Social history

The patient does not smoke, drink alcohol, or use any illicit street drugs.

Physical exam and ancillary studies

- *Vital signs:* the patient's vital signs are as follows: temperature 36.8°C, heart rate 72 bpm, blood pressure 175/86 mmHg, respiratory rate 12, room air oxygen saturation 99%.
- *General:* the patient is confused. He is able to state his name but does not know the date. He is not oriented to place.
- *Head and neck:* the patient's mucous membranes are moist. His neck is supple. Jugular veins are noted at 8 cm above his sternal notch. There are no bruits heard over his carotid arteries. The patient's sclerae are non-icteric. His fundoscopic exam is normal.
- *Cardiovascular:* the patient's heart sounds are normal without murmur, gallop, or rub. His pulses are 2+ and symmetrical.
- *Lungs:* the patient is in no respiratory distress. Basilar crackles are appreciated bilaterally.
- *Abdomen:* the patient's abdomen is soft and non-tender with no palpable masses.

- *Extremities and skin:* his skin is warm and dry with no rashes. His legs are non-tender. Symmetrical 2+ edema to the knees is present.
- *Neurologic:* the patient's pupils are equal, round, and reactive to light. The patient is difficult to arouse and only oriented to self, not place or time. He follows commands and has 5/5 muscle strength in all extremities.
- *Pertinent labs:* his glucose on arrival is 140. His complete blood count is significant for a hematocrit of 28%. His chemistries are significant for a potassium of 6.9, bicarbonate of 15, blood urea nitrogen of 87 and a creatinine of 7.6. His anion gap is 19. All other labs are normal or negative.
- *EKG:* the patient's EKG shows no evidence of ischemia. He has peaked T waves, similar to those in Figure 10.2.
- *Radiographs:* the patient's chest X-ray shows cardiomegally with bilateral basilar vascular congestion. His head CT shows no evidence of traumatic brain injury, intracranial hemorrhage, or masses.

Questions for thought

- What are the appropriate initial actions to take to stabilize this patient?
- How does one urgently treat this condition in the emergency department?
- What is definitive treatment of this condition?
- What is causing this patient's altered mental status?

Diagnosis

Uremia.

Discussion

- *Epidemiology:* according to the 19th Annual Data Report from the US End Stage Renal Disease Program the incidence of end-stage renal disease in the United States is 347 per million person-years. The incidence of uremia is lower than this given that most patients are started and maintained on dialysis prior to becoming uremic.
- *Pathophysiology:* uremia literally means the presence of urine in the blood. This refers specifically to the nitrogen breakdown products that are usually cleared by the kidney building up in the blood. It is the build-up of these waste products as well as the loss of the acid–base homeostasis that leads to an alteration in the level of consciousness. The failure of the kidney is caused by numerous mechanisms. The most frequent causes of kidney failure in the United States include diabetes and hypertension. Other causes of renal failure include membranoproliferative glomerulonephritis, focal segmental glomerulonephritis, IgA nephropathy, polycystic kidney disease, lupus, amyloidosis, Goodpasture disease, multiple myeloma, thrombotic thrombocytopenic purpura, and hemolytic uremic syndrome.
- *Presentation:* patients with uremia will often present with an alteration in mental status. Other findings in uremia include a pericardial friction rub, uremic frost (a skin finding of powdery deposits of urea and uric acid on the skin), and in cases of anuric renal

failure, symptoms consistent with fluid overload including peripheral and pulmonary edema.

- *Treatment:* initial treatment of uremia and hyperkalemia includes stabilizing the myocardium to prevent ventricular fibrillation; calcium chloride or calcium gluconate in addition to insulin (which is accompanied by dextrose to maintain normal blood sugar levels), nebulized beta-agonists, sodium bicarbonate, and kayexalate may be given. Ultimately the potassium and nitrogen waste products will need to be eliminated by renal replacement therapy, usually continuous veno-venous hemofiltration or hemodialysis in the acute setting.

- *Definitive therapy:* renal replacement therapy is the definitive therapy for uremia. This includes kidney transplantation, ongoing hemodialysis, or peritoneal dialysis.

Clinical course

The keys to this patient's diagnosis are careful attention to history, physical exam, and the use of ancillary studies to rule out other pathology.

Historical clues	Physical findings	Ancillary studies
• History of end-stage renal disease	• Bibasilar crackles consistent with early CHF	• Elevated potassium, anion gap, BUN, creatinine
• History of recently missed dialysis treatment	• Presence of bilateral pedal edema	• EKG consistent with hyperkalemia
		• Otherwise negative lab and radiographic workup, excluding other pathology

The patient's clinical picture suggested uremia, especially with a history of end-stage renal disease and the recent history of a missed dialysis treatment. This missed dialysis treatment was especially important given that it was a Friday treatment. Dialysis patients typically receive dialysis three times a week, including every other day during the week with 2 days away from dialysis on the weekend. This patient missed dialysis on a Friday and is now presenting on a Monday, and therefore it has been five days since his last dialysis treatment. He presented with altered mental status and lethargy as well as findings consistent with mild fluid overload, which is not uncommon with uremia. Although not present in this patient, some patients will have skin findings such as uremic frost, asterixis, myoclonus, or pericardial or pleural friction rubs. This patient's EKG showed changes consistent with hyperkalemia.

Our patient also had an anion-gap metabolic acidosis, which is commonly seen in renal failure. The kidney functions not only to remove toxins from the blood but also in the balance of the acidity of the blood. Once the kidneys have failed, the patient relies on renal replacement therapy in the form of hemodialysis to remove the toxins and balance electrolytes, remove excess fluid, and balance the acidity of the blood.

Our patient was treated in the emergency department with IV calcium chloride, nebulized albuterol, insulin, and dextrose to stabilize the myocardium and prevent ventricular fibrillation. Emergency dialysis was arranged and the patient was admitted to the hospital for monitoring. He was discharged a few days after admission with a complete resolution of his symptoms.

Further reading

Alper B, et al. Uremia. Retrieved December 21, 2008, from eMedicine.com.

Tintinalli J, Kelen G, Stapczynski S. *Emergency Medicine: A Comprehensive Study Guide*, 6th edition. New York: McGraw-Hill, 2004.

Marx J, Hockenberger R, Walls R. *Rosen's Emergency Medicine Concepts and Clinical Practice*, 6th edition. St Louis, MO: Mosby Elsevier, 2006.

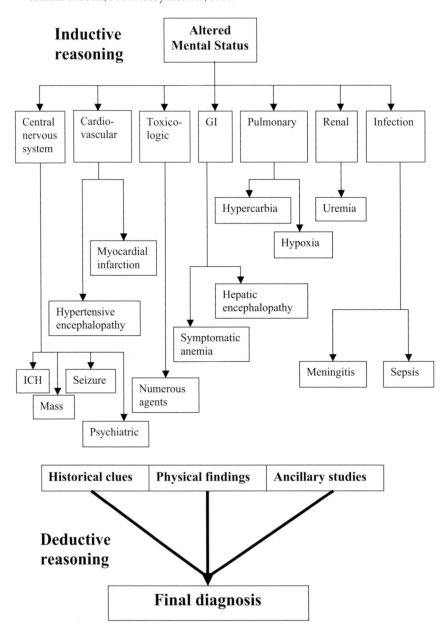

Index